Social Determinants of Health

BScN Program
Grant MacEwan University

Social Determinants of Health

A COMPARATIVE APPROACH

Alan Davidson

SECOND EDITION

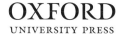

OXFORD
UNIVERSITY PRESS

Oxford University Press is a department of the University of Oxford.
It furthers the University's objective of excellence in research, scholarship,
and education by publishing worldwide. Oxford is a registered trade mark of
Oxford University Press in the UK and in certain other countries.

Published in Canada by
Oxford University Press
8 Sampson Mews, Suite 204,
Don Mills, Ontario M3C 0H5 Canada

www.oupcanada.com

Copyright © Oxford University Press Canada 2019

Library and Archives Canada Cataloguing in Publication
Davidson, Alan (Alan Reginald), author
Social determinants of health : a comparative approach / Alan Davidson.
– Second edition.
Includes bibliographical references and index.

Issued in print and electronic formats.
ISBN 978-0-19-903220-4 (softcover).–ISBN 978-0-19-903224-2 (PDF)

1. Public health–Social aspects. 2. Social medicine. 3. Medical policy–
Social aspects. I. Title.

RA418.D38 2019   306.4'61   C2018-906632-6
                                                    C2018-906633-4

Cover image: © MikeDotta/Shutterstock.com
Cover design: Sherill Chapman
Interior design: Sherill Chapman

Contents

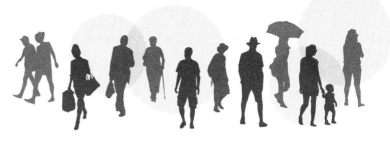

13 ● Social Patterning of Behaviour   303

14 ● The Politics of Population Health   324

Preface

In 1962, my maternal grandfather, age 65, died three weeks after his retirement. Like so many of the men from his birth cohort, born around the turn of the century, he had a massive heart attack. Had he been alive today, his prospects of living longer would not have been much better. He died relatively young because his arteries were choked with plaques and his heart was failing from repeated small assaults. Had he not died when he did, renal problems and incipient diabetes would have become manifest and he would have died shortly thereafter from heart disease, stroke, or multiple organ failure. About all that the medical care available today could have done for my grandfather was relieve some of the symptoms he had suffered from for years—the shortness of breath and angina—but even today's care could not have made him well or materially changed the outcome. Reducing his blood pressure or lowering his blood cholesterol would not have prevented his death. Coronary artery bypass, for example, might relieve angina but not extend life.

My grandfather was always a very active man, but he was overweight and a smoker; was it diet and smoking that caused his (and so many other men's) early demise? This idea, as we shall see, is over-simplistic to the point of being seriously misleading. Yes, the diet of men of my grandfather's generation contained large amounts of saturated fat from meat and dairy products and refined carbohydrates in the form of bleached flour. Men also ate a lot of sugar. High-fat/high-sugar desserts were expected and candy was popular. Combine that diet with smoking and the explanation seems complete.

The problem with this assessment is that men of a later generation maintained much the same diet and smoking habits, while exercising less. Smoking rates, for example, peaked around 1960 and made their most sustained drops after 1980. Yet heart disease rates dropped dramatically from the mid-1960s onward. Deaths from coronary heart disease trended strongly downwards before the implementation of a range of improved treatments from ACE (angiotensin-converting-enzyme) inhibitors (1981) and statins (1985), and have remained on the same trajectory since. Rates of death for men from coronary heart disease fell from 700 per 100,000 population in 1962, the year of my grandfather's death, to approximately 200 per 100,000 in Canada today. No doubt my grandfather's diet and smoking were unhelpful and contributed to his early demise, but the sudden change in rates of coronary health disease suggests that causes run much deeper and are far more complex.

The son of a baker, my grandfather came from humble origins, and worked, in his youth, as a labourer. He remained in blue-collar employment until his death. And it was among people such as himself—relatively poor in childhood, rising to steady but relatively poorly paid manual or semi-skilled work in adulthood—that the heart attack epidemic was most severe. Those men, for some reason, were particularly susceptible to severe cardio-vascular disease and sudden, massive heart attacks.

Rather than simple causes, this book endeavours to show that a complex web of causality is at work over a person's entire life course, from conception to death. Risk factors such as diet and smoking form part of a complete explanation, but, as we shall see, only a small part. From this understanding arises a plethora of reasons to reconsider our health-related policies and programs. Out of those reasons, we can distill important policy recommendations for doing better in the future.

Note on the Second Edition

Since the first edition of *Social Determinants of Health*, epidemiologists have noted the sudden and large decrease in the incidence of several chronic diseases, including dementia and colon cancer. The rate of increase in others, such as diabetes, has slowed or reversed. Like the extraordinary decline in coronary heart disease that began in the 1950s, these more recent changes are inexplicable in conventional terms. Diets and exercise levels have not improved, and environmental risks have worsened. Health care cannot be credited with the changes because decline occurred in the incidence rates—fewer new cases arising—not as the result of better treatment of new or existing cases. The relevant change is in the conditions giving rise to chronic disease. This book attempts to identify what some of those conditions are, and why they have the effects on our biology that they do.

Acknowledgements

I would like to express my gratitude to the University of British Columbia for providing the research leave required to undertake the research supporting this book. I would also like to thank the University of Edinburgh for hosting me while I worked on the first draft, my editors at Oxford University Press, and the reviewers whose constructive criticism substantially improved the end result: Lindsay McLaren, University of Calgary; Janet McLaughlin, Wilfrid Laurier University; Kate Rossiter, Wilfrid Laurier University; Chris Sanders, Lakehead University; Sana Shahram, UBC Okanagan; Audrey Swift, University of Manitoba; as well as those who chose to remain anonymous.

Introduction

The Conventional Understanding of Health and Its Alternatives

How We Understand Threats to Our Health

We are well aware of the significant differences in people's health and longevity. Among the people we know, it is obvious that some succumb to disease, disability, and death, whereas others remain healthy and vital much longer. Mostly, we think of those varying outcomes in terms of innate characteristics—an individual's sex, age, and genes—in interaction with the various threats to health that the individual has encountered, either through choice (for example, too much time spent on the couch playing video games) or through no fault of their own (for example, environmental toxins).

Some threats to health are behavioural. In the research literature, those are referred to as "health behaviours." Examples of health behaviours that increase our risk of bad health outcomes are smoking or riding a bicycle without a helmet. Other risks are environmental. Air pollution, food contamination, and airborne pathogens are examples of environmental exposures that increase our risk of disease or death. We regard the former, behavioural threats, as being substantially within the individual's control, whereas we regard the latter, environmental threats, as mainly outside the scope of any one individual's actions. Changing individual health behaviours through education, persuasion, and incentives is our favoured approach to modifying behavioural risks. Public health intervention, such as clean air and clean water regulations and measures like quarantine of infectious people, form our repertoire of responses to environmental risks.

Of course, the extent to which something poses a risk to us depends on our level of **susceptibility** or our **resilience**. Conventional thinking runs along these lines: Our genes determine our level of susceptibility (or resilience) in the face of various threats. For example, if I am a middle-aged woman with a family history of breast cancer (indicating some degree of heritability or genetic predisposition to that disease), I am susceptible to potentially dangerous changes in breast tissue. Recent case and cohort studies of breast cancer suggest regular alcohol consumption elevates risk of breast cancer. Therefore, as someone with a genetic predisposition to disease, alcohol consumption poses an especial risk to me.

I may, due to my genetic inheritance or because of past exposure to some risk, be susceptible to bad health outcomes. I may have a gene that predisposes me to Alzheimer's disease or a blood lipid profile that predisposes me to heart disease. Health interventions might then include gene therapy, an effort to replace or disable the gene responsible for the susceptibility, or drug therapy to shift my blood lipid profile in a safer direction.

The discussion to this point outlines the common sense or **conventional model of health and disease**. It is built on a distinction between the individual who has various attributes that increase or decrease his or her susceptibility, resilience, or vulnerability, and a set of factors that interact with that individual, generally characterized as potential threats to health or "risks." **Risk factors**, as we saw, may be health behaviours or environmental factors or even specific susceptibilities.

Underlying this familiar view of health, disease, and life expectancy is a theory worked out in the late nineteenth and early twentieth centuries, which in turn echoes an earlier view of "predisposing" and "exciting" conditions. In that pre-scientific view, children, females, the elderly, and the frail are predisposed to poor health outcomes and thus need to be shielded from emotional shocks, sudden changes in temperature, and a range of other "exciting" conditions. Much of this pre-scientific thinking about vulnerability lingers on in today's ideas concerning a healthy person and our notions of variable resilience among various personality types, ages, and sexes. For example, women are often regarded as being prone to emotional distress and hence vulnerable to anxiety and depression. "Type A" men, ambitious and single-minded, are thought to be prone to heart attacks. The idea of exciting conditions survives in various forms, too, such as the fear of catching a cold if you head outdoors immediately after washing your hair. More important, pre-scientific thinking carries over into the modern **medical model** of "host and agent"—the former being us, individuals, and the latter being various threats that might assault us. Health-relevant features of hosts and agents are illustrated in Table I.1 below.

In the modern model of host and agent, if we have a degraded immune response plus exposure to a large dose of common cold viruses, we will fall ill. Similarly, a host may meet a premature death if exposed to a large quantity of a toxic agent such as arsenic or to a smaller dose over an extended period of time. What is considered a significant dose depends on host characteristics such as body size, age, **sex**, and other features that contribute to biologic resilience, features mostly determined by our genes.

Each agent–host interaction is slightly different because of variations among us, among the hosts, and among the agents that assault us. Thus, generalizations about the outcomes of host–agent interactions are *statistical*—they are the usual response observed from a large number of individual exposures. When we say a five-year-old is susceptible to hypothermia, we are implicitly assuming an average size and weight for a five-year-old. A large child may be no more susceptible than a small adult.

Notice that both the older version of predisposing and exciting conditions and the newer one of host and agent centre on ideas about how an individual's health relates to things acting in or on that individual's characteristic features. In other words, modern thinking about risks to health is just as individualistic (or person-centred) as the older conception. The importance of this will be drawn out in the discussion of levels of analysis in Chapter 1.

Notice also how a discussion of health and disease focusing on the condition of the individual, his or her susceptibility, lends itself to moralizing. In the pre-modern view,

Table I.1   Health-Relevant Features of Hosts and Agents

Some Health-Relevant Features of Hosts	Some Health-Relevant Features of Agents
Age of the individual	Virulence (infectious agents)
Sex of the individual	Toxicity (non-infectious agents)
Immune status of the individual	Communicability (infectious agents)
Specific genetic factors	Capacity to damage genes or disrupt DNA

character flaws such as vices (e.g., consuming alcohol, "wantonness" or promiscuity, glut-tony, "intemperance," or risk taking) formed an integral part of the explanation of disease incidence. Vice or virtue made up a big chunk of predisposition to poor health outcomes. Today, under more modern guise, there remains an inclination to blame victims for poor health. Smokers, people who put on weight, and those of us who exercise very little are not only predisposed to poor health outcomes but also are often blamed for them. Men who had sex with men in the late 1980s were blamed for the "gay plague," HIV-AIDS. More re-cently, the media began talking about an epidemic of obesity fuelled by poor food choices, lack of exercise, and overeating. And each of us is inclined to think it is somehow unfair that we fall ill when we have been careful about our diet, have been exercising regularly, and have been watching our weight, whereas we are not surprised and often not very sym-pathetic when someone who we think is careless and prone to poor decisions becomes sick. The importance of moralizing, its ideological basis, and the negative consequences such thinking conveys for health promotion, are themes we will return to later in the book.

The science based on the modern concepts of hosts and agents is known as **epidemiology**. It is the science of explicating the causes and variations in the frequency of various health outcomes. It operates in the context of risks (agents understood as po-tential threats) to individuals and how the attributes of those individuals interact with or relate to those risks. For example, my risk of injury or death in an accident posed by riding a motorcycle depends on whether or not I ride a motorcycle, how much I ride it, where I ride it, the times of day I ride, if I consistently wear an approved helmet, weather conditions when I am riding, my amount and type of riding experience, the mechanical condition of my motorcycle, and much else. In theory, I could collect data on motorcycle accidents by time, place, and weather conditions and work out correlations between rider experience, helmet use, and the mechanical state of the motorcycles to formulate esti-mates of risk based on those factors. That would be a form of **risk factor analysis**, an effort to figure out how probable an injury is given certain factors relating to motorcycle riders and to factors external to those riders such as the condition of their bikes and the roads.

It is important to understand that threats or risks are not the same as causes, although we often speak as though they are. For example, roughly 70 per cent of all cases of lung cancer occur in people who are or were regular smokers. The probability of developing lung cancer is much higher for a person who is or was a smoker compared with a person who never smoked. But this does not mean that smokers, even very heavy smokers who smoke for many years, will develop lung cancer—most in fact do not. Instead it means there is a major threat to smokers' health that does not exist for non-smokers. Smoking *elevates the risk* of contracting lung cancer. That is analogous to the motorcycle example. Riding a motorcycle puts me at significantly higher risk of serious injury, disability, or death compared with people who do not ride motorcycles. But it does not mean that riding a motorcycle will kill or maim me. Obviously, most smokers and motorcycle riders are playing the odds, accepting a higher risk because they perceive benefits just as a person might be prepared to invest money in a risky venture that offers them a 30 per cent return versus a government bond that guarantees them only 3 per cent. People vary in risk aversion just as they do in so many other characteristics. What is folly to one person is an acceptable risk to another.

Risk factor analysis is a useful and powerful way of looking at human health. It was through analyzing populations of people who developed heart disease that we came to learn that high blood pressure and abnormal blood lipid profiles elevate the risk of heart attack.

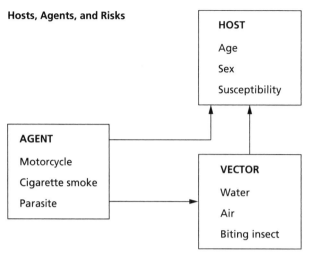

Figure I.1 Classic Model

(In other words, elevated blood pressure and cholesterol levels are consistently associated with more heart attacks, just like riding a motorcycle is consistently associated with more injuries and premature deaths.) We can look backwards to the risks associated with the risks—what raises the risk of high blood pressure? We could test the association of various diets with blood pressure and then (hopefully) show a relationship between some diets and lower (or higher) incidence of heart attack. If we look at a large enough number of cases, we can assign very specific probabilities. For example, regular, vigorous exercise might be found to reduce the risk of heart attack by 15 per cent (or put negatively, sedentary people might be found to face an increase in their risk of heart attack compared with more active ones). This kind of information is obviously very useful. It can help us to give sound health advice and to devise therapeutic interventions (such as blood pressure–reducing medications) with the aim of reducing the risk people face, hopefully altering health-relevant outcomes.

There are, though, several points to keep in mind. The first point is that risks or threats are probabilities, not certainties. Getting more training and always wearing a helmet will reduce my risk of death while riding my motorcycle, but neither the training nor the helmet will prevent accident or death. All we can legitimately conclude is that bad outcomes are *more likely* without precautions. The same logic applies to blood pressure and blood lipid (anti-cholesterol) medications. The risk of heart attack may be lower among people who take medication, but it does not become zero. In fact, meaningful reduction in the risk may be no more than 5 to 10 per cent. This of course means we must always be mindful of the negative impact of any intervention. If the drugs reduce my quality of life or cause bad side effects, the reduction in risk of heart attack may not be worthwhile. And those calculations, whether or not certain risks ought to be run, are personal and each person may make different, completely rational, choices. This, of course, is why health care professionals should always strive for informed consent. A patient should not be directed to one or other course of treatment, but rather should be told the probabilities of various outcomes associated with the choices available and be left to freely choose the one that best suits him or her.

The second point to keep in mind is that the risks we have calculated, the probabilities, are derived from looking at large numbers of cases—what epidemiologists would call a **population**. For example, if we were interested in reducing the risk of heart attack associated with high blood pressure, we would compare a population of people with high blood pressure taking blood pressure–reducing medications with a population of people with high blood pressure who are not. Hopefully we would find there are fewer heart attacks in the population taking the drugs. In other words, the risk of heart attack in a population of medication-taking people is lower than in a comparable population not taking the drug.

If our populations are both of 1000 comparable older adults, each with high blood pressure, and there are two heart attacks in the non-drug-taking population but only one in the drug-taking one, we see a 50 per cent reduction in heart attacks associated with the drug. This seems pretty impressive, but if any one older person's risk of heart attack is only 2 in 1000 (the risk in the older population not taking the drug), is a 50 per cent change in the probability that important to him or her? Moreover, if I am one of those older adults with high blood pressure, can I conclude that *I* will change my personal risk of having a heart attack by taking the drug? Technically, I cannot. Why? Because the probability, the risk, is a **population attribute**, not an attribute of any individual making up that population. Just as I cannot say "I am 150 cm tall" based on the average height—150 cm—of the population of students making up my class (in fact, no individual in the class may be exactly 150 cm tall), I cannot say my risk of heart disease is the same as that of the population to which I belong. But of course it is *reasonable* to take into account the statistical profile of the population to which I belong. Hence, it is also reasonable for me to derive some guidance from the population statistic as to where my risk falls. Thus, where my population's risk is high, it becomes prudent for me to take precautions.

The third, and perhaps most significant, point is that recent research has called into question the ability of risk factor analysis to account for the systematic differences in health across populations. Global findings, in particular, suggest that something else is at work. For example, wherever they reside (Canada, the United States, Australia, New Zealand), populations of Indigenous people live 6 to 18 years fewer than the non-Indigenous people living in the same region (World Health Organization, 2007). The Indigenous peoples in different parts of the world are not genetically similar, and their health-relevant behaviour and diets are not the same. What they share is poverty, racism, and social exclusion. Rates of premature death (below age 75) and infant mortality rates are typically higher for most ethnic and racial minority populations. For example, proportionally more black Americans die prematurely *irrespective of differences in risks between blacks and whites*, including smoking rates, exposure to violence, and drug use. Because they are rooted in social and economic conditions, these differences in death rates have proved to be remarkably resistant to change (Centers for Disease Control and Prevention, 2013).

A New Perspective on Our Health: The Rise of an Alternative View

In April 1974, the Canadian government published a working paper entitled *A New Perspective on the Health of Canadians* (National Health and Welfare, 1974). The paper is often referred to as the "*Lalonde Report*" because Marc Lalonde was the federal minister

Box I.1   Case Study ○ Health Disparities

Average life expectancy for men in Canada is projected to be 79 years in 2017, but only 64 years for Inuit men (Statistics Canada, 2010).

Life expectancy at birth for Indigenous Australians is 59 years for men and 65 years for women. Non-Indigenous Australian men have a life expectancy at birth of 77 years, and women 82 years (Australian Institute of Health and Welfare, 2011).

What factors might explain the premature death of Indigenous people? Which factors might be the same and which might be different in Canada and Australia?

responsible for health at the time of publication. The report is important because it marks the beginning in Canada, indeed in the world, of a shift in thinking away from the conventional view of health toward something considerably more radical.

The *Lalonde Report* argues that health care services are not the primary means of improving health; nor, according to the document, do biological factors alone account for disease. Rather, economic progress has brought fresh threats to health and well-being, notably "environmental pollution, city living, habits of indolence, the abuse of alcohol, tobacco, and drugs, and eating patterns which put the pleasing of the senses above the needs of the human body" (National Health and Welfare, 1974, p. 5). The key risks to our health today, according to *A New Perspective*, are self-imposed—reckless use of natural resources and irresponsible personal behaviour. Consequently, the working paper enjoins Canadians to become more active individually and collectively in maintaining and enhancing their health through adopting healthy lifestyles and protecting air and water quality.

The *report* heartily endorses Dr Thomas McKeown's view (McKeown, 1972) that medical care and biomedical discoveries play very little role in reducing illness and premature death (National Health and Welfare, 1974, p. 13). (That endorsement led some to speculate on the federal government's motives in producing the report because it was engaged, at precisely the same time, in capping financial transfers to the provinces in support of health care services.) From 1974 onward, in Canada at least, federal policy emphasis shifted from health care and a biomedical risk factor understanding of health toward a more social and behavioural point of view. Importantly, *A New Perspective* also brought much-needed attention to social and contextual factors such as the impact of urbanization on eating and exercise patterns, the stresses associated with city living, disorientation arising from rapid social change, and the mental and physical health implications of the modern workplace.

The federal government followed up on *A New Perspective* with the 1986 report *Achieving Health for All: A Framework for Health Promotion* (Health Canada, 1986). This report emphasizes a new vision of health, one embracing physical, mental, and social well-being: "Health is thus envisaged as a resource which gives people the ability to manage and even change their surroundings. This view recognizes freedom of choice and emphasizes the role of individuals and communities in defining what health means to them" (Health Canada, 1986).

Achieving Health for All (the "*Epp Report*," named after the then federal minister of health) identifies the first, and largest challenge: to reduce inequities in health between high- and low-income Canadians. The second challenge is to prevent injury and disease. In *Achieving Health,* "prevention" focuses on lifestyle, but unlike the *Lalonde Report*, the *Epp Report* broadens the analysis to include other factors and explicitly recognizes that choices are bounded by context and resources. The report also speaks of the need to provide better support to individuals and communities, particularly in the areas of chronic disease, mental health, and disability. Social support and the nature of community interaction thus become important health themes. Most importantly, the *Epp Report* introduces the "health promotion framework." Conceptually, health promotion is expanded from health education, and promotion of individual behavioural change, to a multifactoral approach that aims at engaging communities, and governments at all levels, to support individuals in making healthy choices and to create more healthy social and physical environments through coordinated health policy.

The idea of health policy was further expanded by the *Ottawa Charter for Health Promotion* (WHO, 2018), the product of an international conference on health promotion held in Ottawa, Ontario, in November 1986. The Charter calls for coordinated action among all levels of government, non-governmental organizations, communities, and families in pursuit of a physical and social environment conducive to health, access to health information, and the development of life skills and opportunities for making healthy choices.

Following something of a hiatus associated with economic downturn and government cutbacks, a further milestone was reached in 1997 when the Canadian Federal, Provincial and Territorial Advisory Committee on Population Health made the following statement:

> Population health refers to the health of a population as measured by health status indicators and as influenced by social, economic and physical environments, personal health practices, individual capacity and coping skills, human biology, early childhood development, and health services. As an approach, *population health focuses on the interrelated conditions and factors that influence the health of populations over the life course, identifies systematic variations in their patterns of occurrence, and applies the resulting knowledge to develop and implement policies and actions to improve the health and well-being of those populations* (emphasis added). (Public Health Agency of Canada, 2012)

This new way of thinking about public health, derived in substantial part from work by Robert Evans, Greg Stoddart, and Fraser Mustard, all associated with the Canadian Institute for Advanced Research, has not been without its critics. David Coburn and Ron Labonté in particular have suggested it owes too much to the older epistemological foundations of both epidemiology and economics (Coburn et al., 2003). By this they mean it remains reductionist, fails to take adequate account of broader societal determinants and historical forces, and consequently makes it difficult to envisage strategies for change. They encourage an approach more deeply informed by **political economy** and more research effort examining why and how different political and social formations contribute to different health outcomes. Coburn also laments how the new population health agenda, as defined by Health Canada and the Institute for Advanced Research displaces the more politically activist and community focused agenda of the Ottawa Charter. The approach adopted in this book attempts to meet some of those criticisms by explicitly considering public policy and some of the determinants of its formation.

Following the publication of the World Health Organization's (WHO) report of the Commission on Social Determinants of Health (2008) and the World Conference on Social Determinants of Health, attention returned to the conditions that foster or impair the health of Canadians. In particular, health disparities or inequities between populations became the focus of research and policy discussion, at least at the federal government level.

Since 2008, a consensus has emerged that there are a number of major underlying causes of health disparities, *determinants of population health*. The WHO has one list, Canadian researcher and author Dennis Raphael has another (Raphael, 2016, p. 11 and 19), and the Public Health Agency of Canada (2012) has a third, namely:

1. income and social status;
2. social support networks;
3. education and literacy;
4. employment and working conditions;
5. social environments;
6. physical environments;
7. personal health practices and coping skills;
8. healthy child development;
9. biology and genetic endowment;
10. health services;
11. gender; and
12. culture.

All of the determinants listed by the Public Health Agency, save biology, are discussed in this book, with the focus being on *the social determinants of health, in particular income, social status, social support, gender, employment, housing, and neighbourhood.*

Health Inequalities

As we noted, health disparities in Canada are obvious and troubling. The health of Canada's Indigenous people compared with that of non-Indigenous populations is a case in point. Some of the differences in life expectancies between Indigenous and non-Indigenous populations can be readily accounted for by risk factor analysis. For example, housing conditions, access to safe water supplies, diet and nutrition, and health-related behaviour such as smoking and drug and alcohol consumption, all pose greater threats to proportionally more Indigenous men and women than those risk factors do to non-Indigenous men and women. But recent research shows that much of the difference in health and life expectancy cannot be explained by differences in risk exposure. Even taking into account the cumulative impact of known risk factors, only a portion—current estimates vary between 10 and 25 per cent—of the health differences can be accounted for. That fact draws our attention to the social and economic circumstances under which Indigenous populations live and die.

When we look at disadvantaged populations including Indigenous peoples, black Americans, or Pakistanis living in the United Kingdom, we see not only similar differences in life expectancy between them and their host populations, but also disease and disability patterns similar to those we find among Canadian Indigenous people, in spite of large differences in diet, smoking prevalence, housing conditions, exercise behaviour, and use of alcohol. That strongly suggests the context in which populations are living their lives exerts a powerful effect on their health, well-being, and life expectancy. The resulting disparities are very large. For example, if black Americans enjoyed as good health as white Americans, nearly one million deaths would have been prevented between 1991 and 2000. In the same period, medical advances saved only about 175,000 American lives (CSDH, 2008).

Health Inequalities and Health Inequities

Population differences in health may be unavoidable. However, if the variations are avoidable, they are no longer merely **health inequalities** but also **health inequities** (Kawachi, Subramanian, & Ameida-Filho, 2002). In other words, to the extent that it is possible to make changes in society that would reduce or eliminate them, the gaps in health and life expectancy between groups are unjust.

If a child developed a condition that current medical technology cannot diagnose and because of that no effective treatment could be applied and the child died, that would be unfortunate but not unfair. If the child was not diagnosed because her mother could not afford the hospital's fees and, in consequence of not receiving care that would have otherwise been available, she died, that would be not only unfortunate but also unjust.

Differences in people's health are not morally relevant unless we are able to do something about them. If we can do something about circumstances that will lead to someone suffering pain, disability, or premature death, and we do not, we are morally culpable. At the social level, failing to respond to a harmful social circumstance that it is within our collective power to change is an injustice. Health inequalities arise from conditions over which we have no control; health inequities, or injustices, arise from conditions which are amenable to collective action.

The Basis of Health Inequalities

When we look at two countries with very large health differences, say Canada and Cambodia, or two populations in Canada with big differences in life expectancy, like urban Canadians and on-reserve Indigenous people, what is most striking is the level of resources, human and physical, available to the respective populations. These and other comparisons tell us that comparatively more affluent places with more developed health and other services have healthier populations. This suggests that the big differences in health arise from poverty rates and the availability of effective health care. However, as we will see in later chapters, differences in health do not appear only between the poor and the affluent, but also between middle-class and rich people in affluent countries like Canada and the United States. We will also see that health care has clear, positive impacts on people who are injured or at high risk of disease, but that those impacts do not account for the differences we see between healthier and less healthy populations. We are led to the conclusion that the context in which people live their lives, the resources available to them, and in particular their social and economic circumstances are the primary determinants of population health outcomes. How we know this and the consequences flowing from this knowledge are the subjects of this book. We will also address more fully the short-comings and strengths of the conventional view of human health, the importance of distinguishing individual from population levels of analysis, and the consequences for how we should think about health care services and health and social policies. Essentially, we will be following the trajectory from the *Lalonde Report*, through the *Epp Report*, to the Ottawa Charter and the report of the WHO Commission on Social Determinants.

Population Health and Politics

As we have seen in the discussion of the emergence of an alternative view of what makes us healthy or sick, the key concepts have changed from biological states to human capabilities, capacities, and opportunities and how social and physical environments impact on those capabilities, capacities, and opportunities. Alongside this, a shift has occurred from a purely individual level of analysis to a multi-level one that includes population-level and other contextual determinants of health. And, as we have also seen, these shifts in perspective highlight health disparities and draw our attention to the un-equal distribution within society of resources required for human well-being—income, education, social support, housing, and access to quality food and recreation, to name a few. Consequently, advancing the health of populations runs up against power and pol-itics, becoming more a matter of organizing communities, advocating for healthy public policy, promoting effective regulation, and pursuing fair taxation and public services than of simply providing basic health care. In short, health becomes a matter of social justice, where public health and social change merge to create fairer social arrangements.

Had the agenda of population and social determinants of health been set in the 1950s as opposed to the 1990s and 2000s, a good deal more progress on implementation may have been possible. As it stood, the political climate in Canada, the United States, the United Kingdom, and Australia was inimical to population health. The reason for this is that, since the early 1980s, the **liberal regimes** of Britain and its most similar ex-colonies (notably the US) moved toward greater individualism, consumerism, lower taxation, and reduced governmental involvement in society. This **neo-liberal** trend shows very little sign of abating, with the possible exception of Canada, whose citizens elected more progressive governments in Ontario in 2003, federally and in the province of Alberta in 2015, and most recently in BC in 2017. However, Ontario voters turned sharply right in 2018, and it is expected that the Alberta and BC electorate will do likewise in the next provincial elections; thus, even Canada remains under neo-liberal influence. Neo-liberalism is strongly supported by multi-national corporations and the affluent members of society, who are its principal beneficiaries. The ideology aligns well with a conventional view of health that regards health outcomes as mostly a product of genes (about which we can currently do very little) and risks (which are seen as substantially within any person's own control). If health outcomes are a mix of arbitrary and freely chosen variables, there are no grounds, moral or otherwise, for social and political engagement beyond basic health care services and health education, and no compelling reasons to ramp up public services, to tax companies and rich individuals, or to regulate the food industry or the housing and employment markets. Contrariwise, if differences in human health are largely products of how our society is organized and how resources are distributed within it, the defensibility of the status quo is called into question.

Pause and Reflect   What Do the Recent Data Tell Us?

Reflect on the information provided in the following tables and graphs. They draw on recent data from wealthy countries, including Canada. Tables I.2 and I.3 and Figures I.2 to I.5 compare life expectancies among populations. What underlying conditions might account for the differences shown in the tables and graphs?

Table I.2 Variability of Life Expectancy and Child Death in Various Countries: Life Expectancy and Under-Five Mortality, 2016

Country	Life Expectancy at Birth (years)	Under-Five Mortality (per 1000 births)
Australia	83	3
Canada	82	4
United Kingdom	81	4
United States	79	6
Japan	84	2

Source: World Bank, 2017. https://data.worldbank.org/indicator/SP.DYN.IMRT.IN?view=chart and https://data.worldbank .org/indicator/SP.DYN.LE00.IN?view=chart

Table I.3 Different Life Expectancies, White and Black Populations in the US: Expected Life in Years, 2013, United States

White Male	Black Male	White Female	Black Female
76.7	72.3	81.4	78.4

Source: Centers for Disease Control and Prevention, 2015. https://www.cdc.gov/nchs/fastats/life-expectancy.htm

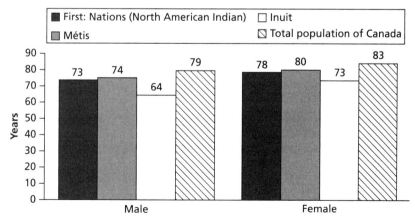

Figure I.2 Life Expectancy in Canada, by Indigenous and Total Population, 2017
Source: https://www.statcan.gc.ca/pub/89-645-x/2010001/c-g/c-g013-eng.htm

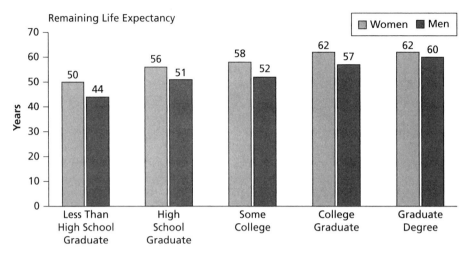

Figure I.3 Remaining Years of Life at Age 25, United States, by Education, 2005
Source: Rostron, Boies, & Arias, 2010.

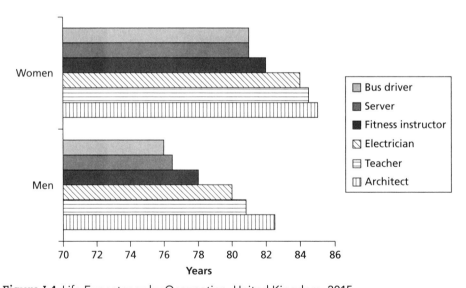

Figure I.4 Life Expectancy by Occupation, United Kingdom, 2015
Source: Redrawn based on: https://visual.ons.gov.uk/most-affluent-man-now-outlives-the-average-woman-for-the-first-time/

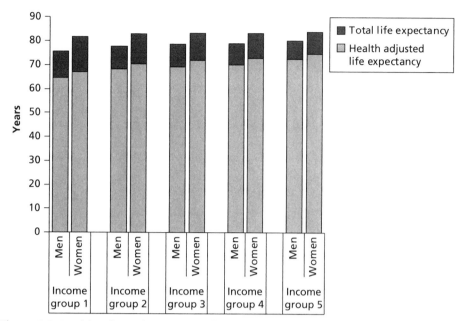

Figure I.5 Health Adjusted and Total Life Expectancies by Income Quintile and Sex, Canada, 2007

Notes: Income group 1 is lowest income. Health adjusted life expectancy is the number of years in *full health* that an individual can expect to live. Total life expectancy includes years estimated to be lived in poor health, based on current morbidity and mortality conditions.

Source: Drawn using data from Statistics Canada, 2012.

What Lies Ahead

As we will see in the chapters that follow, health care is not an important determinant of the health of an affluent country's population. Nor, as is often supposed, are environmental conditions amenable to public health intervention—such things as garbage and sewage disposal, environmental degradation, and air pollution—the major drivers of population health outcomes. For wealthy countries—and it is important to emphasize that the point is true only of industrialized affluent countries—income, education, employment levels, and working conditions, and not health behaviours such as smoking, overeating, and excess alcohol consumption, are the primary determinants of the health of the population (Marmot, 2010; Or, 2000).

Moreover, advanced countries, even advanced capitalist countries, are not all the same in terms of how they deal with incomes, education, and employment. Researchers have fitted these countries to typologies (Esping-Anderson, 1990). This book will focus on Canada, but will also include comparisons with other countries classified as liberal regimes. That grouping includes the United Kingdom, the United States, and Australia. While each of those countries has its unique features, they are importantly alike in terms of the role of government and the nature of most health and social policy. They also have similar economies and levels of economic development. Comparison among the liberal regimes permits drawing contrasts not only among them but also between them and countries that have adopted different approaches. That becomes particularly useful when we examine policy options for improving the health of Canadians.

Esping-Anderson (1990) showed that those countries he grouped together as "liberal" offer assistance only to the most needy, least well-off members of society; characteristically look to the market rather than governments to address issues of employment, income, housing, and health care; and seek minimal taxation on (and maximal liberty for) individuals and corporations. This contrasts with "**conservative regimes**," whose political agendas are shaped by family and traditional community values, and that characteristically look to families to provide requisite support to their members. Portugal is an example. The third classification is "social democratic": these regimes seek non-market, public provision of a range of services such as education and health care because they regard them as rights of citizens, or "universal entitlements." Social democratic countries demonstrate the willingness to use government capacity for taxation and service delivery to create fairer distributions of resources and opportunities. Sweden is an example.

The remainder of the book comprises 14 chapters. Chapters 1 and 3 outline the background, theory, and evidence base for a population health perspective. A primary goal is explicating the relationship between resources available to a person and his or her health. As mentioned above, several chapters go into the social aspects of the determinants of health as identified by the Public Health Agency of Canada (*in particular income, social status, social support, gender, employment, housing, and neighbourhood), as well as the health care system itself.* Chapter 2 covers two related subjects: the health care system and health research. Chapter 4 discusses the relationship between income inequality and population health. Chapter 5 focuses on the importance of early childhood and the transition to adulthood, Chapter 6 covers gender and health, and Chapter 7 deals with the relationship between social support and well-being. Chapter 8 examines circumstances confronting Indigenous peoples, who experience the most social inequalities in Canada, and so who are an illustrative case that provides context for applying the ideas in both the preceding and these next chapters: Chapter 9 deals with employment and health; Chapter 10 discusses housing and neighbourhoods; Chapter 11 examines food, nutrition, and obesity; and Chapter 12 examines environmental factors as determinants of health. The final two chapters move beyond the outlines of the causes of health inequities and examine our attempts at reducing them: Chapter 13 provides an overview of the social patterning of health-relevant behaviour, gives an account of why traditional health promotion fails, and suggests a more effective approach, whereas Chapter 14 deals explicitly with the politics of health-related policy and the implications of globalization.

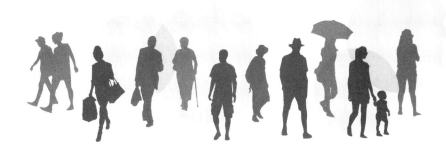

1 Thinking about Individual and Population Health

Objectives

By the end of your study of this chapter, you should be able to
- distinguish between individual and population levels of analysis;
- understand how a shift to a population level of analysis changes our perspectives on
  - treating people for disease;
  - modifying individual behaviour;
  - preventing bad health outcomes through screening and early intervention; and
  - evaluating health programs and services;
- appreciate how broader features of society such as its level of affluence affect the population.

Synopsis

Chapter 1 begins with fleshing out the concept of "levels of analysis" and discusses the variants (biomedical and behavioural) of the individual-level model of disease, illustrating the shortcomings of the biomedical and behavioural analyses. We then introduce the population level of analysis, outlining its genesis and main features. The chapter concludes with a summary of health demography focused on the demographic and epidemiologic transitions.

Levels of Analysis

In the Introduction, we discussed the idea of levels of analysis. The first part of this chapter provides some further context for, and examples of, this important idea.

When we talk about something "being healthy," we need to specify the level of our discourse. When we talk about healthy cells, we are talking at a sub-individual level. In referring to conditions supporting a healthy cell, we might identify satisfactory levels of available oxygen and glucose, among other things. If we move up to talking about the whole body, a functioning individual, different things come into focus. At the individual level, the idea of "being healthy" might focus on vigorous regular exercise, a diet rich in fruits and vegetables, and regular use of seatbelts in cars and bike helmets while cycling. If we were to move up to the population level, once again different things would come into focus. Examples for a healthy population would include effective regulation ensuring the safety of food and water, effective public services, and environmental protection. Table 1.1 lists some cellular-, individual-, and population-level attributes contributing to health.

Obviously there are no cellular counterparts to the healthy lifestyles that support health at the level of the individual. Likewise, many of my cells may remain perfectly healthy, at least for a time, but I may be brain-dead. And individual persons do not have public services, while governments and communities do.

Our concern in this chapter is to contrast analysis at the individual level with analysis at the population level. In general, some variables or attributes are appropriately applied to the individual (income, for example) and some are only appropriately applied to a population (income distribution, for example). Some variables are inherently features of collectivities (neighbourhood security, for example) and cannot properly be applied to persons. Doing so is a form of the "**ecological fallacy**."

When we discuss the health of a person—attributes applying appropriately to her or him—we are by necessity talking about relevant health factors at the level of the individual. Those include age, sex, genetic inheritance, and the **risk factors** arising from the person's behaviour and the environment. Studying the relationships among those individual-level features implicitly excludes features that are not about the individual but rather are about the group to which the individual belongs or about the place where the individual resides or works. Logically, we cannot mix individual features with population and collective ones because, as noted above, they apply to different things.

The example of income is in some ways unfortunate because it introduces a possible confusion. If we are talking about income, can we not talk meaningfully about an individual's income and, in the same way, a population's income? Is not gross domestic product (GDP) a measure of an entire country's income? Thus, we seem to have the variable "income" operating at two levels at once: individuals and nations composed of individuals. How is that possible, given what was just said? The answer is that a measure like GDP is not really a measure of a country's income but rather an adding up (aggregation) of many individual incomes. In other words, there is no content in the idea of GDP that is not included in the income of individuals. Thus the former, GDP, can be disaggregated into the latter, individual incomes, without any loss of meaning. Indeed, "GDP" means the aggregation of individual incomes. But that is not the case with truly collective variables such as income distribution, which is not about an individual's income, either singly or

Table 1.1 Levels of Analysis

Healthy Cell	Healthy Person	Healthy Population
Balanced electrolytes	Eats fruit and vegetables	Effective food safety
Available O_2	Exercises regularly	Good schools and health care
Available glucose	Uses bike helmet regularly	Environmental protection

added together with others, but rather about the relationship among incomes in a population. The concept of income distribution is inherently comparative and relative. Collective variables characterize a whole, not parts, just as my health as a whole person has to be distinguished from the health of my cells.

At the risk of sowing further confusion, an aggregate like a country's income might have an effect on individuals. For example, I may feel secure, but it is my neighbourhood that has the characteristic of security. Security, the absence of threats, is a place or contextual variable, not a personal one. However, the measure of neighbourhood security may be derived by aggregating the sense of security of individuals, although it remains true we cannot infer an individual sense of security from neighbourhood features. But as the example suggests, there is a relationship between collective features and individual ones. One would expect, for example, individuals to feel more secure in a neighbourhood that is well lit at night, relatively open with good sightlines, and so on. But in order to avoid conceptual error, the collective variables and the individual ones must be kept distinct and we must always be careful not to confuse aggregated individual measures with truly collective ones.

Ensuring, when we are trying to determine what affects human health, that we do not inadvertently mix up collective variables such as population and place attributes with individual ones is a daunting task and an important source of error in many studies. An equally daunting task is attempting to determine whether some population and place attributes affect population health or whether, alternatively, everything that is important can be disaggregated down to variables at the individual level. As we will see when we discuss income and health in Chapter 4 and social solidarity in Chapter 7, this is a disputed area. We will also see that the dispute is far from "academic" in the sense of being of little practical importance. Policy-makers decide such things as income-redistribution policies based on their understanding of what variables impact on the well-being of the population.

Levels of Analysis in the Academic Literature

The different levels of analysis are sometimes described in the literature using one of two metaphors as models. The first is the metaphor of "nesting." The individual is nested inside a community, which in turn is nested inside a society comprising a culture, economic and political institutions, and policies and laws (see Figure 1.1).

Societal factors, like the nature of the taxation system and public policy, "condition" community variables such as availability of affordable housing (through, for example, municipal low-cost housing), which in turn affect the quality of housing available to an individual (low-quality housing constituting a risk to his or her health).

On the face of it, this appears to be a more holistic analysis and to incorporate considerations beyond the single dimension of individual factors. But it is problematic because it creates the impression that societal factors are mediated through community ones to eventually influence *the factors that really matter, the ones acting directly with immediacy on the individual*, determining his or her health. It also suggests the pathways of influence/causality are from society down through community to the individual, whereas there is no a priori reason to rule out individual and collective factors (such as collective action by citizens) changing societal variables. Further, the heuristic of nesting implies that action

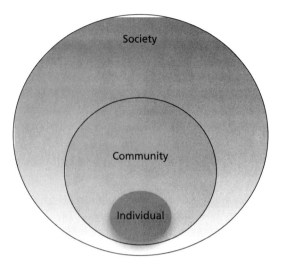

Figure 1.1 The "Nesting" Model of Analysis

relevant to health is most likely to be both appropriate and successful at the individual level. Thus, nesting implicitly gives emphasis to individual risk factors. Interventions such as changing personal behaviour and modifying, through health care intervention, risks like high blood pressure are privileged by this kind of modelling.

A second, and even more popular, approach in the literature is modelling variables in a hierarchy built by judging how "close" the variable is to the health outcome of interest. Variables that are near in time or proximity to the event are "**proximate**," ones distant are "**distal**," and ones in between are "meso" or **intermediate**. For example, my current immune status and the presence of cryptosporidium (a common parasite) in my drinking water are "proximate" and the public policies governing and the funding for water treatment plants are "distal" (see Figure 1.2).

Nancy Krieger (2008) criticized this framework. Like nesting, the "effect cascade" from distal to proximate implicitly assumes **proximal factors** are key, the prime determinants or "causes." They may be conditioned somehow by distal factors that are more distant in time or place (or both), but that are secondary to the principal analysis. This approach lends itself "to focusing on . . . 'proximal factors' ostensibly amenable to control by either individuals or by public health or medical professionals" (p. 223). Moreover, the assumption made by "nesting" is carried over. Effects cascade downward, top to middle to bottom. But as Krieger points out, events or factors at one level can and do affect factors and events at non-adjacent levels. She notes, by way of example, that the US Supreme Court decision (distal) regarding the law on abortion had direct effects on individual women's health (proximate) by creating a personal right to control over fertility, an effect that was *not mediated* through intermediate levels such as the local community.

There is a related problem of logic. The cascade model assumes temporal priority for "distal" factors—they are not only "higher" in level, and "farther away" but also "earlier" in time. But in reality, all levels "coexist simultaneously, not sequentially, and exert influence accordingly" (Krieger, 2008, p. 227).

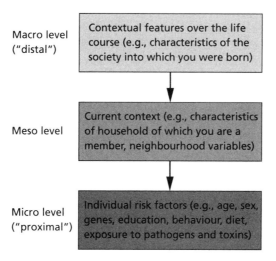

Figure 1.2 Modelling Levels as an "Event Cascade"

While talk of distal, meso, and proximal levels looks like a theoretical advance, it actually generates a conundrum. Conventional health analysis gives a nod to broader determinants like policies and community effects, but only as distant modifiers of the key determinants, the proximal or individual ones. Conventional risk factor analysis is preserved and looks like Figure 1.3.

Public health critics of the emphasis on individual level risk factors try to go the other way, emphasizing the importance of things like social features and policies shaping individual health determinants. To give an example, the same cascade model can be used to advance an argument that because smoking behaviour is so heavily influenced by social

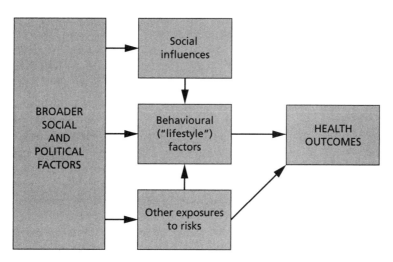

Figure 1.3 Modelling Health as Primarily a Function of Proximate Behavioural and Other Risk Factors

variables, and those in turn are so heavily influenced by public policy, corporate advertising, and so on, the focus should be on changing regulations regarding tobacco production and sales and not on getting individuals to quit smoking. The latter, trying to change individual behaviour, such critics say, is a hopeless, futile activity unless "upstream" variables like promotion of tobacco products are addressed. To take another example, some public health advocates argue the focus on people's eating and exercise behaviour is counterproductive given that people in North America live in an "obesogenic" environment—excess calorie intake in comparison to energy expenditure is straightforwardly the result of food production and marketing in automobile-dominated urban environments. Individual food choices and eating patterns are merely symptoms.

The first of these approaches—reducing everything down to lifestyle and environmental factors—is biomedical individualism. The second approach has been labelled "public health nihilism" (Krieger, 2008). Clearly, something more sophisticated, an analysis that can posit a variety of possible influences between and among levels of analysis, is called for.

One promising direction that has been charted by Maibach, Abrams, and Marosits (2007) is an "ecological model." They describes it thus:

> "The concept of ecology pertains broadly to the interrelations between organisms and their environments. We interpret ecological models of health as positing, in essence, that the health of populations is influenced by (a) the attributes of the people in the population; (b) the attributes of the environments—or places . . .; and (c) important interactions between the attributes of people and places." (p. 2).

The model gives special emphasis to social networks and social support in interaction with social structures, social policy, culture, and physical structures. A similar approach is used here. Social support, social networks, and place, particularly neighbourhood, form significant portions of this book.

Before turning to more of the theoretical considerations, though, we will return to the centrality and ubiquity of the individual-level analysis of health and disease, and further explicate its importance.

Individual-Level Analysis of Health and Disease

In this section, we take a closer look at the individual-level model of health and disease, often referred to the **risk factor model**. There are two variants: a **biomedical variant**, which focuses on the interaction of **host and agent**, and a more recent **behavioural variant**, which emphasizes health behaviour (lifestyle factors). Both are based on risk factor analysis, discussed in the Introduction. We will see in what follows that weaknesses in that model foster interest in alternative ways of theorizing the determinants of human health.

The key considerations regarding the host are age, sex, and genetics. The risk factor model assumes that once we know enough about those individual characteristics, we will understand the host's susceptibility to disease and his or her resilience to the risks to which he or she is exposed. For example, if we know the host is a woman aged 46, she has passed through menopause, and her family has a history of breast cancer, we can infer she is susceptible to (or "at high risk" of) breast cancer.

Behavioural factors such as dietary choices, activity level, use of alcohol or drugs, sexual practices, smoking, etc., interact with host susceptibilities. For example, if our hypothetical

46-year-old woman regularly drinks alcoholic beverages, exercises little, and is overweight, her risk of breast cancer is further elevated (she is now "at very high risk"). Social factors such as support from others, income level, etc., modify the potential impact of behavioural factors. For example, if our hypothetical 46-year-old woman lives alone and is under a lot of personal stress, her risk of cancer may be elevated even more. The various risk factors of alcohol use, activity level, body mass index, personal stress, and social isolation may interact, compounding her risk of disease (making her "at extremely high risk").

According to the risk factor model, external factors, such as pathogens, toxins, etc., interact with behavioural factors and susceptibilities. For example, if our 46-year-old host is a heavy smoker and she was exposed to asbestos fibre, her risk of lung cancer would be much higher than if she were exposed only to cigarette smoke. The behavioural risk factor of smoking interacts synergistically with the environmental risk factor of asbestos fibre. (She is now at "extremely high risk" of developing lung cancer.)

Predictive Capacity and Stability of the Characteristics of Age, Sex, and Genetics

The risk factor model is intuitively appealing and conceptually simple, but it has short-comings. First, there are problems with specifying susceptibility or resilience based on host characteristics of age, sex, and genetics.

Pause and Reflect   Health Predictions Based on Individual Characteristics

What health outcomes can be predicted from knowing a person's age? How reliable are those predictions? Does it matter which population a person is drawn from—for example, Japan versus Jamaica, Sweden versus Sierra Leone?

Host Characteristics: Age

Age is frequently used as a signifier of how healthy a person is likely to be and how much longer he or she will probably live. Unfortunately, age is not a powerful or precise predictor because of (a) substantial variation at all ages in the health, resilience, and susceptibility of people, (b) variability in the potential for healthy living which is steadily extending into ever-older age groups, and (c) the vast differences in health and life expectancy at different ages in different populations. We can make generalizations such as "women over the age of 60 are at increased risk of hip fracture," but those generalizations are not very informative. Many women over age 60 are not at elevated risk of fracture. Much depends on the kind of life they have led, their lifetime exposures, and their current context. For example, a recent high-quality study showed that, at age 38, biological age (measured by physiological markers of aging) ranged from the twenties to the late fifties (Belsky et al., 2015).

Host Characteristics: Sex

Health statistics are routinely reported by sex, based on the idea that sex is a significant determinant of health and life expectancy. However, sex, "the biological and physiological aspects of males and females," is a weak predictor of health outcomes. First, it can be misleading to treat individuals as though they are either wholly male or female. In reality, biologic sex is a spectrum, not two entirely separate states. All people have blends of male and female hormones, and the levels of those vary significantly between and even within individuals. There are some important sexual generalities, but few sex-linked features predict specific health outcomes. Obviously, a person cannot have cervical cancer without a cervix, or prostate cancer without a prostate, and generalizations can be made such as that females tend to outlive males, but the degree of predictability for most health outcomes based on biologic sex is low. Thus, dichotomizing people for predictive purposes based solely on dominant genitalia is not useful, partly because "sex itself is not a biological mechanism" (Springer, Stellman, & Jordan-Young, 2011) and partly because doing so masks broad within-sex variation. It is probable that any two females will differ as much in health as any given female and a male.

Second, sex is confounded with **gender**—the social expectations placed on a person and the roles that person adopts. It is wrong to think the biologic factor "sex" can be separated from socially mediated attributes of gender. In fact, sex and gender are "entangled" (Springer, Stellman, & Jordan-Young, 2011), so treating them separately can be misleading. Although difficult to separate, we can readily see that many health-related differences between men and women are more gender- than sex-related. For example, in our society men take more risks, engage in more health-damaging activities, and seek less support from others than do women. Those behavioural attributes carry greater significance for health and longevity than physiology. Moreover, unlike strict biological attributes of sex, gender is composed of features closely aligned to the kind of society in which men and women find themselves. Socially assigned gender roles and behaviours are highly variable from place to place and from one historical period to another. But remember, gender is not detached from sex; the two are "entangled." Gender is partly sexually determined, structured, and supported by physiological and hormonal differences. Thus, a proper analysis of health should take into account both biology and social context. The biomedical variant of the risk factor model will emphasize sex, whereas the behavioural variant will emphasize gender. Neither is right, because both variants are partial and incomplete. It is vitally important to recognize the *interaction* between sex and gender.

Host Characteristics: Genetics

In the past decade, research on the human genome has generated enthusiasm for the idea of "personal medicine." Because of the influence of the risk factor model, it is widely assumed that detailed knowledge of an individual's genome will tell us his or her precise susceptibilities as well as how that individual's biologic mechanisms will react to specific drug treatments. In theory, genetic knowledge will inform us of who needs treatment (or preventive measures regarding a susceptibility) and allow us to tailor the treatment to that person. Discovering host genetics will thus be the great leap forward long anticipated in medicine—safe, effective interventions for those at risk of disease. However, this enthusiasm for genetics in general, and personal medicine in particular, is largely misplaced.

At this point, we will stand back and review some basic genetics. In the 1950s, Watson and Crick famously discovered that the deoxyribonucleic acid (DNA) molecule has a double helical structure, a bit like a twisted ladder. DNA, of course, has a very interesting property. Its double helical structure allows it to "unzip." Each strand is a template for the creation of its partner, yielding two identical DNA molecules, the secret of replication.

The rungs in the DNA ladder are made up of a code comprising a sequence of four bonded chemicals: adenine, cytosine, guanine, and thymine (labelled As, Cs, Gs, and Ts). The combinations of the four letters ("condons") code for a specific amino acid, and the arrangement of those condons, a chunk of the DNA, codes for a protein. That DNA chunk is called a "gene," the basic unit of heredity.

DNA is crammed into structures referred to as "chromosomes." Humans have 23 pairs of identical chromosomes, one-half of each pair from each parent, residing in every cell of the body. Only one of the pairs, labelled "23," differs between males and females. Chromosome 23, the sex chromosome, has an identical pair of X chromosomes in females but an X and a Y chromosome in males.

Building on the old idea from Mendel's groundbreaking nineteenth-century work explaining heritability of traits in plants, Crick declared "the Central Dogma"—each gene codes for a specific protein and the cumulative result is the living organism. We are straightforwardly functions of the genetic code embedded in our DNA. Or to put it another way, our bodies and biologic processes are completely programmed by our genes. It follows that if we can decode the genetic sequence, we can understand an organism's biology. The quest was on to sequence the human genome, what scientists, in a rather unscientific flush of enthusiasm, referred to as the "Holy Grail" (Rose & Rose, 2012).

The Human Genome Project, as it reached completion in the late 1990s, threw up many surprises. First, humans have a measly 22,000 genes. Thus, it became obvious that each cannot be producing one and only one protein—that would require a million or more genes. Second, the human genome varies little from apes, indeed even earthworms. Clearly, sequencing the genome did not explain the complexity of human life; rather it raised more questions than it answered. Belief that knowledge about our specific genetic code is the key to improving our health was replaced by widespread skepticism, as illustrated by the following comment:

> Rapid improvements in "next generation" sequencing mean that people will soon be able to carry their genome on a memory stick at an affordable cost. What scientists have yet been unable to provide, however, has been a compelling reason why anyone would want to do so. (Kitsios & Kent, 2012)

In 2018, Kaplanis, Gordon, and Shor (2018) published a paper that reported on the results of studying 13 million individuals' life expectancies as functions of their ancestry ("pedigree"). The study shows that *less than 16 per cent of life expectancy is heritable and therefore can be predicted by genetics.*

Recent discoveries show that a gene or sequence of genes does not code proteins (or specific amounts of a given protein) simply because it exists in the genome. A gene codes the amounts of protein it does only because it has been "expressed," and when it is active and how active it is are processes controlled extra-genetically, mostly in response to the environment. The study of gene expression comprises the rapidly growing field of **epigenetics**. Epigenetics tells us that the correct answer to the "nature versus nurture" question is "neither." Neither our genes nor the environment decisively determines who we are and how healthy we will be. Underlying this is an important fact: biological entities adapt to the conditions in which they find themselves.

A classic study conducted in Finland in the 1970s illustrates human biologic adaptability. A person's height is heritable, and we know the genes that determine how tall a person will grow up to be. But the Finnish study shows that the heritability of the trait "height" is variable. Children with genes for tallness will not become tall under stressful conditions, whereas under conditions of plentiful food and low stress they will (Silventoinen et al., 2000). Or to take another example, researchers have found that the ADH2-2 gene is protective against alcoholism. People with this gene are less likely to enjoy the effects of alcohol and thus are less likely to become alcoholics. The ADH2-2 gene is relatively rare among New Zealanders of European descent but relatively common among the Maori. But alcoholism is relatively rare among European-descent New Zealanders and relatively common among Maori (Pearce et al., 2004). Environmental and social conditions modify not only behaviour but also genetic expression—which genes are active and how active each is. In sum, genetics, like age and sex, must be understood contextually, not abstracted from biologic, environmental, and social processes.

Another compelling example of environmental factors interacting with genes is a Canadian paper examining French-Canadian populations of identical genetic ancestry, which shows very different disease risk profiles due to differences in environmental exposures. The paper conclusively demonstrates that environmentally triggered epigenetic changes overwhelm genetic inheritance (Fave et al., 2018).

A further reason why genomics is not likely to be the answer to health and disease is the fact that there are very few unambiguously genetic diseases. Cystic fibrosis, Duchenne muscular dystrophy, and hemophilia are among the more common ones, and even those are rare conditions. Nor have we found, at least to date, specific features of the genome that might be health conferring. Pharmaceutical companies are continuing to investigate the possibility that certain gene sequences might enhance or detract from the effects of drugs, but "designer drugs" may also prove to be a dead end. Genetic testing for individuals' susceptibility to, or the usefulness or safety of, some drug is problematic because not one gene or a single genetic variant is involved. Instead, most physiological processes involve thousands of genes, the activity of each regulated, some in unison, some independently. Even the much hyped matching of breast cancer therapy to genetic type has been called into question.

In May 2013, the issue of genetic susceptibility to disease hit the front pages of the world's newspapers and virtually every television talk show. Celebrity actress Angelina Jolie announced she had had both of her breasts removed. Ms. Jolie had been found to have defective or missing BRA1 protein, a situation associated with elevated risk of ovarian cancer in women and breast and pancreatic cancer in both men and women.

Investigation of mutations in the family of genes involved in BRA1 and 2 proteins is an area of major, billion-dollar research by pharmaceutical companies. The current test for the mutation is monopolized by a patent held by Myriad Genetics. The strength of the link between a specific range of mutations and "hereditary breast-ovarian syndrome," a rare condition that most frequently occurs in women of Eastern European Jewish origin, is contested. With a family history of the disease and a positive test for the genetic defects, some, but by no means all, cancer specialists recommend prophylactic surgery. Others think stepped-up surveillance, such as regular mammograms, is more appropriate. Even in this extremely limited area, there is by no means consensus on the value of the genetic testing and there is a great deal of controversy regarding cancer-preventive mastectomies.

Also researching the case of breast cancer treatment, Nancy Krieger (2013) shows that the assumption that breast cancer estrogen receptor (ER) is a genetically determined, invariant (i.e., never-changing) characteristic of the patient and the tumour is false. ER is actually a flexible characteristic with variable expression dependent on time and context. Each of us embodies our history and context as "an emergent phenotype," not as an innate product of genetics. Thus, oncologists basing treatment on ER are mistaken in their approach.

The enthusiasm around disease prevention through genomics is even more misplaced than the effort to genetically customize treatment. For example, twin studies show that people with identical DNA develop different diseases from each other and have different life expectancies. Even having a gene that predisposes twins to a disease such as early dementia or coronary heart disease is only weakly predictive of outcome. That should come as no surprise because there are so many other factors at work besides potential genetic vulnerability. The best commercial enterprises can do in terms of providing health advice to people who pay to have their genome sequenced is to recommend exercising, eating more vegetables, and getting adequate sleep. The rest is mostly conjecture.

Box 1.1   Case Study ○ Genetic Health Conditions

A high-quality study of genetic determinants of autism concluded susceptibility to autism spectrum disorder (ASD) has "moderate genetic heritability and a substantial shared twin environment component" (Hallmayer, 2011). Autism is considered one of the most heritable conditions, yet even here recent discoveries show the conditions to which the fetus is exposed in the womb and the circumstances of his or her early childhood have decisive implications for how genes are expressed and what the ultimate outcomes will be for the child. (Hallmayer has shown that environmental factors are decisive, but has not yet discovered precisely which environmental conditions interact with genetic predisposition.)

Cystic fibrosis is another example of a genetic disease. Unlike autism, it does not appear to require an environmental trigger, just the misfortune of a particular genetic inheritance. But the health condition does not determine how ill a child will be or how long he or she will live. Rather, the health and life expectancy of a cystic fibrosis patient depend on the socio-economic circumstances of his or her family. The effect does not appear to arise from differential access to treatments but rather arises directly from the circumstances under which the child lives (Barr et al., 2011).

What conclusions flow from these recent findings?

Recent discoveries prove the "evolution of genes is less important than the evolution of regulatory sequences upstream of genes" (Sapolsky, p. 228, 2017). Scientific founders of the field of genetics, such as Crick, were wrong to think genes are the autonomous determinants of biology; rather, genes are themselves regulated by complex processes that depend on a host of contextual variables. An example is "gene–environment" interaction, wherein a particular genetic variant has an effect only when exposed to an environmental factor and, similarly, an environmental exposure has an effect only in interaction with a specific genetic variant. It's a mistake to think it's only the exposure that matters, just as it's a mistake to think it's only the genetic variant that matters. Sapolsky (2017, p. 246) notes that the FADS2 gene is associated with high intelligence, but only in breast-fed children. Neither the gene nor breastfeeding is associated with high intelligence in the absence of the interaction between them. Similarly, genes associated with high intelligence reliably produce that result when combined with being raised in families with high socio-economic status; poverty and adversity can trump genes. In general, genetics isn't a predictor of health outcomes—some straightforward determinant of health—but rather is "about context-dependent tendencies, propensities, potentials and vulnerabilies" (Sapolsky, 2017, p. 265). Consequently, our health is significantly a product of our personal histories and context.

Behaviours Portrayed as Individual Risk Factors

In addition to problems with predictions based on host characteristics of age, sex, and genes, there are problems with specifying individual behaviours as "risk factors." The most serious one arises from seeing behaviour as an individual attribute, implying that health-relevant actions are (at least largely) chosen. But apart from the trivial sense in which I must have decided to have a drink in the pub, it is by no means clear that behaviour is a straightforward function of individual choice. Studies demonstrate, for example, that the likelihood of me staying in the pub and having one or two more drinks critically depends on whom I am with at the time and the specific context (Demers, 2002; Kalrouz et al., 2002). I may well know that I should not drink any more tonight, determine I will call it quits, but go ahead and have those extra drinks. While we tend to think of health behaviour as choices not unlike deliberating over whether we will choose the brown or the black shoes, a surprising amount of our behaviour turns out to be more like the pub example.

Pause and Reflect   Context and Behaviour

If you are visiting your parents during a break in the university term, do you talk about the same things and use the same language as you do when you are with your friends? If your parents offer wine at a family meal, are you likely to consume as much alcohol as you would at a party with friends? Why might you modify your behaviour?

We all realize our behaviour is largely context dependent, but we rarely see the implications. To the extent that health-relevant behaviour is socially determined and not simply socially influenced, an individual-level description is inadequate. Given that some of our behaviour is virtually inexplicable without reference to the group we were with and without interpreting the specific context, an individual-level analysis will either fail or at best mislead. The study of the social determination of health behaviour is emerging as an important field—the **social patterning of behaviour**.

We will take up the subject of social patterning of behaviour in Chapter 13; however, it is worth pointing out, at this stage, two other weaknesses of the individual-level approach to health-relevant behaviour. The first is that the approach draws us into trying to change individual behaviour as our key strategy for improving health. As we will see in the upcoming discussion of the MR FIT study, modifying individual behavioural risk factors is no easy matter. The second weakness is that the approach lends itself to blaming the victim of disease. If it is a person's choice to exercise too little or to eat too much or to choose unhealthy foods over more nutritious ones, then that person has no one to blame but him- or herself for his or her diabetes or heart disease. As we noted before, the conclusion we draw is either the person is ignorant (needs educating) or is irresponsible (needs behavioural modification). We must always bear in mind that changing individual behaviour is difficult, people are more aware of health-relevant information than we often assume, and blaming people for illness is counterproductive and unfair if significant factors are beyond their individual control.

As attractive as the risk factor model appears at first sight, it should now be clear why the individual-level characteristics of age, sex, genetics, and behaviour provide an inadequate conceptual platform for considerations of human health.

As a final set of comments on the individual level risk factor analysis (whether the biomedical or behavioural formulation) relates to its inherent reductionism, or to put it another way, its methodological individualism. It's easiest to show this through looking at a central concept in risk factor analysis: "**relative risk**."

Relative risk (RR) is the measure of probability that a factor contributes to a disease or premature mortality. A variable that has no effect on health has an RR of 1.0, a variable with a negative impact on a health outcome has a value greater than 1.0, and a variable with a positive impact on health has an RR less than 1.0. Most health-relevant variables have RRs between 0.5 and 1.5, meaning they have a relatively small probability of shifting an outcome. An important exception is long-term heavy smoking, defined as 20 pack years (one package of 20 cigarettes smoked every day for 20 years), which has an RR of 4.0. That means a heavy smoker has a 400 per cent (four times) greater risk of lung cancer than a non-smoker.

RRs are calculated by examining outcomes in cohorts (populations of similar people) who are exposed to some variable such as tobacco smoke. The logic of cohort studies and the mechanics of calculating relative risks are discussed in Chapter 2. Cohort studies provide useful information such as whether it appears worthwhile to reduce blood pressure in order to prevent heart attack. (RR of elevated blood cholesterol is roughly 1.15, indicating that if blood cholesterol in a group with elevated blood lipids could be brought down to "normal," a 15 per cent reduction in heart attacks could be achieved.)

However, reductionism—the elimination of life history, contextual, and other environmental variables from the analysis—skews assessment of risk. Again, an example helps. The calculation of relative risk of heavy smoking applies in the United States. If researchers draw cohorts representing the US population, an RR of about 4 would be found. But Americans have patterns of early childhood development, diet, and drinking behaviour, a given level of exposure to viruses and air pollution, a typical work setting, and are exposed to US neighbourhood features, the stress of living in a competitive, high-crime society, with limited social programs, and the societal features of extreme income and wealth inequality. For those reasons, a different RR would be found in Japan or Sweden (both around RR = 2). In other words, RRs are not stable artifacts, but products of context. Because so many of the existing data for relative risks are measured in the US, they tend to be biased upwards. In other words, relative risks are typically exaggerated because of conditions unique to the United States. That raises serious questions about the wisdom of trying to modify small relative risks, including ones like elevated blood cholesterol, particularly if the means to modify the risk, often drugs, also bear health risks (more on this in Chapter 2).

Box 1.2   Case Study ○ The Enigma of Healthy Japanese Men

Japanese men are among the longest living in the world and have a remarkably low incidence of coronary heart disease. The natural way for us to look at this situation is at the individual level, trying to make sense of how different risk factors might be at work in Japan versus North America.

One candidate stands out as obvious: diet. The Japanese diet traditionally has been low in saturated fats, contained very little red meat and included a large amount of cereals (mostly rice) and vegetables. Diet turns out, however, to be a poor explanation of differences between Japanese and North American health for three reasons. First, people with Japanese-like diets in North America do not enjoy the same health advantage as the Japanese. Second, Japanese men have been eating increasingly more meat and American-style foods for decades. The average volume of vegetables, fruit, and seafood consumed has fallen, and meat, instant noodle, and American fast-food consumption has risen (Ministry of Health, Labour and Welfare, 2018). Yet Japan's heart disease rate continues to fall and its life expectancy continues to rise. Third, in spite of Herculean efforts by health researchers, the evidence that high-fat diets contribute to heart disease in North America is not very compelling.

We know that heart disease is associated with heavy drinking and especially with smoking. But heavy drinking and smoking are more prevalent among Japanese men than among North American men.

If the answer does not lie in behavioural differences, perhaps it lies in differences in susceptibility to heart disease. It might be that Japanese men have genes protective against coronary heart disease. But genes provide no better explanation than diet. Studies of migrants show that Japanese men's health is closely patterned by where they are living. Japanese men living in California, for example, will have a health profile closer to other Californians, including heart disease rates, than to other Japanese still living in Japan (Marmot et al., 1975).

How might we account for the difference in coronary heart disease incidence between North American and Japanese men? What other risk factors might be at work? Might context or population-level differences, rather than a singular factor or a set of risk factors, play an important part of the explanation? What contextual differences are there between Toronto and Tokyo? How do the Canadian and Japanese populations differ? Why might the differences matter?

Shifting Gears: From an Individual Risk Factor to a Population Approach

A change of focus from an individual level of analysis to a population level has practical public health implications. It is obvious that getting individuals to change their behaviour in order to improve their health is a very difficult and slow process, full of reversals, even when backed by government regulations, incentives, and sanctions. Careful studies, such as the Multiple Risk Factor Intervention Trial (MR FIT)(1982) study in the United States, show that even with intense education, group support, and a range of incentives, health-related behaviours and the health outcomes associated with them fail to shift significantly.

The MR FIT study is a classic in the field of research illustrating the problems associated with individual risk factor modification. MR FIT launched in the United States in 1972. The study was a clinical trial composed of a control group and an experimental group, each randomly drawn from a pool of 12,866 middle-aged men at high risk for heart disease. The control group received normal care in the community, whereas the experimental group was given stepped-up care to reduce blood pressure and blood cholesterol; counselling and support to quit smoking; dietary, shopping, and cooking advice to make weight-losing, heart-healthy meal choices; and support and training for increased exercise. Seven years into the trial, no significant differences could be found in health behaviours or health outcomes between the experimental and control groups, and the experiment was abandoned. Two conclusions may be drawn: (1) it is extremely difficult to change people's habits, at least in a lasting way; and (2) the risk factors the trial focused on—exercise, diet, smoking, and reducing blood pressure and blood cholesterol—account collectively for only a minority of heart attacks. The study must be interpreted cautiously, however, because of the problem of **secular change**. The behaviour of both groups could have changed over the study not only in response to the interventions of the researchers but also in response to broader changes in American society regarding smoking, diet, and exercise. Secular change, factors associated with developments that had nothing to do with the experiment, may have "washed out" some of the differences between the experimental and control groups, making the effects of the trial's interventions harder to find.

MR FIT is not a "one-off" finding. For example, findings consistent with the MR FIT study were published in 2009. The Women's Health Initiative Dietary Modification Trial, a concerted effort to shift the eating habits of women in order to improve health, failed to show positive results. Like MR FIT, the study suggests that targeting individual behaviour, particularly at mid-life or later, is not a very productive strategy (Michels & Willett, 2009).

Research study after research study provides little reason to believe that current campaigns in Canada, Australia, the United States, and the United Kingdom targeting obesity and inactivity through education and a variety of incentives will make much difference. This raises the question as to why governments and public health authorities continue to rely almost exclusively on individual-level measures intended to change personal behaviour. Part of the answer may be that we have been misled by the example of smoking into investing too much time, effort, and money into changing individual behaviour.

It is true that a mix of strategies, including punitive taxes, regulations prohibiting smoking in public places, and education on the health impact of smoking, applied mostly in the two decades from 1990 to today, helped reduce the prevalence of smoking. But it is unlikely those strategies were the root cause of the social change in smoking. This can be seen by the fact that smoking rates have declined in most places around the world, even where these public health policies have not been applied (including China, where use of tobacco products continues to be promoted). Smoking decline has occurred not only in Canada and the US, the countries that most aggressively targeted tobacco use, but everywhere around the world. The principal reason appears to be secular change, also known as a "temporal change." In the case of smoking, after its peak in 1960, using tobacco increasingly fell out of fashion, just like disco music, mirror balls, and the "big hair" of the 1970s fell out of fashion. It is changes in fashion that explain the fad in the late 1990s of rich people starting smoking (fancy cigars) while the general population was quitting smoking (cigarettes). More widespread knowledge of the health damage done by smoking, advocacy group action, and government-sponsored anti-smoking policies accelerated and reinforced a trend, but it is a mistake to think they caused it.

Box 1.3 Case Study ○ Secular Change and Tobacco Use, United Kingdom

Figure 1.4 shows the downward trend in smoking in the United Kingdom. The UK was a late adopter of smoking control measures, not implementing restrictions on smoking in enclosed work spaces until July 2007, not printing health warnings on cigarette packages until 2008, and not banning tobacco displays (Wales) until 2012.

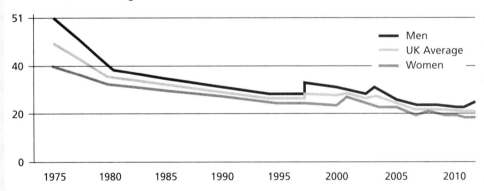

Per cent of Individuals Aged 16+

Figure 1.4 Smoking Rates in the United Kingdom

Source: "Unemployed and Single?" (2013). Copyright Guardian News & Media Ltd., 2013.

Oddly, smoking rates plateaued as control measures ramped up, before resuming a slow decline. Buried inside the aggregated figures shown in the graph is the fact that smoking rates have changed very little among socially excluded populations including prisoners, people experiencing homelessness, and those living with serious mental illness. The big changes have taken place among the privileged, the more affluent and the more highly educated, a feature true of Canada and United States as well as the United Kingdom. What might account for these findings?

One easy way of seeing that cultural variables and the norms of given groups are more influential than education, regulation, and pricing strategies is to compare smoking across countries (World Bank, 2012). Rates of smoking among men in Asia are very high (66 per cent in Indonesia) but very low for women (8 per cent in Indonesia), and that pattern holds irrespective of whether countries have more aggressive or less aggressive public health approaches to smoking (Singapore versus Vietnam or Japan). Africa, by and large, has low smoking rates, especially among women (13 per cent men/5 per cent women in Cameroon), in spite of heavy marketing by tobacco firms and little or no public health intervention by African governments. Some years ago, France implemented moderately strong bans on smoking, but its rates are higher than Germany's (36 per cent versus 33 per cent smoking prevalence among males) in spite of the fact that Germany has a lax approach to tobacco use. Greece has strong tobacco pricing and smoking regulations in place, but smoking rates remain stubbornly high (63 per cent men/41 per cent women). Mexico has relatively weak public health intervention, but low smoking rates (24 per cent men/8 per cent women), whereas the US has strong public health interventions but fairly high smoking rates (33 per cent men/25 per cent women). But pretty much everywhere, smoking rates are trending downward, irrespective of public health measures, mostly because the fashion for consuming tobacco is dying out.

Modelling public health interventions on what is widely regarded as successful anti-smoking measures can and does lead to wasted effort and misspent resources. Educational, pricing, and regulatory strategies may have the desired effects, but their impact is limited and, more often than not, these measures cannot play much more than supportive roles. Systematic failure to modify drinking behaviour, from the sixteenth century to today, through bans, licensing measures, purchasing regulations, education, and punitive pricing illustrates the point.

But if we target context rather than individual behaviour, important health-related changes become feasible. One example is serious injury and death due to road accidents. Engineering safer roads, improving intersections, ensuring better signage, and including more safety features in cars have made an enormous impact on motor vehicle injury and death, all without any effort on the part of individual drivers. Likewise, improving sightlines and lighting has bigger impacts on residential safety than increased policing. These are examples of population-level interventions, as opposed to targeting individual-level risk.

Origins of Population Health

Antecedents

In this sub-section, we will look at the significant theoretical contributions made by three seminal nineteenth-century thinkers: John Snow, Friedrich Engels, and Rudolf Virchow. All three brought to the forefront the importance of context for human health and well-being. We will also make passing mention of Émile Durkheim, a social scientist whose work greatly influences our understanding of human behaviour.

John Snow
John Snow (1813–58) was a physician who contributed significantly to the development of surgical anesthesia. He was highly regarded by Queen Victoria and provided her with pain

relief during labour and childbirth, pioneering the use of anesthetics in obstetrics. But it was John Snow's hobby for which he is most famous; Snow discovered the cause of cholera.

At the time that Snow practised medicine, the prevailing model of disease was the predisposing and exciting cause model discussed in the Introduction. One of the significant exciting causes was thought to be "miasma" or bad air. It was believed that if vulnerable people were exposed to mists or bad smells they would fall ill. That belief lay behind a variety of odd practices, such as royalty sleeping propped up to prevent their mouths falling open (and thus allowing foul vapours to enter them in their sleep). Fear of miasmas also lay behind the habit of ladies covering their mouths with perfumed hankies when confronted by strong smells. The rich built their homes on high ground to avoid fog and to enjoy the health advantage of breezes. They also built upwind from the smelly activities of slaughterhouses and tanneries. Ironically, it was fear of miasmas that motivated Victorian reformers in England to build sewers (to end the "Great Stink" of London). Other measures we would regard as related to public health, such as prohibiting the practice of driving livestock into town centres for slaughter and butchering, were also motivated by fear of the associated smells.

Miasma was blamed for the outbreaks of cholera in London. The evidence seemed strong as most cases occurred among people living in low-lying parts of the city, and cases were concentrated in poorer areas where stench truly was a problem. Snow, however, thought the cause lay elsewhere and undertook a detailed investigation. He painstakingly tracked cases of cholera and developed maps relating place to disease incidence. Those maps implicated sources of water supply as the cause of the outbreaks, establishing for the first time the idea of water-borne disease. Snow had no knowledge of micro-organisms as pathogens. While microscopic life had been discovered over a century before Snow's time, Snow died before the germ theory of disease would be formulated and a half-century before it finally displaced the model of predisposing and exciting causes.

The implications of Snow's approach are profound. Instead of looking for flaws in the person combining with some external factor, Snow saw cholera as arising from the context in which people were living, in particular the neighbourhood source of drinking water. Snow saw no moral dimension to the epidemics, unlike many of his contemporaries. Victims were simply unlucky to be living where they were. Florence Nightingale, in contrast, opposed admitting prostitutes suffering from cholera to hospital because in her opinion, they had brought on their condition. Beds should be reserved, in most Victorian minds, for persons of good character who could not be faulted for contracting disease. Snow's idea that people were victims of circumstance simply could not get any traction with his contemporaries.

In spite of Snow's flawless research, his hypothesis that cholera arises from impure drinking-water supplies was rejected in his own day. When the germ theory finally gained acceptance, Snow's emphasis on context was still lost because the germ theory carried over the old individualist bias of the predisposing and exciting cause in the new form of host and agent. Although his work failed to have an immediate impact, today Snow is credited with inventing both modern epidemiology and health geography.

Friedrich Engels
Friedrich Engels (1820–95) was the son of a German industrialist who owned textile mills in Manchester, England. Between 1842 and 1844 Engels studied the circumstances under

which working people lived in Manchester. The result was the publication of *The Condition of the Working Class in England* in 1844.

Engels produced data to show that the death rates of poor people in urban centres were much higher than the death rates of poor people in rural settings. He was also able to show that the death rate among children was lower in the town of Carlisle before industrialization than it was afterward. Engels sought to demonstrate that social and economic change can substantially affect health and longevity and that living and working conditions are the major determinants of human health and well-being. Engels also advanced the argument that health-harming behaviour among the working classes (family violence and alcoholism are examples) was a product of the conditions under which people live (a legacy of the "satanic mills" and squalid slums), not a consequence of character flaws or bad choices on the part of working-class men and women. Indeed, Friedrich Engels and Karl Marx later took great pains to demonstrate that, rather than being chosen by individual men and women, the appalling conditions under which they lived and worked were imposed on them. And those appalling conditions in turn determined the high rates of disease, disability, and early death.

Rudolf Virchow

Rudolf Virchow (1821–1902), like Engels, was German. Unlike Engels, he spent his entire life in Germany. Like Snow, Virchow was a physician, and he is now regarded as the father of modern pathology. Among many other things, Virchow developed what remains to this day the standard approach to conducting autopsies.

Virchow is important to the development of population-health thinking because of his groundbreaking analysis in his *Report on the Typhus Outbreak of Upper Silesia* (1848). Virchow argued that additional medical care, drugs, improved food supply, or any other combination of ad hoc interventions would not enhance the health of the population of Upper Silesia. Instead, radical political, economic, and social reforms were required to transform the living conditions of the inhabitants. Remarkably, Virchow explicitly linked civil and human rights to health outcomes, a very dangerous thing for him to do in authoritarian Germany.

Virchow went into politics later in life. He campaigned until his death for improved living conditions for less well-off Germans and for public health improvements, such as potable water systems and effective sewage disposal.

Émile Durkheim

A fourth nineteenth-century figure bears mentioning in the context of antecedents to population health—Émile Durkheim. Durkheim (1858–1917) is regarded as the father of sociology, and he developed the concept of "social facts." **Social facts** are human artifacts in the sense that they arise from the interaction of people in groups. But social facts also have the capacity to act as determinants of human behaviour. Durkheim noted, for example, that every individual has his or her own reasons to commit suicide, but rates of suicide are stable and predictable from features of the society in which those individuals lived and died (Durkheim, 1897). Social norms—what is expected of the individual by the group—are particularly powerful in this regard. It follows from Durkheim's analysis that we should understand health-relevant behaviour as arising from the individual's social context, not as freely chosen activity.

The social environment, according to Durkheim, is an important force shaping individual beliefs and norms of behaviour, providing or denying individuals opportunities, and increasing or decreasing the stress experienced by them. In short, features of the society in which we live shape our understanding and behaviour because social structures embed opportunities and constraints, many of which we remain oblivious to, much as a fish remains oblivious to the constraints imposed by living in water. It follows that what we experience as "choice" is substantially conditioned by our social setting.

Box 1.4	Case Study ○ Naming of Children

Each mother thinks she is choosing a unique and appropriate name for her child but, in any given time or place, many mothers end up choosing the same names. Table 1.2 shows the top 10 Canadian names for boys and girls, collectively accounting for a significant proportion of births in 1980 and 30 years later in 2010–2011. Notice that none of the popular names in 1980 are popular in 2010. What might account for these findings?

Table 1.2   Popular Children's Names

1980 Boys	1980 Girls	2010 Boys	2011 Girls
Michael	Jennifer	Liam	Olivia
Christopher	Amanda	Ethan	Emma
Jason	Jessica	Jacob	Sophia
David	Melissa	Logan	Ava
James	Sarah	Owen	Chloe
Matthew	Heather	Noah	Abigail
Joshua	Nicole	Alexander	Emily
John	Amy	Nathan	Madison
Robert	Elizabeth	Benjamin	Lilly
Joseph	Michelle	Lucas	Charlotte

Source: Based on: BabyCenter, https://www.babycenter.com/babyNameYears.htm.

The Revival of Population-Health Thinking

Two modern figures are closely associated with the revival of a population-health perspective. The first is the medical epidemiologist and health demographer Thomas McKeown. The second is the eminent British epidemiologist Geoffrey Rose. We discuss the work of McKeown (and related work in health demography) in this chapter, then launch Chapter 4 with a discussion of Rose and population health.

Thomas McKeown and Demographic Studies
McKeown is perhaps best known for his controversial book *The Modern Rise of Population* (1976). He argued that medical measures such as immunization and treatment played little or no role in the improvements in health evident in Western European populations

since 1700. Rather, according to McKeown, the sharp decline in mortality in Western Europe after 1850 was entirely due to changing social and environmental factors, notably the availability and affordability of more diverse and nutritionally rich foods.

McKeown based his work on observations that infectious diseases such as tuberculosis (TB) and pertussis had begun their spectacular decline, both in terms of incidence and death rates, long before the development of modern medical measures. In Canada, for example, the TB mortality rate dropped from 165 per 100,000 population in 1908 to less than 1 per 100,000 by 1985 (Grzybowski & Allen, 1999). Data from England and Wales show a three-fold drop in tuberculosis mortality between 1851 and 1935 (Wilson, 1990). US data show precisely the same trend. No evidence supports the possibility that the virulence of the TB bacillus weakened, and no evidence supports the possibility that population resistance strengthened due to genetic selection. It is important to recognize that the deaths dropped not because people continued to get the illness but for some reason—better care or more resilience—survived in spite of having TB. Rather, the death rate went down because the number of people newly acquiring infection went down. Moreover, in Canada, immunization only began in 1948, and antibiotics effective against TB did not become widely available until the mid-1950s. Thus, the main factor reducing TB incidence appears to be, as McKeown claimed, social change, not improved health care.

English mortality rates from scurvy, a nutritional disease caused by lack of vitamin C in the diet, and of measles, a highly infectious viral disease, changed at roughly the same rate and time (see Figure 1.5). While that relationship does not necessarily prove anything, it certainly suggests a common underlying cause. The nutritional status of the population is the most obvious candidate.

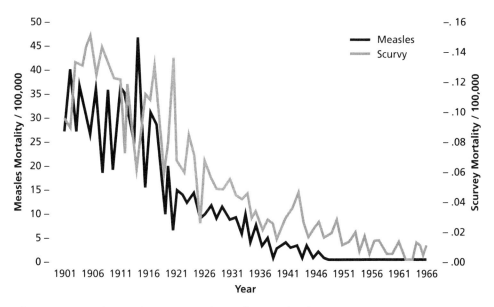

Figure 1.5 Death Trends, Scurvy and Measles, England

Source: Adapted from Keith Montgomery, n.d., http://pages.uwc.edu/keith.montgomery/Demotrans/demtran.htm.

McKeown's strident rejection of health care as a determinant of human health and his rather singular focus on nutrition understandably attracted a good many critics. His work has been criticized for failing to recognize the ambiguity and potential complexity of the ideas of rising affluence and social change. McKeown produced no evidence that the key variable in rising living standards is nutrition. Worse, McKeown completely discounted the measures that were taken to reduce diseases like TB, which included isolating patients and thus containing the pool of infection (Wilson, 1990).

There remains a strong political element to the dispute over the role of health care in general, and vaccination in particular, in reducing mortality. Anti-vaccination activists (e.g., Obomsawin, 2012) have seized upon McKeown's data, claiming vaccines make no difference to public health—a proposition that is patently false. Incidence rates of measles, for example, have dropped dramatically in Canada, the US, and the UK since the introduction of universal vaccination in the 1970s.

But after what appeared to be a near total demolition of McKeown's ideas, more recent research has, at least in part, vindicated him. It is now widely recognized that health care and even public health interventions, such as piped drinking water and sewage systems, played a relatively small, albeit important role in the reduction of disease incidence, infant mortality, and the extension of life expectancy. Attention in research has been drawn away from medicine and public health and toward the social and economic factors underpinning human health and development.

Thomas McKeown was further vindicated by health services research focused on the effectiveness of medical and hospital interventions. Many studies in the 1980s and 1990s confirmed that the impact of health care on the health of populations is actually quite small. Paradoxically, studies often found, especially in the United States, that more health care leads to worse population health (Or, 2000), presumably due to unnecessary or inappropriate services. Today, health researchers generally agree with the following statement:

> Medicine's much hailed ability to help the sick is fast being challenged by its propensity to harm the healthy. A burgeoning scientific literature is fueling public concerns that too many people are being overdosed, overtreated, and overdiagnosed. Screening programmes are detecting cancers that will never cause symptoms or death. . . . With estimates that more than $200bn may be wasted on unnecessary treatment every year in the United States, the cumulative burden of overdiagnosis poses a significant threat to human health. (Moynihan, Doust, & Henry, 2012)

Overall, though, it would appear that in the last 30 years, in advanced countries, health care is making a more positive impact on population health than in the past. Thus it should be noted that McKeown could be correct about the limited role of health care in the past but wrong about the present. Arguably, modern medical interventions are more effective than older ones and it is possible they may exert more influence over the health of today's population than they once did. However, admitting this still leaves us with the conclusion that factors other than health care have far more impact on the health of populations.

The Demographic and Epidemiologic Transitions

Closely associated with the work of Thomas McKeown are two core ideas in the field of health demography, the study of birth and death rates in human populations. These are the **demographic** and the **epidemiologic transitions**.

The Demographic Transition

It has long been noted that death rates, especially in the early years from birth to age five, have fallen sharply from historic norms. People who survive childhood have also been living longer. More recently, at least in affluent countries, birth rates have fallen sharply. What is interesting about these trends is that they appear related. Health demographers have shown that as a place becomes more affluent, measured in terms of average per capita income, death rates drop. Initially birth rates remain high causing the population to grow very rapidly. This is the principal cause of the world's population doubling since 1968, and the consequent pressure on the planet's resources. But as death rates have continued to decline and income to rise, birth rates have begun to fall. Eventually, in the most affluent places, birth rates may decline to match or even end up lower than death rates, marking a period of zero or even negative population growth. This is the phase of the demographic transition that Canada, Japan, and Western Europe currently find themselves in (but not the United States, due to the large number of young immigrants and high birth rates among African Americans and Hispanics). The demographic transition is illustrated in Figure 1.6.

The demographic transition comprises three phases, which may be expressed as historical epochs when referring to advanced wealthy countries such as Canada or as representative of different standards of living when comparing contemporary countries.

Phases of the demographic transition are as follows:

1. From a stage of low economic development characterized by high birth and death rates and hence near-zero population growth (the way the entire world was for thousands of years from 5000 BCE to roughly 1500 CE) to a stage of increased wealth and urbanization characterized by declining death rates but continuing high birth rates (modern Africa is an example);
2. From a stage characterized by high birth rates to a stage of relatively advanced economic development characterized by declining birth rates (modern China is an example);

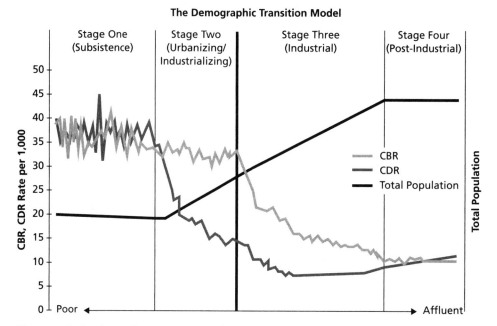

Figure 1.6 Crude Birth Rates (CBR) and Crude Death Rates (CDR) at Various Societal Developmental Stages

Source: Adapted from Keith Montgomery, n.d., http://pages.uwc.edu/keith.montgomery/Demotrans/demtran.htm.

3. From a period of declining birth and death rates to an advanced stage of economic development characterized by near stability of the population—very similar birth and death rates (modern Canada is an example).

    By examining historical records and comparing contemporary countries at different levels of affluence, demographers have calculated that the key transition to the simultaneous decline in death and birth rates occurs somewhere between $6000 and $10,000 per capita (Preston, 1975), roughly the position of contemporary China or Brazil.

Box 1.5	Case Study ○ Demographic Transition

The demographic transition model arose out of studies of Western European countries and Japan. Recently, it has come under attack because it presupposes an invariant relationship between rising societal affluence and declining death and birth rates. While the relationship between economic development and life expectancy appears robust (because infant mortality declines as per capita income rises), the relationship between economic development and birth rates is more uncertain. Birth rates remain stubbornly high in some moderately affluent countries.

1. What are the underlying factors that drive down death rates as countries develop economically?
2. Why might birth rates respond to higher levels of social and economic development?
3. Why might the demographic transition model be accurate with respect to death rate trends but fail to predict birth-rate trends?

Epidemiologic Transition

Another feature that is obvious when we compare the situation in rich countries today with that of poorer ones (or, alternatively, compare the situation today in rich countries with the situation that existed in those countries in the past when they were less rich) is the causes of disease and death are different. In Canada, the United States, the United Kingdom, and Australia, people commonly suffer from diabetes, heart disease, and cancer, but in poorer parts of the world people commonly suffer from malaria (a parasitic disease) or infectious diseases like TB or HIV-AIDS. If we look backwards in time to a century ago, the most common causes of death in Canada, the United States, the United Kingdom, and Australia were infectious diseases like TB and measles, but those are all rare today. Just as is the case with changes in birth rates and death rates, health demographers have charted the epidemiologic transition. The epidemiologic transition is the change from infectious and parasitic diseases in poorer places to chronic diseases in richer ones. Once again, this transition appears to occur when societies reach a level of affluence equivalent to roughly $6000 to $10,000 per capita income. The epidemiologic transition is illustrated in Figure 1.7.

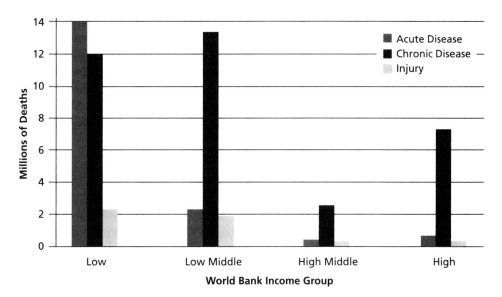

Figure 1.7 Epidemiologic Transition from Low- to High-Income Countries
Source: WHO, 2005, p. 4.

Like McKeown's claim about the priority of nutrition in determining the health of populations, the demographic and epidemiologic transition models have been criticized for oversimplifying complex relationships and underplaying factors other than affluence that may explain part of the process. But the recent work of health demographers has firmly established that a relationship does exist both between birth and death rates, the kinds of diseases that afflict a population, and the level of resources that are available to that population. The fundamental finding that improved health derives from rising wealth drives much of the contemporary research into population health.

Some Notes on Terms

The discussion to this point has introduced some concepts found in the health demographic and epidemiologic literature. A few of those key terms are explicated in this sub-section.

Morbidity means any departure from a normal state, such as illness or disability. It is often used, not quite correctly, as a synonym for "disease."

The incidence of a disease, such as sexually transmitted chlamydia, is not the same as its prevalence. **Incidence** is the number of new cases that arise in a specified population in a specific period of time. For example, we might be on the lookout for the number of new chlamydia cases that arise in the next year among students on campus. Incidence is expressed as a number per 1,000 (or if the condition is rare, 10,000) people. It is a rate because of the inclusion of a time interval, usually one year. Because we know the numbers arising out of a specified population in a specified time period, incidence is also a probability, a way of expressing risk. If the chlamydia incidence on campus is 20 new cases per 1,000 students a year, that amounts to a 12-month risk of 1 in 50 of infection.

Prevalence is not a rate, but rather a simple count of the number of cases in a population at a point in time. For example, "Today we estimate 200 cases of chlamydia on campus." The count includes old cases, people who have been infected for a while, as well as newly arising cases. Prevalence has some odd characteristics. Breast cancer prevalence, for example, might be rising even if the incidence of the disease is falling. How? People who come down with the disease may be living longer because of improved treatments.

Prevalence is useful as a measure of the burden of disease on the population (and how much it may be costing to manage that burden), but it tells us nothing about probability or risk.

Prevalence is easy to confuse with incidence because it is often expressed in a similar way. For example, the current prevalence of diabetes in Australia is estimated to be 73.9 per 1,000 people. The 2009 calendar year incidence of insulin-dependent diabetes in Australians over 70 years old was 3.89 per 1,000 people (Australia Institute of Health and Welfare, 2012). The prevalent cases of diabetes in Canada in 2000 were 1.4 million, rising to 3.5 million in 2015 and an estimated 5.0 million in 2025, 12.1 per cent of Canadians or approximately 121 per 1,000 people (Ohinmaa et al., 2004 Canadian Diabetes Association, 2018).

Crude death rates are simply counts of the number people who died within a given period, usually a year. They cannot be used to compare one place with another or a place at one time with the same place at a different time. The reason for the lack of comparability is differences in the characteristics of the people making up the population. Proportionally more women or proportionally more younger people in one population than in another will skew the results, making it appear one population has proportionally fewer deaths than the other. Rates, to be comparable, have to be standardized for age and sex.

Life expectancy is normally an average lifespan for the men and women in a given population. That implicitly assumes life expectancy from birth because every live birth is included in the population count. Life expectancy from birth can be quite misleading. For example, one might assume people in the eighteenth century lived short lives because life expectancy was only around 37 years. But the reason for such a low life expectancy was very high infant and childhood mortality. Once someone reached 20, the odds were they would live to over 60; and once over 60, the odds were they would live to 75. Generally speaking, it is wise to separate out under-five mortality from over-five mortality to avoid skewing the results. Moreover, the causes of death of infants and children are different from the causes of death later in the life course. For that reason, portions of the lifespan should be treated differently.

Figure 1.8 shows life expectancy at age 40, which is a much more reliable measure for comparing populations than life expectancy at birth, especially in higher-income countries. Notice that the most affluent people live longer in the UK than in the US, whereas middle- and lower-income earners have similar life expectancies in both countries.

Premature mortality is a calculation of years of life lost before age 70.

Health adjusted life expectancies (HALEs). Only years spent in good health are counted in calculating life expectancy. The disability adjusted life year (DALY) is a related measure that discounts years of life spent disabled.

Infant mortality, deaths of children less than one year old, is generally regarded as a reliable summative measure of the health of a population combined with the availability and quality of health care. The rate is calculated by dividing the number of infant deaths by the total number of live births occurring within one year and multiplying the result by 1000. The resultant measure is an indicator of the health in the community because it reflects maternal and infant nutrition, the living conditions into which the baby was born, and the availability of effective maternal and child care. Canada and Australia have an infant mortality rate of approximately five, the US over seven, and Japan just over two deaths per thousand births.

Theoretical Considerations

Chapter 1 discusses the importance of maintaining clarity about the level of analysis in general and the nature of the independent (possibly causative) variables in particular. It is possible that individual-level factors—characteristics of the person or specific things that interact with that person—individually and jointly influence

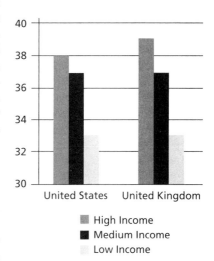

Figure 1.8 Remaining Life Expectancy at Age 40, US and UK
Source: de Looper & Lafortune, 2009, p.18.

health outcomes. Features like my age, what I eat, whether or not I smoke, and the like, are individual-level independent variables. Even when we introduce relatively complex chains of influence such as low birth weight interacting with poor diet in early life interacting with negative school experiences, we are still dealing with individual-level variables, but incorporating their possible interactions into our analysis.

It is crucial to recognize that factors of a more general nature might also affect the individual's health. Such contextual, collective, or ecological variables include things like societal features (degree of inequality or hierarchy or amount of **social capital** are examples) or other features of social interaction in groups (nature of a person's social network is an example).

Sometimes a contextual variable can be translated into individual variables. For example, a person's housing situation might be disaggregated into exposure to moulds, indoor smoke, overcrowding, and poor hygiene. Indeed, reductionism of this type might be the only way we can understand what is going on and postulate the probable causal pathways. However, reductionism can be dangerous; social entities like neighbourhoods, populations, groups, and networks have characteristics that apply only to the collectivity and cannot be applied to its parts. And those collective or ecological features might be important to health, provided, of course, that they impact on the individual and somehow find their way into that individual's biology. Moreover, it is theoretically possible that collective variables (such as the level of social capital in a given place) might modify the effects of individual-level variables (such as smoking). For example, it is possible that places which have high levels of interpersonal trust and robust social networks reduce the risk to the people living there arising from risky individual behaviours like tobacco use. Evidence suggests this may be true in Japan.

To the extent that we fail to take note of how collective variables may influence individual outcomes, we may misunderstand some important phenomena. A good example of this is health behaviour. To the extent that individual behaviour is socially determined, significantly shaped by the context in which the person finds him- or herself, the idea of choice becomes problematic. We assume the presence of choice when we reach for behavioural change strategies, such as education, incentives, or punishments—all individual-level interventions. But if the behaviour is substantially socially conditioned, those individual level interventions will prove ineffectual.

These and other considerations underlie the trend toward undertaking multi-level analyses—efforts to identify both individual-level and collective-level variables, the attempts to estimate the effects of both, and the struggles to sort out their interaction effects. This work is complex, expensive, and still in its infancy, but it is the heart of the social determinants of health research agenda.

Summary

The conventional approach to health and disease is the risk factor approach. Broadly, the model gives special importance to the interaction between genetic susceptibility (or resilience) and behaviour. If you are susceptible to diabetes, and you overeat and exercise little, you are at high risk for the disease. If you are resistant to viral infection, and you eat properly, exercise routinely, and maintain regular sleep habits, you are at low risk of catching a cold.

But risk factors at the individual level account for only a small proportion of the incidence of disease. Most cases arise among people of low to moderate risk. Evidence has been building that knowledge of a person's educational level, level of income, and relative social position is much more strongly predictive of health than knowledge of their genetic susceptibility and health behaviour. For example, a recent high-quality study of reported differences in health among—and between—Canadians and Americans shows that health inequalities are mostly attributable to education (up to 16 per cent of the difference in people's health), household income (up to 50 per cent of the difference in health status), and unmet needs (up to 10 per cent of the reported health differences). Smoking, body mass index, and physical-activity level have very little to no effect on health inequalities (McGrail et al., 2009).

Health-related behaviour must be interpreted carefully. The extent to which behaviour affects health varies depending on context and social, economic, and educational status. Smokers and drinkers in Osaka, Japan, do not do as much damage to their health as smokers and drinkers in Ottawa, Canada. The context makes a difference. Studies as far back as the 1960s found that doctors who smoke are less likely to develop lung cancer than nurses who smoke, who in turn are less likely to develop lung cancer than hospital support staff who smoke. Socio-economic position makes a difference. Incidence of most diseases is higher among people with lower incomes.

Health-related behaviour is socially patterned. For example, in Canada, the US, and Australia, obesity and smoking are most common among the rural poor, whereas good nutrition and regular exercise are most common among the urban rich. Typically, health promotion activities broaden the gap between the health status of the richest, most educated and the poorest, least educated. That is because uptake of information and its translation into action are both faster and more thorough among those who are better off. It is also because richer people usually have more sources of information and resources for making lifestyle modifications than poorer people. It is much easier for more affluent people to translate health education messages about the value of physical exercise into gym memberships, golfing greens' fees, skiing holidays, home gyms, and so on, and incorporate these things into their lifestyle. Their friends and associates will similarly be making the lifestyle trend sustainable and self-supporting. But if you are less affluent and your neighbourhood is not conducive to walking or jogging, you cannot afford a gym membership, and you have to take a bus to get anywhere, you face a lot of obstacles making it unlikely you will change your activity level.

All the modern emphasis on healthy lifestyles is somewhat misplaced. As we saw in this chapter, healthy lifestyles may have a more limited effect on human health than we suppose. Ironically, positive effects from lifestyle changes are greatest for people already living in favoured economic and social circumstances. Blaxter (1990), for example, showed that healthy lifestyles have little measurable effect on the health of people living in less favoured circumstances, such as a poor neighbourhood.

We saw that the focus on "lifestyle factors" implies individual choice, which all too readily lends itself to blaming the victims of illness. It may also limit our success. Focusing on people's choices inclines our efforts toward informational and educational strategies—approaches that are "notoriously ineffective" (Evans & Stoddart, 1990).

Lifestyle factors actually have remarkably little explanatory power. We are inclined to think we can readily change our risk of heart disease and premature death if, for example, we reduce the salt and fat in our diet. Everyone has heard dietary salt contributes to high blood pressure, which is a risk factor for heart disease. Equally, everyone has heard fatty diets contribute to heart attack, stroke, and cancer. But recent high-quality studies show that neither of these things, reducing salt or reducing overall fat in your diet, will influence heart disease or life expectancy (Hooper et al., 2011; Taylor et al., 2011). Indeed, reducing salt may even increase risk of death from congestive heart failure (Taylor et al.). No wonder the outcomes of most lifestyle interventions aimed at reducing risk of disease or premature death are disappointing.

We also saw in Chapter 1 that health care is not a large determinant of human health. Affluent Americans who have unimpeded access to the best health care technology in the world have worse health than less-affluent people in Canada, the United Kingdom, and Australia. Fair access to health care is a social justice issue because it obviously matters if you can obtain good-quality care when you are ill, but achieving fair access to good-quality health care will not close the health gap between rich and poor (more on this in Chapter 3). Moreover, good, accessible health care will not substantially alter the health of the overall population because, as Geoffrey Rose shows (also in Chapter 3 as well as 5), only a small minority benefits from treatment.

The distribution of health care is, however, a resource for population health even though its population level impact is less than determinants like income. It raises special issues of equity because there is a strong correlation between disease (and thus the need for health care) and low income. People with low income have the greatest difficulty accessing health care *and are most affected by government policies respecting the financing of health care services.*

Critical Thinking Questions

1. Chapter 1 noted that a number of carefully run trials have tried to induce health-relevant behavioural change in experimental groups. However, the expected differences in behaviour and health between the experimental and control groups have failed to ensue. Why might experiments intended to support healthier behaviour fail?

2. In what ways does life for the average person living in Toronto differ today from 100 years ago? How might those differences affect infant mortality? Life expectancy? The patterns of disease and disability?

3. At lower stages of economic development, infectious, parasitic, and nutritional diseases afflict predominantly the less well-off, while the rarer chronic diseases such as coronary heart disease afflict mostly the rich. As social and economic change advance, infectious, parasitic, and nutritional diseases become rarer, but chronic diseases become more common, among the less well-off, not the rich. What lies behind

these important changes? What features of our modern society are driving coronary heart disease, diabetes, and renal failure, particularly among the less well-off members of our society?

Annotated Suggested Readings

Those interested in the John Snow story would enjoy reading Steven Johnson's fascinating *Ghost Map* (New York: Riverhead, 2006). Johnson has many resources posted on his website, including replicas of the maps Snow developed in his research into cholera. See https://stevenberlinjohnson.com.

Steve Wing ("Whose Epidemiology, Whose Health?") provides an incisive critique of risk factor epidemiology as well as an outline of an alternative approach, which he argues offers much greater potential for positive change in human health (in Vincente Navarro and Carles Muntaner, editors, *Political and Economic Determinants of Population Health and Wellbeing*, Amityville: Baywood, 2004).

Part One of *Healthier Societies: From Analysis to Action*, edited by J. Heymann, C. Hertzman, M. Barer, and R. Evans (New York: Oxford University Press, 2006) discusses in detail the complicated relationship between biology and social factors. The book provides one of the best general introductions to the field of social determinants of health.

Annotated Web Resources

TEDSalon: "How the 'Ghost Map' Helped End a Killer Disease"
https://www.ted.com/talks/steven_johnson_tours_the_ghost_map
As noted above, Steven Johnson wrote a fascinating summary of the work of John Snow and the London cholera epidemics. This is his 10-minute TED Talk on the subject.

"The Demographic Transition Model"
www.youtube.com/watch?v=0dK3mL35nkk
The demographic transition is clearly explained in this animation.

"A Glossary for Multilevel Analysis"
https://deepblue.lib.umich.edu/handle/2027.42/56188
Ana V. Diez Roux provides an overview of multilevel analysis and a glossary of terms associated with using multi-level modelling in epidemiological analysis.

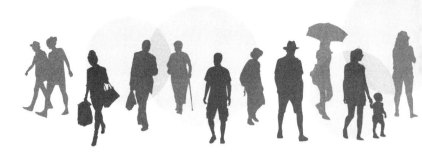

2 Health Care Services as a Health Determinant and Health Research Methods

Objectives

By the end of your study of this chapter, you should be able to
- understand the complex relationship between health care and health;
- appreciate the strengths and limitations of various health research methods.

Synopsis

Chapter 2 begins by clarifying the relationship between health care services and health, pointing out that this relationship is both contingent and complex. Health care services do not address all health needs; and even when they do so, the results for health can be mixed. Issues of access to health care are discussed, and why these give rise to equity concerns is explained. Health services are distinguished from public health before the chapter moves on to an overview of health research methods and how those inform, and sometimes fail to inform, health care and health policies.

Health Care as a Determinant of Health

We typically regard health care as a determinant of health, indeed perhaps the most important determinant. Access to good-quality health care is one of the most salient political issues, both domestically (with Canadian rural and Indigenous populations expressing concerns regarding inequitable access to treatment services) and internationally (particularly in the United States, where health care access is bound up with financial barriers—i.e., who pays?).

In this chapter, we will attempt to get a better understanding of what health care is and isn't, how it relates to health, and how diagnostic and treatment services differ from public health. Because health care is to a greater or lesser extent informed by health research, the chapter will end with a survey of health research methods and their implications for health care services and policies.

Health Care or Health?

Pause and Reflect   Health Care or Health?

"The health care industry . . . is one of the largest clusters of economic activity in all modern states. Such massive efforts reflect a widespread belief that the availability and use of health care is central to the health of individuals and populations" (Evans and Stoddart, 1990, p. 27).

Out of every dollar spent in Canada, about 12 cents goes to health care products and services. How much health is purchased via this massive annual expenditure of $228 billion (Canadian Institute for Health Information, 2017)?

On the face of it, people want health care. Otherwise, why would there be such a fuss over financial barriers to accessing it, wait times to see a doctor or have a procedure, and the amount of it on offer? But as long ago as the 1980s, health economists questioned the underlying assumption that health care equates to health (Evans, 1986). Do people seek out waiting in a doctor's office or the emergency room or having an operation to remove their gall bladder? Of course not. What people want is to be healthy, free of pain, and as functional as possible. They only want health care as a means to an end: health. Health care, unlike health, is not good in its own right.

The Relationship Between Health and Health Care

What is the relationship between what the health care system offers—principally medical and hospital services—and health? This question proves to be more complex and troublesome than might be expected.

Scope of the Health Care System: Which Health Needs Are Included?

First, what is the scope of organized health care? In Canadian society, the health care system is limited by two constraints. There must be a known, trusted treatment, and doctors must accept that the problem is medical in nature.

It's important to note that many health-related issues are not amenable to treatment, and thus are excluded from the formal health care system. Grief, anxiety, personal distress, and chronic pain syndromes are not only poorly understood but also beyond simple medical intervention. They are the reason why many people show up in doctors' offices, but doctors do not see them as their responsibility. Doctors report that one-fifth of their time spent with patients has nothing to do with an illness (Citizens' Advice, 2015); anxiety—and conditions associated with it such as headache—rank in the top 10 reasons for visits to the doctor (Advisory Board, 2013). Distress drives the system but is not managed by the system; feeling unwell or being distressed is part of a large class of largely unmet health-related needs, essentially orphaned by the mainstream health care system. Caring for those abandoned by conventional medical and hospital services are an enormous array of alternative care providers, from naturopaths to homeopaths, and social services, from counsellors to community mental health agencies. This array lacks coordination and robust government regulation. Moreover, it is riddled with gaps and financial barriers to access.

If a condition is not clearly biomedical (in a doctor's view), then it doesn't fit the mandate and scope of the health care system. Care is shunted off to the twilight world of self-care, alternative care, and social services. By and large, non-biomedical and psychosocial needs are met by families (**informal care**), not-for-profit voluntary organizations (charities), and a host of for-profit consumer services (private counselling, wellness centres, nutritionists, etc.). A person may choose a service—a counsellor, for example—but he or she will likely have to pay out of pocket, because non-medical health needs fall outside the mandate of the publicly financed health care system.

But the boundary between the health care system and social and consumer care services is flexible. If a drug company claims a product is effective for anxiety, for example, the condition is transformed from the social to the medical, and care moves from social service provision to become part of conventional medical practice. Depression took this trajectory with the discovery of MAO inhibitors and, later, SSRIs, both classes of drugs based on a re-description of depression from a psychological malady to a disturbance in serotonin levels in the brain. To take another example, impotence was considered an unfortunate situation facing some men, and, like male baldness, not a medical problem. But when drugs were (accidently) discovered that promoted erections in otherwise impotent men, a medical condition was born—"erectile dysfunction"—and visits to doctors' offices and pharmacies for the complaint became a normal part of health care. These are examples of a process called *medicalization*.

Different societies draw the boundaries between the health care system and social and consumer care services differently. In Germany, for example, massage and spa treatments are considered by doctors to be legitimate medical treatments and are thus covered by German health care insurance plans ("sickness funds"). In contrast, in Canada, in the 1990s, doctors questioned the treatment efficacy of community-based physiotherapy, leading provincial governments to end health care insurance coverage and rendering physiotherapy (offered outside of hospitals) a consumer service.

Boundary shifting is commonplace, and it turns out to be more a political than an evidence-based process, driven by lobbying by health care providers and citizen coalitions. For example, optometry, chiropractic, and naturopathy became health care services in Canada only after extensive political lobbying by optometrists, chiropractors, and naturopaths (and considerable political resistance by medical doctors). They moved uneasily and only partially from being consumer services to being encompassed by the health care system. Physiotherapy in Canada moved the other way—still firmly in the health care system when part of a rehabilitation unit in a hospital, but now mostly outside of it when provided in the community.

In general, in Canada, any given health-related service is a genuine health care need if and only if a medical practitioner says it is. Thus, correcting a crooked nose (rhinoplasty) is assumed to be a cosmetic, not medically necessary, procedure. Consequently it is treated as a consumer-driven choice and is undertaken at the person's expense as a commercial service. Alternatively, if a medical practitioner is prepared to argue that the correction is "medically required" (for example, breathing is impaired), the surgery will be paid for by provincial health care insurance. In the former case, "cosmetic surgery," the *consumer* pays. In the latter case, the *patient* pays nothing. A medically necessary procedure will be undertaken in a provincially regulated health care facility; cosmetic surgery will be undertaken in the commercial world of a private clinic. The procedure is exactly the same, but it can be delivered inside or outside the health care system, depending on whether a doctor deems it medically necessary. Thus, in Canada, *medical practitioners exercise an (often decisive) influence over issues including health care need, status as a patient, venue for care, and who pays.*

It is clear that health care services do not map neatly onto health-relevant needs. Many such needs are excluded from the health care system, and boundaries are arbitrary and contested. At best, the health care system deals with some health-relevant matters, as determined by doctors—in particular, accidents and illnesses amendable to medical intervention. The actual content of the health-care-system package depends on the current views of doctors regarding their roles and the scope of medicine; the current state of science; the technology available to doctors; physician and hospital funding; the number of doctors, nurses, and other personnel; and political pressure from interest groups and health coalitions.

Is the Health Care System Really about Health?

Paradoxically, the health care system isn't obviously about health. A healthy person doesn't normally seek health care. There is no reason to think that consulting a doctor or spending time in a hospital will improve our health, unless we are ill. Sick people, people in pain and distress, or those confronted by fresh limitations on their capabilities seek health care. Thus, the health care system isn't about health, but rather about illness. Health care's role is to manage illness and disability, mitigate pain, restore or maintain function, and prolong life in the face of risk of premature death.

The health care system thus deals with a minority of the population: the injured, the sick and the dying. To the extent that the health care system is successful in restoring function or mitigating pain, it indeed improves health, but it is important to recognize that these successes pertain only to individuals who are already ill. The implication of this set-up is that the (successful) function of the health care system will not have a very large impact on the population as a whole.

But of course the health care system may have a decisive impact on sick individuals. If a bus hits me, I want immediate ambulance service and a well-staffed, well-equipped emergency room, even though my personal fate won't make a discernable difference to the national health statistics. Buses only hit a few of us, but we all have an interest in emergency services, just in case we're one of them.

Do Health Care Interventions Promote Health?

As noted in Chapter 1, it isn't obvious that all health care interventions have positive health outcomes. Plainly, some do. The discovery and use of antibiotics, for example, meant that thousands of people who would otherwise lose limbs to gangrene or their lives to bacterial infection no longer do so. Hip replacement surgery means that many older adults are now pain free and more mobile than they otherwise would be. Removal of cataracts restores eyesight. Trained birth attendants and aseptic practices mean that today few women die in childbirth, and their babies are much more likely to survive.

Pause and Reflect   Iatrogenesis: When Treatments Go Wrong

It is very difficult to estimate how many diagnostic and treatment services are unnecessary, and of those, how many episodes of patient harm occur. We do have good estimates of medical error, however. Medical error occurs when the wrong procedure or drug is administered, or a procedure goes badly, or the correct drug or treatment is administered but done so incorrectly. In the United States—and a similar pattern applies to Canada—medical error is the third leading cause of death, causing more than 250,000 deaths annually (Makary & Daniel, 2016).

What steps might reduce the rate of unnecessary or inappropriate treatments? How might hospitals better protect their patients from the consequences of error?

But surgery and taking drugs carry risks, and undertaking unnecessary surgeries or prescribing inappropriate drugs for extended periods of time substantially damages health. The key scientific problem is determining who is most likely to benefit from a given intervention. Medical researchers typically think that this problem is best solved by conducting better clinical trials (more on this later in the research section of this chapter).

The reality is that many medical interventions lack a solid scientific basis, evidence regarding risk and benefit is conflicting, medical technologies disseminate and proliferate without proper testing and evaluation (Evans & Stoddart, 1990; Wootton, 2006; Welch, 2011; Cassels, 2012), doctors are more likely to do what their colleagues in the local setting do than follow the scientific literature or practice guidelines from their professional bodies, and drug manufacturers aggressively promote drugs for which the relevant evidence for effectiveness and safety is missing.

What About the Health Care System's Preventive Medicine Services?

Rather than concentrating on diagnosis and treatment, the historic core of health care, perhaps a larger impact on health may be found in looking at the newer, and now burgeoning, field of **preventive medicine**. Preventive medicine aims to identify health risks, the earlier the better, and to execute interventions that modify those risks, thus reducing the probability of adverse health outcomes. There are two parts to this: screening individuals for risk factors, and then applying some therapy believed to change the risk profile. We see this most in evidence in "general practice" or what in Canada is usually called "family practice." Today's family physicians, the usual first point of contact people have with the health care system (and therefore categorized as **primary care**), are expected to monitor their patients' blood pressure and blood-lipid profiles, irrespective of the patients' self-perceived health.

The story of family practice preventive medicine is intertwined with health research and the pharmaceutical companies. The famous Framingham heart disease study, a **prospective cohort study**, launched in Framingham Massachusetts in 1948, was the first to introduce the modern concept of risk factors, discussed extensively in Chapter 1. The researchers claim (the studies are ongoing) that several factors contribute substantially to coronary heart disease—in particular, high blood pressure and elevated blood cholesterol. In other words, populations of people with either or both high blood pressure and elevated blood cholesterol are at substantially higher risk for coronary heart disease than are populations of people with normal blood pressure/normal cholesterol levels. These findings kicked off a race within the pharmaceutical industry to come up with drugs that could reduce blood pressure or reduce blood concentrations of cholesterol, with a view to ending the coronary heart disease epidemic among American men (and, of course, making a lot of money for investors). By the 1960s, a range of drugs for blood pressure reduction, a range much expanded in the 1980s, came onto the market. And, in 1987, Merck launched the first anti-cholesterol drug, the statin lovastatin. Statins are now the most widely prescribed class of drugs in the world.

There is no doubt that blood pressure medications, and statins, reduce the total number of heart attacks in a population; studies have proven this over and over. But it is worth bearing in mind that approximately 70 per cent of heart attacks occur in people who have neither high blood pressure nor high cholesterol levels. It follows that if everyone at risk, those with high blood pressure or high cholesterol, was correctly identified and prescribed the correct drug, and that drug worked with 100 per cent effectiveness, less than one-third of heart attacks would be avoided. But, of course, not everyone will be identified, the drugs are not effective in all cases, and patients may not tolerate the drug or may have adverse side effects, so at the end of the day a more realistic estimate is about one-half that rate. Perhaps one-sixth of heart attacks are meaningfully avoidable by means of **prophylactic** drug therapy. But then, of course, patient compliance has to be factored in: Do patients always take the correct dose at the correct time? Do they continue with their therapy forever? (a necessary condition because the reduction in risk is contingent on continuous use).

It's easy to see such preventive medicine strategies, even when they work, will not have a substantive effect on the overall health of the population. A thoroughgoing, rigorous screening and drug program, with good compliance, is likely to have an effect on total heart attacks of 10 per cent or less. That doesn't mean it is not worth doing; but it does mean the overall impact on the population is small, while the cost will be great. (Canadian health researcher Alan Cassels (2012) goes further in his analysis of medical screening and early intervention in disease, arguing that people are over-diagnosed and rendered ill by a profit-driven health care industry that systematically exaggerates benefits and downplays risks.)

Box 2.1	Case Study ○ Adverse Side Effects: Might Drug Treatments Do More Harm than Good?

All drugs have unintended side effects. This problem is illustrated by the case of statins. It has been demonstrated by high-quality studies that if 10,000 high-risk (high-cholesterol) women take statins every day for 10 years, there will be 271 fewer heart attacks than if none of them did. But 307 of these women will develop cataracts, 73 liver dysfunction, 39 muscle pains and weakness, and 23 kidney disease *directly associated with taking the drug* (UBC Therapeutics Initiative, 2014). Because of this, a controversy rages over whether only those with extraordinarily high blood lipid levels should take the drugs, or only those who, in addition to elevated cholesterol, have other risk factors such as high blood pressure, or if anyone at all should be taking these drugs, because of recently discovered links between

continued

statin use and cancer, diabetes, and even sudden death. But other medical researchers, and some cardiologists, think everyone should reduce their blood cholesterol level, by drugs if necessary. In 2014, the National Institute for Clinical Excellence in the UK recommended substantially reducing the risk level for prescribing statins. Through inaction, we are inching toward that situation. Nearly one-third of Americans over age 45, and over 50 per cent of men over age 65, are now taking a statin every day (Centers for Disease Control and Prevention, 2010). And Canadians aren't far behind. The *British Medical Association Journal* asked a good question: Is it wise to place otherwise healthy people on complex, powerful drugs hoping to reduce their risk of disease (Godlee, 2016)? Is it?

Modifying Risks versus Modifying Health Outcomes

Regardless of where the research on the effectiveness and safety of statins ends up, several points can already be made. One is that modifying risks, even if successful, doesn't necessarily modify important outcomes. Statins do reduce cholesterol—that is a fact—and reduced cholesterol in a population is associated with fewer heart attacks—that's also an established fact. But what we want to know is whether people who are put on "preventive" drugs live longer, healthier lives. This is where it gets interesting. Clinical trials, as we shall see, depend on some measure between the experimental and control group, a measure such as change in blood cholesterol or change in blood pressure. But those measures are "proxies" for health outcomes. We assume lower cholesterol means greater health, but *high cholesterol is not a disease*; it is simply a metabolic feature associated with heart disease. This distinction is critical because we cannot assume that reducing the special risk of high cholesterol will yield a positive health outcome. First, we have to prove that not only does cholesterol go down when the drug is taken, but so does the frequency of heart attacks. Studies on statins have done that. But, second, we have to prove that people with the altered risk profile, lower cholesterol, actually live longer or better lives. Surprisingly, there is no evidence to support this second statement in the case of statins. In fact, researchers have found no difference in mortality rates between those treated and those not (UBC Therapeutics Initiative, 2014).

Pause and Reflect   Treating Risks as Though They Are Diseases

In what sense do statins or other preventive drugs "improve health"? Are high blood pressure, or elevated cholesterol, or mildly elevated levels of blood glucose "diseases"? Should we be treating them as though they are diseases by prescribing powerful drugs that people can expect to take for their entire lifetime?

How Much Do Modifications in Risk Change Health Outcomes?

Closely related to the issue of the extent to which health outcomes are changed is the question of whether the magnitude of change in outcomes attributable to a change in risk is significant or worthwhile. The National Institutes of Health produced a risk assessment tool based on the Framingham research (see the Annotated Web Resources list at the end of the chapter). According to the tool, 65-year-old men in the United States who have both high blood pressure and high cholesterol have a 19 per cent risk of heart attack over the next 10 years. Assuming that successful therapy with statins reduces blood pressure by 20 per cent, that risk drops to 17 per cent—a 2 per cent change. In other words, if 100 65-year-old men took a blood pressure medication such as an ACE inhibitor every day for 10 years, two fewer heart attacks would occur than if no one took ACE inhibitors over that 10-year period. What if the men took both a statin to reduce cholesterol by 20 per cent and the ACE inhibitor to reduce blood pressure by 20 per cent? After 10 years of 100 men taking both drugs daily, five fewer heart attacks would have occurred. Two questions arise: Is that significant? And if so, in whose eyes?

Screening and Early Intervention

Screening for disease is another dimension of preventive medicine and, like reducing risk by therapeutic intervention, is intuitively very attractive. The seductive feature of screening is that it holds the promise of discovering disease early. That could be important because it is widely assumed that early detection is important for successful cure.

Screening is most widespread in the case of cancer, because it is here, with cancer, that the belief in the importance of early detection is strongest. The most successful example of cancer screening is the PAP smear. Named after the Greek doctor Papanikolaou, the test involves harvesting some cells from the cervix and examining them for pathological changes indicative of cervical or uterine cancer. For many years, the screening has been routinely done on women between the age of 21 and 65 by their family doctors. PAP smears are credited with reducing the fatality rate from cervical and uterine cancers; 92 per cent of women whose cancer was found through screening were cured, versus 66 per cent whose cancer was diagnosed from symptoms (Andrae et al., 2012).

Other forms of screening, however, are more controversial. Problems arise for several reasons. The first problem is that all tests yield false positives, often a very large number of false results. False positives are an issue because they cause needless worry (i.e., people given a cancer diagnosis when in fact they don't have cancer), but worse, they initiate progressively more invasive testing to confirm or discount the findings of the screening. Apart from the cost and inconvenience associated with the medical follow-up, real harms, including death, can occur.

For example, in 2016, the BC Cancer Agency introduced FIT tests, a benign but slightly icky fecal test for blood in the stool. Blood in fecal matter might be indicative of cancerous changes in the bowel. But the immediate rash of positive results, many—indeed most—ultimately proving false, necessitated follow-up colonoscopies on thousands of people. Because of widespread screening, gastroenterologists were overwhelmed, colonoscopy clinics experienced rapidly growing wait-lists and ever-lengthening wait times, costs ballooned. Patients already known to be ill with colon disease were caught up in delays. Consequently, people with positive FIT results have waited anxious months to find out if they really do have cancer. But worst of all, a small but not insignificant number of people receiving colonoscopies will suffer major harms such as perforated bowels. It remains to be seen how many lives are saved from early detection of colon cancer through FIT/colonoscopy and how many people are harmed. (Note: the BC Cancer Agency subsequently withdrew the original FIT test and changed its screening protocols. As of 2018, the balance of benefits and harms remains unknown.)

Obviously, tests that are more reliable, that detect real cases (true positives), and that do not report non-cases (false positives), wouldn't create this problem. But in reality, if tests are tweaked to reduce false positives, then they fail to find true positives, and vice versa. Thus, there is always a trade-off. The main way of dealing with this issue is to apply the screening test only to people known to be at very high risk, because that reduces the problem of false negatives. But attempting to define the high-risk population raises another problem. How do we best establish the cut-off for high risk to maximize the benefits of screening and minimize the harms? There is no consensus on this question. Additionally, if a test is limited to high-risk groups, political problems arise. Younger women and cancer care advocates, for example, lobby for a younger age for mammography screening, while many oncologists argue for restricting mammography to older women in order to reduce false positives. In reality, guidelines get shaped as much by politics as science.

Box 2.2   Case Study ○ The Controversy over Mammograms

Since the 1980s, controversy has swirled around using mammography—X-rays of women's breasts—to detect early-stage cancer. First, there are concerns about exposing otherwise healthy women to ionizing radiation because X-rays are not benign. Second, there is an awareness of different types of tumour in the breast—some grow very slowly and others extremely fast; some tumours are localized and others are invasive. Screening is more likely to discover the slow-growing tumours and miss the fast-growing ones. Slow-growing tumours are much less likely to cause serious near-term illness or death, so discovering them earlier may yield very little or no health benefit. Third, abnormal findings are common due to innocuous variations in density of breast tissue, benign growths, cysts, and the like. That means many women who do not have cancer will be labelled as suspected cases and subjected to painful biopsies when they are in fact healthy. Finally, there is no hard proof that life years are saved by screening. Women who are screened positive for cancer and treated may appear to live longer, but that may only be because they were diagnosed earlier—i.e., we merely set the clock back.

If the evidence suggests that screening might be worthwhile, the question remains: Whom should we screen? Plainly we should not screen girls and young women because their risk of cancer is very low and the risks of exposing them to radiation and unnecessary treatments are high. So, should we target women over 40? Over 45? Over 50? Or should we screen only women with a family history of the disease? Different studies and different clinicians continue to come up with different answers. It appears women over 45, especially those with a family history of breast cancer, might benefit, but the answer is far from certain.

The discussion raises two obvious questions: Why is screening mandated in Canada, the United States, the United Kingdom, and Australia? And why might governments launch and heavily promote expensive screening programs when the evidence is weak, the outcomes uncertain, and the groups who might benefit difficult to identify?

Tests that have low reliability, such as the PSA screen for prostate cancer, are particularly contentious. Canadian health care insurance plans don't insure the PSA because government medical advisors believe the test does more harm than good by triggering unnecessary (and health-damaging) biopsies of the prostate when in fact there is no cancer to be found. Most screening tests are like the PSA; they have pretty low reliability, making early detection, and effective early intervention, more goals than realities.

Faith in early detection is also a bit misplaced, at least in the case of cancer. A serious confounding circumstance in cancer care is that there is no standard tumour or predictable natural history for the disease. In fact, it's not a disease at all but a dizzying array of cellular malfunctions, each with variable manifestations. Some tumours are remarkably aggressive, arise out of nowhere, and spread very rapidly; others are what oncologists call "indolent" and may stay pretty much unchanged, doing little or no harm, for years or even decades.

Cancer screening tests such as mammography tend to pick up the latter, long-term indolent tumours, and miss the former, invasive tumours, because by the time they're detectible they're spreading rapidly. There is thus a mismatch: we want to find the dangerous deadly cancers, but our only available approach finds instead a preponderance of less dangerous tumours. In both breast cancer and prostate cancer screening, this feature raises the legitimate concern that we end up treating, very aggressively with surgery, highly toxic chemotherapy, and radiation, cancers that may not be posing much threat to the person. In other words, screening can, and does, lead to overtreatment, and thus harm health.

The Agenda of Managing Risks

The modern medical agenda of managing risk factors, seeking risk reduction through the modification of risk factors, and screening high-risk people in the hope of detecting disease early is fraught with difficulties. Clearly progress is being made, therapies improved, interventions more wisely targeted, tests improved, drugs made safer, but nothing is straightforward and very little should be taken for granted. Perfectly rational people reject blood pressure–and blood lipid–modifying medications on the grounds that the benefit to risk profile is not as clear as it should be; equally rational people do not participate in screening programs because of ambiguity regarding benefits and harms. But it would not be rational to reject treatment with antibiotics in the event of a bacterial infection, or being put on a drip in the event of blood loss, or having a surgeon sew up a wound. Medicine is a powerful discipline, and appropriate care, if we're seriously injured or sick, can and does save our lives. Medicine is far less successful, however, in managing risks. But even with greater success in that regard, it's unlikely the health care system can yield substantial population health benefits.

Issues of Access and Equity

As noted, for a given individual, timely access to health care, especially urgent health care, can be a matter of life and death. This is obvious in the case of a serious accident, stroke, or heart attack. Even in less urgent cases, harm can arise from delays in being diagnosed and offered treatment. That's true in the case of many infections, and in situations such as diminished renal, liver, or heart function. Yet health care resources are unevenly distributed; emergency response times of ambulances and medical transport by air vary wildly from place to place; and physicians and other health care providers are concentrated in the more affluent areas in larger cities, and are often in critically short supply (or missing entirely) in rural and remote settings.

Pause and Reflect	Commission on the Future of Health Care in Canada: Rural Health

Canadians in rural communities often have difficulty accessing primary health care and keeping health care providers in their communities, let alone accessing diagnostic services and other more advanced treatments. In some northern communities, the facilities are limited and in serious need of upgrading.

People in rural communities also have the added burden of paying for the high costs of travel in order to access the care they need. This often means days or weeks away from family and social support as well as the added cost of accommodation and meals. (Romanow, 2002, p. 162)

Does Canada's distribution of its health care resources constitute a health inequity or is it the inevitable outcome of a sparse population occupying a massive landscape?

Barriers to Care

Some populations, notably Canada's Indigenous population, are significantly disadvantaged by the absence of qualified health care personnel in their communities. Compounding this problem are issues of **cultural safety**: cultural barriers, racism, language differences, and legacies of abuse of Indigenous people by medical researchers and public health personnel who, in the 1950s and 1960s, rounded up First Nations and Inuit suspected of having TB and incarcerated them in southern sanitoria (sometimes thousands of kilometres from their homes). Thus, health care services, when they are available, may be far from appropriate for, or acceptable to, a community. The redress of these injustices, and issues of equitable access to services supporting health, are discussed in Chapter 8, on the health of Indigenous peoples.

Stigma is another major barrier to care. Drug users; people with mental health issues; those with problems managing their weight, including people with eating disorders; people who suspect they have a sexually transmitted infection; people experiencing homelessness; transgender people; and many others may be deterred from seeking health care because of anticipated adverse reactions from care providers.

In general, poorer populations and ethnic minorities have far less access to health care services than do more affluent Canadian populations. Poorer Canadians are unlikely to have a family physician; indeed, over 4.5 million Canadians currently have no doctor (Gionet & Roshanafshar, 2015). Consequently, emergency rooms and urban walk-in clinics are disproportionately used by the poor and by ethnic and racial minorities.

Unfortunately, emergency rooms and walk-ins are the worst venues for providing comprehensive primary care, due to their inherently chaotic nature; the need to triage cases into the most urgent, leaving others to wait for hours; the chronic shortage of doctors and nurses; and the lack of a mandate or capacity to do any follow-up after basic treatment. There is no overall assessment of the patient and his or her context, no comprehensive care plan, no contact once the person is discharged. Patients experience the care offered in walk-in clinics as dehumanizing.

Recognizing this, many regional health authorities in Canada have established outreach clinics to make appropriate services more readily available to marginalized and hard-to-reach populations (such as IV drug users or those experiencing homelessness). Service providers have begun to improve co-operation and collaboration across agencies such as community mental health services, poverty charities, ethnic organizations, urban Indigenous organizations, and Indigenous peoples' friendship societies. Nevertheless, the facts of inequitable access, poor coordination, and inappropriate services stubbornly remain.

Community health services in general, and community mental health services in particular, remain underdeveloped and fragmented. Some populations, particularly youth and First Nations people on reserve, are underserviced. Likewise, addictions services, from community support for people suffering from addiction and their families to residential treatment facilities, are in very short supply in Canada. Many addiction and eating disorder treatment programs are private and charge substantial fees.

Pause and Reflect   Access to Mental Health Services

"Timely access to needed mental health services is a critical issue facing consumers nationwide. Numerous barriers to service access include stigma; poverty; lack of integration between mental health and health services; shortage of mental health professionals; regional disparities and cross-cultural diversity. As a result, demand for services often exceeds supply. Some community-based services considered essential for recovery (e.g., prescription drugs, psychological services) are not publicly funded, and some populations (children/youth, seniors, and people with severe and persistent mental illness) are in particular need" (Canadian Mental Health Association, 2017).

Do you think prescriptions and psychological services, when essential for recovery, should be publicly funded?

Health Care Financing and Access to Services

Another social justice issue stemming from a society's approach to taxation, redistribution, and providing support for the least well-off—all macro-level considerations—is health care financing. Whether health-related goods and services are publicly financed or require partial or whole payment from the user is a key determinant of who can access those goods and services. But before turning to the issue of how different societies approach taxation and health care financing, a few words on the concepts of "public goods" and "needs" versus "wants" are necessary.

Public Goods and Health Needs

Economists divide goods into public and private ("commodities"). A public good is, in principle, shared. It cannot be divided up and appropriated by individuals as their own property. A textbook example is a streetlight. Everyone benefits from streetlighting; the street is safer to drive on, safer for pedestrians, and less likely to harbour criminals. My benefit does not take away from yours; everyone can benefit from the light without taking anything away from anyone else. Moreover, I cannot scoop up the light and take it away as mine. A public park, in principle, is similar. We can all enjoy it (unless too many of us show up at once!). Because they are held in common, public goods cannot be bought or sold.

Private goods ("commodities") are different. They are subject to appropriation—becoming someone's property—and when they do so, they are no longer available to anyone else. A cake is a commodity. If I take a piece, you cannot have it. Private land is a commodity; if I own it, you can't use it for your purposes without my consent. Because they can be appropriated for private use, commodities can be bought or sold.

So what is health care? Is it more like a public good or a private one? The question is amenable to quite a number of answers. If I regard my health to be at least partially contingent upon yours, we have a degree of solidarity; I have an interest in your health because it affects mine and vice versa. Collectively, we have an interest in the health of the population of which we are members and thus are prepared to support measures that enhance population health, even if we may not receive an obvious direct benefit in the here and now. This doesn't extend to everything health care–related, but it does extend to things that we regard as real, substantive threats to health, such as accident and disease. Sharing the cost of health care may thus be analogous to sharing the cost of streetlighting or a park.

But some aspects of health care are very difficult to separate from things we regard as pure commodities, or private goods. Medication for a stuffy nose is hard to distinguish from menthol candies; both make it easier to breathe and neither can be argued to be critical to human health. We're happy to treat both as commodities, appropriately bought and sold, and denied to anyone who cannot or will not pay. We are more troubled by cases like therapeutic massage versus a spa treatment, but in general we decide they're so alike they can be freely bought and sold as commodities and made available only to those who can pay. Dental care poses a challenge: is it mostly cosmetic, and therefore like going to the hairdresser, or mostly about dental health and like going to a family physician? Some dental services (cleaning and brightening) look more like the former; some (extractions of infected teeth) more like the latter. Should people be able to get dental care only if they can pay? Should they be able to get extractions but not tooth brightening?

Cutting across this discussion is the concept of need. If I genuinely need something, there's a prima facie case for it to be made available to me. But if I merely want something, there is no apparent obligation on anyone to make it available. If the need is extreme—that is, I could die in this something's absence—it is morally wrong for others to deny it. But if the need is less extreme, the obligation on others lessens.

Different Political Responses to Public Goods and Needs

When we put these two themes together—public goods and solidarity on the one hand, and need on the other—we can readily see a variety of public policy responses with respect to health care. In Sweden, for example, there is a strong sense of solidarity (my well-being hinges in part on yours; we can only have a prosperous, healthy society if everyone has an opportunity to be prosperous and healthy) aligned with broad support for public goods. Consequently, most Swedes support high levels of income tax and substantial investment of those taxes into public goods, including a comprehensive public health care system that is free for all people (apart from some minor fees), like a public park. The Swedish health care system reflects Swedish beliefs and preferences regarding solidarity and public goods. In the United States, in contrast, a significant portion of the population is less inclined than the Swedes to see their situation as being linked to the situations of their fellow Americans, and they are more likely to see themselves occupying their social position or having the health they enjoy because of their own personal efforts and merit. Americans are also much more likely than Swedes to see health care goods and services as no different *in principle* from cosmetics and personal care services such as hairdressing or spa treatments—i.e., as commodities appropriately bought and sold in the marketplace.

But Americans do acknowledge that *extreme need* has moral force, and therefore most believe that arrangements should be made for access to essential life-and-death health care services, irrespective of ability to pay. The public policy result of attitudes and beliefs in the US isn't a broad public health care system like Sweden's, but rather a private marketplace in health care. However, recognizing the force of extreme need, American law prohibits the private system of health care providers from turning away a person who might die if denied treatment. (That person will still get a bill after the fact, and a collection agency on their doorstep after that.)

Canada, as in most things, falls mid-Atlantic, right between Sweden and the US. In the 1970s, Canadians put in place a public health care insurance system—slightly different but similar in all provinces and territories—which pays for health care services on behalf of every legal resident. The purpose is *to ensure there are no financial barriers to health care access*. However, public financing was—and still is—limited to medical services provided by doctors and hospitals, and then only to services certified to be "medically necessary." This term was cast, on the one hand, broadly to include things that look more like commodities (such as advice from a doctor on lifestyle), but, on the other hand, narrowly, to exclude all dental services, drugs no matter how essential to our health, and all services provided by anyone other than a hospital employee or a doctor providing "medically necessary services" (as defined by the doctor). This approach captures all the extreme life-and-death services, apart from ambulance services, which Canada treats the same way as the Americans: service won't be refused, but you'll get a bill. In short, the approach in Canada is a mishmash of American-favoured markets and Swedish-favoured public goods.

Continuing Financial Barriers to Health Care in Canada

Canadians face significant financial health care access issues despite universal provincial health care insurance. Public financing of health care extends to only 70 per cent of the total cost of that care, unlike the roughly 90 per cent typical in countries like Sweden. Canadians must find private means of financing a substantial portion of their care needs. In consequence, Canadians are two to three times more likely than the British *to not receive needed care*, to fail to comply with treatment, or to encounter serious problems paying for their care, because coverage under Canadian health care insurance is narrower and shallower than under the UK's National Health Service (Soril, Adams, & Phipps-Taylor, 2017).

In particular, dental services and prescription drugs are a major expense, and in some instances, dentistry or drugs can prove critical to our health and well-being, as in the case of a child with an infected tooth. As in the US, wealthier Canadians, people employed in the public sector, and people working in unionized larger-scale enterprises can avail themselves of private health care insurance, and about two-thirds of Canadians do so. That insurance, called *supplementary health insurance* (i.e., supplementary to the provincial health care insurance plans) covers, at least in part, dental and drug expenses. Of course, less-affluent Canadians do not have private insurance and in most cases can neither qualify for it nor afford it. Consequently, they receive little or no dental care and frequently do not fill their prescriptions because they cannot afford to do so. Very poor Canadians may qualify for support for drugs and dentistry through provincial social assistance ("welfare") programs. First Nations people are eligible for a federally funded *non-insured benefits program* (i.e., benefits non-insured by provincial health care insurance) that includes prescription drugs and dentistry. Most lower-income Canadians, however, are simply denied access because of lack of funds to purchase the relevant health goods and services.

Pause and Reflect   Inequitably Access to Prescription Drugs

One in ten Canadians does not fill his or her prescription because of cost (Law, Cheng, Dhalla, Heard, & Morgan, 2012). Canadians whose spending on prescription drugs amounts to 5 or more per cent of household income or higher are three times more likely not to adhere to their doctors' prescriptions (Hennessy et al., 2016). How might these financial barriers affect the distribution of health in Canada?

Proposals to incorporate drugs and dentistry into provincial health care insurance have been born and died repeatedly since the 1960s. At the time of writing, there is renewed hope that the current federal Liberal government will work out a deal with the provinces for some form of extension in health care coverage to include prescription drugs. Some provinces already have partial drug coverage, often for specific diseases such as cancer or chronic conditions like cystic fibrosis, but coverage is patchy and subject to change under fiscal constraint or changes of provincial government.

Social Care
Also left out of comprehensive delivery and uniform public financing is so-called **social care**, non-health-care-system services that are nevertheless central to people's health and well-being. These services include nursing homes; group homes for the disabled and developmentally delayed; community mental health services; child development centres; home support services for the frail, elderly, and disabled; and a whole raft of other community services. Some are partly integrated into the provincial health authorities, many are quasi-autonomous, most are poorly funded and uncoordinated. Almost all depend at least in part on fees paid by users, again raising issues of access and equity. Quality of services and accountability to users across social care services are variable.

By the 1990s, the grand efforts by some Canadian provinces to pull the full range of health-relevant services into some kind of coherent, community-based whole, integrated with hospitals and public health, stalled out due to complexity, cost, resistance by health care providers and unions, and lack of support from the public, who generally failed to understand what was being attempted (Davidson, 2004). Consequently, gaps, omissions, delivery problems, and financial access barriers remain an enormous problem in Canada. That problem disproportionately affects less well-off Canadians because they are the most dependent on health and social care.

In short, there are many social justice issues arising from the Canadian approach to health and social care. Poorer Canadians, rural Canadians, Indigenous peoples, and minorities typically have less access to the resources required for healthy living than do urban affluent Canadians. Provincial health care insurance was a major political achievement and reduced many, but unfortunately not all, financial barriers to access. In Canada, health and social care remain very much works in progress.

Does Equity Matter?

Given our earlier discussion of the somewhat mixed value of health care services, and the lack of a strong connection of such services to health and well-being, do inequity and the problem of access matter? The short answer is "yes." Problems accessing services arising from availability or cost are associated with poorer health outcomes. For example, the absence of universal health care insurance in the United States is associated with worse outcomes for American cancer patients than Canadian ones because so many Americans have no, or poor-quality, health insurance (Guyatt et al., 2007). In the case of social care, it is even more obvious that health outcomes depend on access and quality.

Public Health

Conventionally, the organization of health services is divided into primary care (first point of contact such as doctor's offices and emergency rooms), secondary care (community hospitals and diagnostic services), tertiary care (specialist resources like teaching hospitals and cancer care facilities), and public health. Unlike the health care components, which are an amalgam of public goods and commodities, public health is just that: *public*, an unalloyed public good. Public health programs and services exist *not for the benefit of any identifiable person needing care or treatment but for the good of the general public*. The benefits do not accrue to identified persons, cannot be appropriated, are inherently shared, and the programs themselves are publicly funded and publicly administered. They are, and have been for well over a century, a core responsibility of government.

The Example of Immunization Programs

Immunization programs are not designed and funded to make it less likely that you or I will get measles or whooping cough or polio. They are designed to boost immunity in the community to a threshold *beyond which a pathogen no longer spreads through the community*.

Communicable diseases are spread by an infected person mixing with people who have no immunity to the particular pathogen causing the infection. If the chain of infection between infected and susceptible people can be broken by making it less probable that infected and non-immune individuals mix, the disease cannot spread.

The proportion of the population that needs to be immunized to stop future spreads of infection depends on how communicable the particular pathogen is. In the case of the most communicable pathogen we know of, the measles virus, a very large proportion of the population, somewhere around 90 per cent, must be immune to stop the infection from occurring. The goal of blocking the spread of pathogens by reducing the probability of infected and vulnerable people mixing is an attempt to achieve "**herd immunity**." That is the principal purpose of immunization programs.

Thus, from a public health standpoint, getting an individual immunized has nothing much to do with his or her present or future health. It is part of working up to the numbers needed to create herd immunity in the population. In short, immunization isn't done only for the sake of the person being immunized and is not merely an individual-level health intervention. Rather, it is conducted on behalf of the community in general (and on behalf of vulnerable members of the community in particular). Some children, because of a pre-existing disease or the status of their immune system, cannot be immunized. For them, it is vital that everyone else is, so that they never encounter an infected person. Otherwise, that encounter could kill them. Parents who refuse to immunize their children because of (the demonstrably tiny) risks associated with vaccination are therefore undermining public health and threatening the well-being of vulnerable children in their communities.

Of course, those who are immunized gain too. Their personal risk of disease is reduced alongside the risk of disease in their community. But that's not why we conduct immunization programs. The primary purpose of such programs is to stop disease spreading in our community. Getting immunized against tetanus or for diseases encountered in foreign travel is different in principle. Such immunization is intended to prevent the individual him- or herself from getting ill. Because immunization for travel purposes is for personal and not public benefit, Canadians have to pay for vaccinations associated with their own personal disease risk (such as yellow fever shots for foreign travel), but not for vaccination against infectious diseases, such as measles or rubella, that threaten our fellow citizens.

Public immunization, ensuring clean potable water, proper management of sewage, and regular organized rubbish collection are obviously public goods, just like streetlighting or parks. So is the inspection of the food supply and regulation of restaurants, all core public health functions. None of these processes are undertaken with the health of any particular individuals in mind; rather, they are instituted for the health of the overall community. Individuals, of course, gain in the sense that everyone in the community is a beneficiary of the reduced risk of disease in the population. *Public health initiatives have as their target some population, whereas health care (diagnostic and treatment services) targets a specific individual.*

The Example of Food Supplementation

When Health Canada decided, in 1998, to put additional folate (folic acid) into a range of consumer foods as a supplement, it did so without any individuals in mind. Rather, the goal was to reduce the number of fetal spinal anomalies caused by low-folate maternal diets. An alternative program could have been rolled out based on risk, and pregnant women could have been screened for their blood folate levels, with those having low levels being given supplementation (a preventive medicine program as described earlier). But instead, folate was added to food for the whole population, ensuring the entire Canadian population would not be deficient. Thus, this is a classic public health initiative.

A public health approach such as food supplementation has its critics because it means that people with adequate folate in their regular diet may consume, as a result of the program, too much. To the extent that excess folate in the diet might harm some people's health (and it might), a program that improves the public's health by reducing birth defects associated with folate deficiency could simultaneously harm some individuals. Consequently, we are less likely to see public health initiatives like folate supplementation or fluoridation of water supplies in the future. Lobby groups today are much more likely to point to possible individual harms. The scope of broad-based public health interventions is shrinking because, culturally, Canadians are becoming more concerned about individual rights and personal impacts, and they have a weaker sense of solidarity with their fellow citizens. From a population point of view, this is unfortunate because it is very difficult to match the impact and cost-effectiveness of public health interventions.

Health Research Methods

In order to understand the reach and impact of health care interventions and to identify potentially important public health initiatives, we must undertake research of at least two sorts: epidemiologic research examining the patterns and probable causes of health and disease in populations; and health services research evaluating the effectiveness and efficiency of treatments, interventions, programs, and services. In this section, an overview will be given of some forms of health research, and the major strengths and weaknesses of various methods will be touched on. It is important to recognize that it's possible in such a short space only to scratch the surface of this vast topic.

There are two large classes of population health research study, **observational studies** and **experimental studies**. Observational studies do not intervene in the study setting, but merely collect information about what already exists. They are essentially descriptive. Experimental studies, in contrast, are interventionist. Events are manipulated in order to test one or more hypothesis about the relationships among the variables of interest. Observational studies are able to identify **associations** among variables; experimental studies can test the nature of the relationship between variables, attempting to ascertain **causation**.

Cross-Sectional Studies

The simplest and most common observational study is the **cross-sectional study**. Data from a specified point in time are collected, then statistical methods are applied to determine the strength of association between variables of interest. For example, a survey may be used to determine how frequently employees cycle to work. The same survey may ask for self-reported body mass index (BMI). Simple statistical techniques can be applied to determine whether there is a correlation between cycling to work and BMI (more cycling, lower BMI) and the strength of the association between those two variables (frequency of cycling and BMI). If a strong association is found, the study may conclude that it appears frequent cycling is associated with lower BMI.

This oversimplified example illustrates some limitations. Because the data (cycling frequency and BMI) are collected at the same time, there is no way of knowing which came first. Low BMI people might be more inclined to cycle than high BMI ones—so perhaps BMI influences likelihood of cycling. Or, on the other hand, cycling might limit weight gain—so perhaps cycling influences BMI. *Nothing can be said about causality without knowing temporality*—which variable came first.

The second obvious limitation is **confounding**. It is difficult in cross-sectional studies to rule out variables that might be the real reason for the association. In our imaginary study, there is no way to measure prior physical fitness, for example. It could be, and indeed probably is, true that fitter people are more likely to both have lower BMIs and cycle to work. Cycling, per se, might have nothing to do with influencing BMI. The real associations are with physical fitness.

Cross-sectional health studies may be purpose-designed surveys or questionnaires, or may draw data from existing sources such as a national census, or national or international health and mortality data. Typically, data include measures of geographic, demographic (age and sex), socio-economic (income and education), dietary, behavioural, and morbidity and mortality variables. Most are large scale, using large data sets, and they apply statistical techniques, most commonly linear regression, that identify which variables are associated with each other. It is through such studies that it can be shown that moderate to vigorous exercise is associated with better health outcomes, a Mediterranean diet is associated with lower risk of coronary heart disease, and drinking red wine is associated with lower incidence of fatal heart attack. This is very useful because the results indicate relationships that *might* be significant for health.

But *correlations are not causes*, and the results have to be treated cautiously. Because two things consistently occur together doesn't make one the cause of the other. As Bertrand Russell pointed out many years ago, roosters always crow at dawn, but they do not make the sun rise.

Moreover, confounding is a very serious and common problem. If we take the Mediterranean diet as an example, many things might contribute to both the choice of diet and low rates of heart disease—the Mediterranean climate, the active lifestyles of people in Mediterranean countries, or cultural and social dimensions of life such as levels of social support or strong family ties. The positive health outcomes observed may have nothing to do with olive oil and avoiding red meat.

An even clearer example is the notorious association of red wine drinking with heart health. Cross-sectional studies yielding this result compared moderate wine drinkers with non-drinkers. The first problem with this approach is bias arising from the fact that people who are non-drinkers may have had previous problems with alcohol and therefore had to abstain completely or they may be people who have pre-existing health problems and so avoid alcohol. The second problem with the approach is that heavy drinkers are excluded, introducing another bias. If only moderate drinkers are included, effectively the study (through the twin biases in its design) includes only healthy people because most healthy Western European and North American people have the occasional alcoholic drink. Thus the findings come down to "healthy people are healthier than unhealthy ones"!

Worse still is the problem of confounding. Moderate wine drinking correlates strongly with high income and high income correlates strongly with heart health. In other words, consuming wine may not have anything to do with heart health. The meaningful relationship may be between income and heart disease. A final problem here is that such studies don't include other health outcomes. In the case of wine studies, only heart health is included. But drinkers, even modest ones, have an elevated incidence of cancer. All these considerations might leave you wondering why the wine studies are such poor quality and why they arrive at such unsupportable conclusions. The answer is that many were funded by the alcoholic drinks industry. For example, it has come to light that the US government and alcohol producers are partnered in a large-scale study in the United States intended to show that daily alcohol consumption is part of a healthy diet. An investigation has been launched into the roles of Harvard-based researchers and officials in the National Institutes of Health in receipt of industry funding (Rabin, 2018). (Note: the resulting political fallout ultimately led to the cancellation of the study.)

A final example comes again from the field of diet studies. It was observed through cross-sectional studies that vegetarians such as Seventh Day Adventists have lower rates of heart disease than non-vegetarians. By now you may see the problem. Vegetarian groups like Seventh Day Adventists, in addition to being vegetarian, are non-smokers, have lower BMIs than the general population, and are more physically active. Plainly, smoking, BMI, and fitness are significant determinants, and the findings regarding vegetarianism are now seen to be spurious. It appears there is little or no meaningful relationship between vegetarianism and health, heart or otherwise, despite the strong association. In short, confounding proved to be a serious problem in many, if not most, dietary studies.

Identifying correlations between lifestyle factors—such as diet and exercise—and health is a very weak form of science, subject to significant doubt and frequent error. More rigorous studies with better controls are needed to get beyond the exploratory stage set by cross-sectional studies.

Pause and Reflect   Dietary Fat as a Risk to Health

Cross-sectional studies persuaded many doctors and public health advocates that fats in general, and saturated fats in particular, constitute major risks to health, especially heart health. Results of dietary studies appeared to dovetail with the Framingham finding that elevated cholesterol in the blood is a major risk factor for heart attack, because it was believed blood cholesterol was largely determined by the amount of fat in the diet.

We have known for quite a long time that the assumption that blood cholesterol is a product of dietary factors is wrong (mostly it is the liver that determines cholesterol levels). Recent studies have also shown that associations between dietary fat and cancer are also spurious. But medical advice and food producers have continued to claim that dietary fat is a health risk and low-fat foods are "healthy."

A recent high-quality cohort study shows that vilifying fats as risks to health is completely wrong. In fact, high-fat diets are associated with a *23 per cent reduction* in the risk of death. The researchers found a similar reduction (18 per cent) in the risk of stroke associated with high-fat diets (Dehghan et al., 2017).

Given the low quality of dietary health studies, and the way those studies are hyped by the media and misleadingly reported by the food industry, how should we decide on a sensible diet?

In general, the approach of treating food types and food components as though they are risk factors, and claiming meaningful health implications from simple associations (positive or negative) between a food and a health outcome, is looking less and less like sound science. Foods are chemically complex, and so are the biological processes involved in their digestion, absorption, and cellular uptake and conversion. Moreover, those biological processes are heavily conditioned by environmental factors, a whole host of variables that influence how health-relevant events unfold. The reductionism inherent in risk factor analysis, especially in observational studies, can and does seriously mislead.

Case-Control Studies

A second kind of observational study, much stronger than those relying on a cross-sectional approach, is the **case-control study**. Case-control studies look specifically at the association between a factor and a disease. Researchers do so by recruiting two study populations. One population has the disease of interest (for example, lung cancer), while the other does not. The two populations are often matched by age, sex, place of residence, income, and education. Interviews or questionnaires are used to determine the "exposures" (things the study participant has encountered that might be associated with the disease of interest). The level of exposure, the frequency and duration of that exposure (for example, amount smoked over how long a period), is then compared between the group with the disease and the group that does not.

In its simplest form, a two-by-two-cell table can be constructed of cases and non-cases ("controls"), exposed and not exposed, with the number of each placed in the relevant cell. The "odds" of disease given exposure can then be calculated as shown in Figure 2.1.

An **odds ratio** of 1.0 indicates there is no association between cases and controls. In other words, the exposure has no discernable effect on disease outcome. An odds ratio greater than 1.0 indicates that exposure is associated with more disease. Famously, in 1955, Richard Doll, a British epidemiologist, published a case-control study that first established the link between smoking and lung cancer.

Odds of being exposed, if a case; a/c.
Odds of being exposed, if not a case: b/d.
Odds Ratio: a/c ÷ b/d = ad/bc
OR = 1 no difference between exposed and
unexposed regarding disease
OR > 1 exposure is associated with disease

| | Disease | |
	Cases	Controls
Exposed	"A" number with disease who have been exposed	"B" number without disease who have been exposed
Unexposed	"C" number with disease who have not been exposed	"D" number without disease who have not been exposed

Figure 2.1 Logic of Case Control

An odds ratio less than 1.0 (<1.0) means that there is a meaningful association between the exposure and the outcome, but the association is inverse. In other words, the exposure has a protective effect.

Case-control studies have weaknesses and limitations, which render them, like all observational studies, more suggestive of important health-relevant relationships than definitive. In particular, because of their retrospective design, looking backwards to see if some exposure is relevant to disease, they are subject to **recall bias**. People who become sick are much more likely to remember behaviours or events that preceded their illness, whether they are relevant or not, than people who remain well, especially if those who are sick suspect some exposure to have contributed to their disease. A person with brain cancer, for example, is much more likely to report extensive cellphone use than someone who is well. Misidentification of the relevant exposures is thus a problem with case-control studies.

Cohort Studies

The most powerful observational studies are cohort studies. Researchers recruit a more or less uniform population, and gather baseline information on their health status, biomarkers associated with their current state of health such as blood pressure and BMI, past exposures that may be relevant to their future health, and health-relevant behaviour such as smoking, alcohol use, exercise, and diet. The entire "cohort" (group or population enrolled in the study) is then followed up over time ("prospectively,"—that is, into the future). Data on changes in health are collected at intervals as the study progresses, and so too are data on changes in exposures, behaviours, and other variables thought to be important drivers of health outcomes. Researchers sift the enormous mass of data collected to find associations between exposures (e.g., environmental exposures, behavioural variables like smoking and diet) and the observed health outcomes. Because the research is conducted over time, and the sequencing of exposures is known (i.e., which variable occurred first), it is possible to identify not only associations between variables but probable causal pathways (see Figure 2.2). We will be examining some of the most important prospective cohort studies, the Whitehall Studies, in some detail in Chapter 3.

Prospective cohort studies are powerful. But they are extraordinarily time-consuming, complex and expensive. Often, studies like birth cohort studies, which follow up on all the babies born in a particular place in a particular year, have to run 50 or even 80 years to yield the significant relationships among the variables. They are, for obvious reasons, quite rare.

Relative risk is a more powerful measure than the odds ratio, because a prospective study has time as one of its dimensions. Cohort studies don't just count total number of cases at a point in time (**prevalence**) but instead calculate **incidence**, how many cases *occur over a specific period of time*. Time is essential for probability, the determination of how likely something will be. Relative risks are true measures of probability; odds ratios are merely measures of association. Thus, when we see a very large relative risk—for American men, smoking yields a relative risk of 4.0—we can say with confidence that for this population there is a 400 per cent greater likelihood for these men to develop lung cancer than for non-smoking American men to develop the disease.

Like the odds ratio, a relative risk of less than 1.0 (<1.0) indicates that the exposure is inversely associated with the outcome.

Incidence rate in exposed population (I_e) = a/a + b.
Incidence rate in unexposed (I_u) = c/c + d
   Relative Risk = I_e/I_u = a/a + b ÷ c/c + d
   RR = 1 no difference between exposed and unexposed
      incidents regarding disease
   RR > 1 exposure is associated with disease
      (smoking as an RR of 4)

	Disease occurs	No disease
Exposed	"A" number with disease who have been exposed	"B" number without disease who have been exposed
Unexposed	"C" number with disease who have not been exposed	"D" number without disease who have not been exposed

Figure 2.2 Logic of Cohort Study

Experimental Studies

Experimental studies are, at least in theory, the most powerful type. They move beyond measures of association between variables to testing hypotheses about the nature of the relationships between those variables. An experiment, unlike observation, involves intervention by the researcher in order to perform a test.

In health research, the usual form of experiment involves the creation of an experimental group that will be exposed to some intervention (e.g. a drug, an exercise modality, a particular diet) and a control group that will not be exposed to that intervention. Differences in outcomes between the experimental group and the control group are measured, and if the differences exceed what is likely to have occurred by chance alone, the difference is considered "**significant**."

Because the differences observed between the experimental group and the control group must be attributable to the intervention, and not some other extraneous variables, it is critical that the two groups, experimental and control, are strictly comparable. The most common way of achieving this is through **random selection**. If the number of study participants is large enough, randomization ought to make the distribution of characteristics such as age, health status, and so on similar in both groups. It is obvious why this is important: if by chance the experimental group is younger and fitter than the control group, an experiment showing a higher level of fitness following an exercise intervention would be worthless due to selection bias. But randomization is not an easy fix. For example, randomizing hospital patients by putting Monday and Wednesday patients in one group and Tuesday and Thursday patients in another is hopelessly biased because a variety of variables affect which days patients arrive at a hospital. For technical reasons, matching study participants by age, gender, and socio-economic background raises other methodological concerns. In short, ensuring comparability of groups is critical but not at all easy. Selection biases are very common, even in good quality studies.

Demonstrating that the groups are indeed comparable is one issue, but not the only one. To be valid, an experiment must have a clear hypothesis regarding the variables to be studied, a clear definition of those variables, a defensible method of measuring the variables, and clear outcome measures—specifically, what is the difference the intervention is hypothesized to cause? An experiment that is ambiguous about how variables are operationalized and/or measured and that doesn't have specified endpoints is a poor quality experiment. Unfortunately, many clinical trials, especially drug trials, fail on one or more of these counts (Goldacre, 2012).

An example of a common failure in clinical trials is the inappropriate use of proxy measures. A proxy measure is a measure that represents something else. For example, blood pressure may be used as a proxy measure for cardiovascular health. In clinical trials it is possible that a drug or other intervention—say, exercise—truly changes the proxy measure—say, blood pressure. The error is to assume that the reduction in blood pressure is equivalent to an improvement in cardiovascular health. It isn't. It is possible that people taking the drug remain at the same—or are at an even higher—risk of death from cardiovascular disease. Some blood glucose–reducing drugs, for example, have been shown to work, but they actually increase the risk of death. The measure should always be the health outcome and not some proxy, which may or may not truly represent it. Proxies are handy because they're easy and quick to measure, but they do not substitute for proof that health has been improved.

More important is the generalizability of the findings of an experimental study, assuming selection was sound and the methods rigorous. A study that compares types of fitness intervention—for example, interval training versus aerobic training—and draws its study participants from among university students (using carefully considered randomization methods) might find that interval training has a greater impact on heart function than aerobics. But this is a study that has shown a difference between two groups of *university students.* There are absolutely no grounds for inferring that the findings apply to children, old people, or even university-aged people who are not attending university. Why? Because those populations are not comparable. The findings are interesting, and *might apply* to other population groups, but additional studies would have to be conducted to confirm that.

In the case of clinical trials for drugs, generalizability is a huge problem. Trials are often done on men (because the menstrual cycle in younger women may affect the findings and there has been, since the **thalidomide scandal**, concern about drug experiments in women who might be pregnant). But then once the drugs are licensed as effective and safe, they are freely prescribed to women. There is no science to support their safety and efficacy, the appropriate dose, and so on, in women versus men. Likewise, drug companies will recruit people with a common form of arthritis—say, osteoarthritis in the hand—who are otherwise well, and then randomize them into control and experimental groups. A drug being trialled may have a positive effect measured by better outcomes in the experimental than in the control group. But this is not a good reason to approve the drug for treatment of arthritis of the hip, or cervical spine, or knee, because the study can only be properly generalized to cases involving arthritis of the hand. Worse, because the trial patients are all healthy apart from the arthritis, we have no understanding of what might happen if unhealthy people take the drug, or people who are concurrently taking other drugs. Again, more studies across different populations are required (but are expensive and resisted by the drug companies). We can see why drug safety and efficacy are such big problems, and why licensed prescription drugs can do as much—or more—harm than good.

Chance findings cannot be discounted even if an experiment involves large numbers and is properly randomized. In science, an experiment has to be replicated to ensure the findings are valid and not just a fluke. Replication means the experiment must be conducted in precisely the same way under precisely the same conditions. Outside of the area of clinical trials for drugs, this never happens. Similar experiments looking at similar or closely related variables are commonplace, but careful replication is not. For this reason, compounded by the fact that many health experiments involve small numbers and poorly specified variables and endpoints, the majority of studies fail to establish what they purport to establish, or are just plain wrong (Ioannidis, 2005).

These observations are not intended to denigrate Health research. Quite the opposite: they are intended as a plea for better-quality research, more attuned to the methodological challenges and more modest in terms of the claims based on their findings. But they are also a cautionary tale. The findings of both observational and experimental health research need to be treated with extreme caution, even more so once they've reached the media, where they are further misinterpreted, distorted, hyped, and extended beyond the populations to which the findings might properly apply.

Theoretical Considerations

It is important not to confuse or to **conflate** health care with health. Health care bears a contingent relationship to health. Some health care supports health; some health care has unintended, and all too often unfortunate, outcomes. Health care systems address only a small subset of health needs, specifically managing diseases for which there are known and accepted therapeutic interventions.

Attempting to manage risks to health at the individual level through health care interventions is a challenge, at least partly because each individual has a different history imprinted on his or her biology, different genetic attributes, different exposures arising from behaviour and context, and much else that makes responses to therapies quite different from person to person. The knowledge about effects of interventions and the various risks to health, on the other hand, is all population based—derived statistically from groups of people. The attributes of a single person, and an intervention's effects on him or her, may or may not align with the generalizations drawn from the population studies, particularly if the individual comes from a population group other than the one(s) in which the research was conducted. Clinicians, whether doctors or physiotherapists or dentists, must be alert to the idiosyncratic reactions of individual patients, including the possibility that a well-tested therapy might prove harmful in a given patient.

Public health raises some theoretical issues, but not the one just discussed. For example, at the population level, unlike at the individual level, we can be confident that reducing smoking will yield a large health benefit (more on this in Chapter 3).

Health research methods and statistics are themselves enormous disciplines, and we barely scratched the surface of the subject in this chapter. The goals of research are **validity** and **generalizability**. Validity is the truth-value of the findings; do they accurately and truthfully apply to the phenomenon under study? The main threats to validity are various biases: selection biases, recall biases, poorly defined or poorly operationalized variables, etc. Generalizability (or reliability) is the issue of whether or not the findings can legitimately be extended to other cases. Mostly, this is ensured by replication of the research across different study populations.

Summary

The health care system addresses only a small portion of health care needs, and tends to do that quite arbitrarily. Physicians define what constitutes a need amenable to health care intervention, and those definitions are narrowly biomedical. Consequently, the health care system is really about disease management.

Preventive medicine attempts to manage risks, mostly risks associated with coronary heart disease because that is the most thoroughly researched area and the one with the most drugs on offer purporting to shape risk profiles. Some success is evident, but there are risks associated with managing risks. Drugs and other interventions are not risk free, and in some cases the balance of risk and benefit is contested.

Overall, health care interventions will not, and cannot in principle, substantially shift the health of a population (because sick people, and people at high risk of disease, are a minority, and not all of them will be helped). Nevertheless, individuals can and do benefit from diagnosis, treatment, and efforts to reduce their risk of disease. Health care services associated with trauma, heart attack, stroke, infection, cancer, and managing serious cases of diabetes, kidney, liver, and lung disease extend lives and improve the health of patients. They are socially important, and equitable access to such services is an important goal for social justice.

In Canada, there are many gaps in services intended to meet the health needs of the population. There are also serious problems with coordinating existing services, issues of distribution and availability of health care, and financial barriers, particularly with respect to prescription drugs and dentistry. Numerous obstacles to care, such as availability, cultural appropriateness, language, and financial barriers, confront poorer Canadians, rural Canadians, ethnic minorities, and Indigenous peoples. Those limitations on access to effective health care adversely impact on their health, compounding other sources of disadvantage.

Countries differ regarding the extent to which health is considered a public concern and health care a public good. Some countries support high levels of taxation and high levels of publicly funded, health-relevant services. Others regard health as more of a private concern and health care as a commodity not unlike other commercial goods and services. Consequently, taxation is resisted and public health care services are few. Canada falls in the middle with respect to these two extremes.

Public health is recognized pretty much universally as a public good. Every society has an interest in preventing the spread of infection. Public health services are different in principle from health care because the target is populations, not individuals, and the goal is to prevent the occurrence of disease, not manage it once it has occurred.

Health research is a complex field, and good-quality health research is very difficult to conduct. Each study design has its own strengths and weaknesses. In general, findings have to be taken as tentative and subject to revision by further research.

Critical Thinking Questions

1. If counselling and social support are resources for health, should the health care system incorporate their provision to Canadians who might benefit? Is the current mandate of health care too narrow, too medical?

2. Fluoridation of municipal water supplies is quite common in Canada. Fluoride is added before the water is pumped into the water supply to ensure children have sufficient stores of fluoride in their bodies to grow and maintain tooth enamel, and to thus reduce the number of cavities and teeth lost to dental decay. But some Canadians object strongly to a chemical, which in large quantities is clearly toxic, being added to their drinking water without their express consent. How should such public health matters be managed? Is it right for public health officials to decide based on the evidence?

3. Over the years, Canada's Food Guide has been subject to negotiations between dietitians, food scientists, epidemiologists, and representatives of the food industry. Recently, cultural, religious, and ethnic considerations have been added in order to align recommendations with people's values. Is that the right approach? Should dietary recommendations be based solely on the science? Why?

Annotated Suggested Readings

Public Health and Preventive Medicine in Canada is a comprehensive and reliable guide to its stated subject. The book covers virtually every aspect of health and disease, as well as the organization and delivery of public health and treatment services in Canada. (Chandrakant Shaw, *Public Health and Preventive Medicine in Canada*, Toronto: Elsevier, 2005).

The essay "Producing Health, Consuming Health Care," by Robert Evans and Greg Stoddart, is considered a classic in the field. It is included in the excellent collection *Why Are Some People Healthy and Others Not?*, edited by Robert Evans, Morris Barer, and Theodore Marmor, New York: Aldine de Gryter, 1993.

Overdiagnosed: Making People Sick in the Pursuit of Health, by Gilbert Welch, Lisa Schwartz, and Steven Woloshin (Boston: Beacon Press, 2011), is a well-researched and easily accessible book on the problem of overdiagnosis and treatment.

Bad Pharma: How Drug Companies Mislead Doctors and Harm Patients (Toronto: McClelland & Stewart, 2012) is a well-researched and entertainingly written book by British doctor and epidemiologist Ben Goldacre. The term "Bad Pharma" is a parody of "Big Pharma," which refers to the multi-billion-dollar global pharmaceutical industry. In his exposé, Goldacre details the ways in which clinical trials and the regulation of prescription drugs go wrong.

Annotated Web Resources

Audio from *The Lancet*
http://www.thelancet.com/lancet/audio
The prestigious medical journal *The Lancet* has an excellent podcast on the PURE study and cardiovascular disease (August 29, 2017), also available through iTunes or your podcast app. The PURE study proves that the claim that saturated fats from animal sources contribute to coronary heart disease is poorly founded, arising from inadequate and poor-quality research. Despite the lack of evidence, low-fat and vegetable-fat diets continue to be heavily promoted as "healthy."

"Management of Blood Cholesterol in Adults: Systematic Evidence Review from the Cholesterol Expert Panel"
https://www.nhlbi.nih.gov/health-pro/guidelines/current/cholesterol-guidelines/quick-desk-reference-html/10-year-risk-framingham-table
A tool for calculating the risk of heart attack based on Framingham data, produced by the US National Institutes of Health.

"Battling Bad Science"
https://www.ted.com/talks/ben_goldacre_battling_bad_science
Physician and epidemiologist Ben Goldacre delivers an excellent and amusing TED Talk on problems in health research.

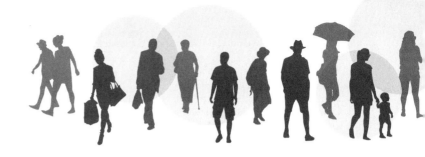

3 Population Health and Social Epidemiology

Objectives

By the end of your study of this chapter, you should be able to
- understand the origins and meaning of key concepts in population health and social epidemiology;
- understand how preventive medicine differs from the pursuit of improved population health;
- describe and compare the principal theoretical frameworks that link an individual's context to his or her health;
- appreciate the significance of the "**gradient in health**."

Synopsis

Chapter 3 discusses the field of social epidemiology and its principal characteristics. We continue on with a detailed discussion of the population-health perspective and the reasons why preventive medicine and treatment have a limited effect on the health of populations. The chapter then provides an overview of the seminal work in population health, summarizing the Whitehall Studies, the *Black Report,* and the work of Richard Wilkinson. We conclude with a brief look at some of the competing theories that try to explain the socio-economic gradient in health and life expectancy, which will be further examined in the following chapters.

The Emergence of the Field of Social Epidemiology

Social epidemiology is the branch of epidemiology that studies how social position and context influence human health (in contrast to **clinical epidemiology**, which focuses on risk factors within a host–agent model). There are several developments that contributed to the knowledge base and research interests of social epidemiology. This sub-section will provide a sketch of a few of those key developments. Later in the chapter we will look at how a set of related ideas emerged regarding population health by examining the work of Dr Geoffrey Rose and then look at the recent history of thought respecting social determinants of health and life expectancy by reviewing the Whitehall Studies, the *Black Report,* and the work of Richard Wilkinson. We will then see what theoretical frameworks have evolved within this tradition of research.

In the 1970s, sociologists explored the consequences of bereavement. They found that the odds of the surviving spouse dying increased dramatically following the death of his or her spouse (Martikainen & Valkonen, 1996). Later research showed that not only the death of a spouse but also a serious illness or an episode of hospitalization could affect the health and life expectancy of the sick or deceased person's partner (Christakis & Allison, 2006). Evidence mounted in support of the idea that social support and the nature of a person's relationships with others could influence his or her health. More recently, a branch of social epidemiology has grown up around concepts of social inclusion and exclusion, social support, and social networks. We explore this branch in Chapter 7.

Also in the 1970s, several studies linked social disintegration to disease processes. The evidence mounted in support of the idea that a lack of predictability of results from your actions harms your mental and physical health. It was later shown that having compensatory supports such as well-functioning friendships, social support, and other personal resources to fall back upon might mitigate harm to health (Cassel, 1976).

In the 1990s, first Meryn Susser and then Ezra Susser, both in the epidemiology department of Columbia University, argued on theoretical grounds that risk factors could not account for disease. Their papers *"Choosing a Future for Epidemiology" parts I and II* (1996) laid out clear arguments, showing that health researchers must treat the person's context and his or her environment as critical variables.

Unrelated work led to a breakdown of the mind/body distinction. Researchers became much more aware of placebo effects (real health outcomes occurring as a result of a person's beliefs), **psychosomatic illnesses**, and **social epidemics**. For example, Dr Andrew Malleson in his highly entertaining book *Whiplash and Other Useful Illnesses* (McGill-Queens, 2005) shows that the number and extent of disabilities such as whiplash correlate not to the kinds of accidents people have but rather the availability of insurance, paid time off, and legal compensation. He also documents epidemics of diseases, ranging from the nineteenth-century "railway spine" to twenty-first-century carpal tunnel syndrome, arising from social conditions, prevailing attitudes, and entrenched beliefs. Dr Malleson emphasizes that evidence supports the contention that most people suffer genuine pain and disability even though the cause of their distress is not physical. Their condition arises out of personality characteristics and the context in which they are living their lives (although there may be a trigger such as minor injury).

Such work has made it increasingly obvious that humans are exquisitely attuned to their social context, and cues from the environment can lead to significant changes in people's state of health.

Pause and Reflect   Dying of a Broken Heart

Can the sudden loss of a loved one kill you? The surprising answer is "yes." "Broken heart syndrome" (stress-induced cardiomyopathy) is the abrupt seizure of the heart muscle,

continued

similar to a massive heart attack, but without occlusion of the coronary arteries. It is the most dramatic emotion–biology interaction we know of. In addition to a loss such as a death, a breakup, or rejection by someone important to us, broken heart syndrome can be triggered by positive shocks (winning the lottery) or negative ones (losing a fortune on a horse race).

Can you think of some other examples of health-related outcomes arising from emotional reactions?

Recent work in psychology and neuro-endocrinology also boosted interest in, and the credibility of, social epidemiology. Emotional stress arising from a context can now be shown to affect hormone levels that in turn can lead to biologically relevant outcomes, such as plaque deposits on arterial walls or increased resistance to insulin, a precursor to diabetes. We discuss those findings in more detail when we examine the psychosocial hypothesis in Chapter 4.

Finally, the emerging field of neuroscience demonstrated that brain development and cognitive function are highly dependent upon experience. The discovery of how neural pathways are laid down, and how the brain sculpts itself depending on what is required of it, revitalized the field of early childhood development and reinforced the message that social context and environment are critical to health-relevant outcomes. We explore those developments in Chapter 5.

Social Epidemiology

Four main features characterize social epidemiology:

1.   Social epidemiology takes a population-level perspective.
2.   Social epidemiology concerns itself with the social context of behaviour.
3.   Social epidemiology relies on multi-level analyses.
4.   Social epidemiology takes a developmental, life-course perspective.

As we will see when we examine the work of Geoffrey Rose, a population-level perspective requires us to recognize that an individual's risk of disease is not independent of the population to which she or he belongs. A normal level of blood cholesterol in Finland would be alarming in Japan. The various health outcomes we see reflect complex interactions of many social forces and they can only be properly understood in their context. We should always ask "Why does this population have 'x and so' characteristic?" not simply "Why does this individual have 'x and so' characteristic?"

Social epidemiology adopts the sociological stance that human behaviour is largely determined by the social context. It explores the question of how and why certain health beliefs, attitudes, and actions arise in a population and how health-relevant behaviour is influenced by an individual's membership in a social network.

Since they recognize the importance of context and population attributes, social epidemiologists build models that test the relationship between individual-level variables and population-level and collective variables. For example, a social epidemiologist might be interested in the question of whether the effects of being unemployed (individual level) are modified by the level of unemployment in the individual's community (collective level). The interest in individual-level variables is complemented by recognition of contextual and population-level factors (Syme, 1996). In other words, social epidemiologists contend that contexts are important because they determine the individual's opportunities and set the constraints under which they live and work.

Social epidemiologists are sensitive to the dimension of time. Exposures or experiences may be cumulative over time with different effects than a single, one-off exposure or experience. For example, it matters not only if you are poor, but for how long you have been poor, at what stage of life you became poor, and so on. Some events may have latent (existing but not yet discovered) effects. As we will see later in the book, being born small for gestational age predisposes the newborn to heart problems in later life. Events might form part of a pathway. Being born into poverty may lead to impaired early childhood development, which may lead to problems in school, which may lead to dropping out of school, which may lead to adult unemployment and poverty. Social epidemiologists are thus interested in how experiences may operate to expand or contract opportunities later in life, or increase or decrease resilience to health challenges over time.

Geoffrey Rose and the Population Health Perspective

The eminent British epidemiologist Geoffrey Rose is regarded as the father of population health. In 1992, he pointed out that "the scale and pattern of diseases reflect the way people live and their social, economic, and environmental circumstances, and all of these can change quickly" (Rose & Arthur, 2008, 35). He was writing about coronary heart disease. Had he lived longer, he would have seen that he was right that the terrible epidemic of heart disease of the 1960s and 1970s was giving way to new epidemics of diabetes and obesity. And this shift from one "scale and pattern of disease" to quite another one has nothing to do with health care, and surprisingly not much to do with health behaviour either. Heart disease began its monumental decline before smoking rates and dietary practices had shifted in a more healthy direction. Why we have seen such a big shift in scale and patterns of this disease remains unknown, but it is clearly not due to genetics, health-relevant behaviour, or medical care. Something else is at work on the population.

Rose drew attention to the fact that important health attributes like height, weight, blood pressure, blood lipid levels, and blood glucose profile are not categorical things, but rather points on a distribution (the measured frequencies of occurrence). My height, weight, or blood pressure is "normal" only in the sense that it lies in the common range of values for the population of which I am a member. No absolute standard exists.

When plotted on a graph, the range of values for a population, for most but not all health-relevant attributes, form a normal or bell-shaped distribution (see Figure 3.1). This means the most common values cluster toward the centre, with low values representing roughly the same number of measurements as high values. If we were to measure every student's height at a university, we would find in North America the average height for men to be somewhere around 173 cm, with most men's height coming just above or just below this value. For women we would find average height to be somewhere around 163 cm. We would expect to have roughly similar numbers of short people as tall ones, a symmetrical distribution of values. With an average height of 173 cm, we would see "normal height" for men to be somewhere in the 169–177 cm

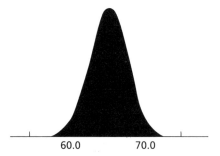

Figure 3.1 The Normal Distribution

The distributions of heights of American women aged 18 to 24 is approximately normally distributed with mean 66.5 inches and standard deviation 2.5 inches. Therefore, 68 per cent of American women are between 66.0 inches and 68.0 inches tall.

Source: www-stat.stanford.edu/~naras/jsm/NormalDensity/NormalDensity.html.

range. But if the university were in Vietnam instead of North America, we would expect a lower average height. "Normal" for men might be in the 164–172 cm range.

When we say someone has high blood pressure, Rose points out, all we are saying is that the person's blood pressure reading is in the high-value range of the distribution—the right-hand side of the bell-shaped normal distribution (what statisticians call the right-hand "tail," Figure 3.2). Exactly where the cut-off is for "high" is a judgment call, not a feature of either the distribution or of blood pressures. A case of high blood pressure—having a value calling for medical intervention—is, Rose pointed out, equivalent to a clinician's decision to treat. For systolic blood pressure, a value of 140 mmHg is considered by North American doctors to be elevated, and a value over 160 mmHg is high. But that of course is relative to the distribution of blood pressures in our population, and the values chosen are more or less arbitrary. Blood pressure distributions or distributions of other health factors such as blood cholesterol will be different for different population groups, just as height is (see Figure 3.3).

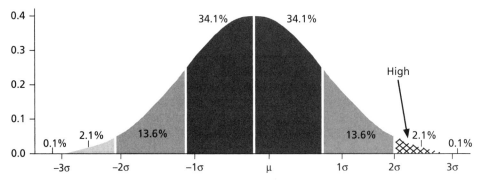

Figure 3.2 Example Distribution with Part of the Right Tail Crosshatched and Labelled "High"

The dark grey area is less than one standard deviation away from the mean. For the normal distribution, this accounts for about 68 per cent of the set, while two standard deviations from the mean (medium and dark grey) account for about 95 per cent, and three standard deviations (light, medium, and dark grey) account for about 99.7 per cent.

Source: http://tabmathletics.com/welcome-to-tabmathletics/normal-distribution.

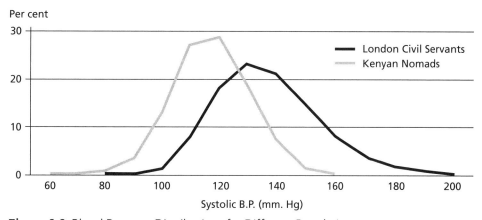

Figure 3.3 Blood Pressure Distributions for Different Populations

Source: Geoffrey Rose, "Sick Individuals and Sick Populations," *International Journal of Epidemiology*, Vol. 14, No. 1.

Not all health-relevant characteristics follow a normal distribution. An important exception is **body mass index (BMI)**, a measure of obesity. (BMI = kg/m2, weight in kilograms divided by height in metres squared.) Because a small number of people with very high body mass indexes affect the average, distributions of BMI tend to be skewed, pulled in a rightward direction. This is illustrated in Figure 3.4.

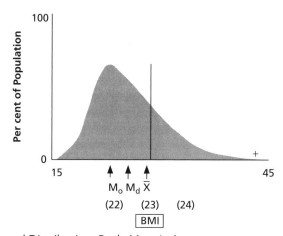

Figure 3.4 A Skewed Distribution: Body Mass Index

Pause and Reflect The Distribution of Body Mass Indices

What feature of the distribution of BMIs in our population gives rise to the skewed result? How are the average and median (most frequently occurring) values affected by the rightward skewing of the distribution of BMIs?

One of the important features of a distribution is that the population mean, the average value for that population, will predict how many cases will fall in the tail of the distribution. If the average BMI goes up in a place, then we know the number of people with high BMIS, the obese, will also go up. In short, the entire distribution is shifted to the right. A non-health example from England illustrates this point. Every increase of one British pound ($1.60 Cdn) per week per household spent on gambling is associated with a 1 per cent rise in the number of problem gamblers, defined as those spending more than 10 per cent of their income on gambling (Rose & Arthur, 2008). Likewise, if the average grade in a university class goes up, the number of A's awarded will go up with it.

This is very important to understand from a health-promotion point of view. More people will become obese if the average BMI in their community continues to rise. More people will smoke or drink more alcohol if the averages shift upwards in their communities. More people will exercise or stop smoking if the norms, the averages in their communities, move toward more exercise or less smoking.

It is also important from a health point of view to recognize that relatively few cases occupy the extreme tail and most people fall toward the centre of the distribution. That means if we concentrate our efforts on the high-risk individuals in those extreme positions, even if we are successful in lowering their risk, we will make little difference to the health profile of the overall population. Moreover, if we examine the incidence of disease, we will quickly discover that most disease occurs in the lower-risk range of the distribution simply because that is where most of the population is.

For example, if we screen men between 40 and 59 years old, we will find about 15 per cent have elevated risk factors for disease, such as high blood pressure, abnormal blood lipid profiles, and so on. The percentage of heart attacks that will occur in this high-risk group within the next five years is 32 per cent, roughly one-third. In other words, two-thirds of the expected heart attacks will occur in men without elevated risk factors (Rose & Arthur, 2008, 84).

In short, Rose reminds us that the large number of people at low risk will give rise to more cases of disease than the small number of people at high risk. But, of course, there are some exceptions to this important rule, such as HIV/AIDS in North America. HIV incidence in North America remains highly concentrated among two sub-populations, gay men and intravenous drug users. Thus HIV/AIDS, unlike most health conditions, is closely associated with specific risk-related activities.

Rose thus explains why it is that even effective medical management of all high-risk individuals leads to limited change in overall population health—though obviously it makes quite a difference to those patients. If we could somehow shift the averages for the population, though, we would make an enormous difference in the burden of disease in that population. A great many potential cases, individuals with the elevated values, would be shifted downwards to lower values along with the overall distribution. Overall incidence of the disease or condition, that is new cases arising, would decline.

Rose's Paradoxes

Rose's conclusions are sometimes referred to as his paradoxes. If, on the one hand, we treat only high-risk people, we will not do much to improve the overall health of the population. If on the other hand we change the average-risk profile, we will not have much effect on the average individual. Recall the example of improving roads and car safety standards versus getting high-risk drivers to change their behaviour. The former, improved roads and safer cars, will reduce the overall number of accidental injuries but probably have little or no effect on the health of you or me as individuals (because our individual risk was already low). The latter, stepped-up policing and traffic law enforcement, if effective, will reduce the risk of serious injury or death among the high-risk drivers (whose risk was very high), but will do little to change the overall accident-injury rate in our society.

The obvious question arises: Should we continue to emphasize individual-level high-risk interventions or move toward more population-oriented approaches? Rose gave a clear answer. As a rule, a population-based approach is preferred partly because it is difficult to determine in any objective sense who is at high risk. Remember, high risk is always a more or less arbitrary cut-off point on a population distribution. Notice, for example, the controversy that has raged on and on as to whether all women, some women, only women over 50, all women over 40, or indeed any women at all should have screening mammograms. This is an example of determining who is truly at risk. In light of this problem, Rose suggests, we should first consider whether there is any feasible strategy of moving the entire distribution rather than focusing our efforts on those who seem most at risk.

Rose thought that because focusing on high-risk groups is intuitively attractive for reasons such as that it might keep costs down and allocate resources where most needed, targeting high-risk groups should not be ruled out. He concluded the high-risk approach may be feasible and effective, but only where cases are highly concentrated and the causal links to the risk are well understood. An example is HIV/AIDS in North America (but not Africa). Cases are concentrated in two small populations, gay men and intravenous drug users, and the risks in both cases are well understood. Here, focusing on changing behaviour in those high-risk groups rather than shifting population norms makes more sense.

Pause and Reflect   Why Was the HIV/AIDS Campaign Not Targeted?

Given that it was known that HIV infection was limited to gay men, people who received contaminated blood products, and their sexual partners, why did public health authorities initially (in the late 1980s and early 1990s) respond to HIV/AIDS with a safe-sex campaign directed at the general population? Did that approach make sense?

The situation is quite different where risks are small and widespread, such as the risk of serious injury or fatality as a driver or passenger in a car or the risk of heart attack. Here we must, according to Rose, be mindful of the fact that most accidents do not occur among the high-risk drivers and most heart attacks do not occur among people with known coronary heart disease risk factors. Risky drivers have proportionally more accidents, but most accidents occur among people who are not speeding or drinking and driving. And as we have already seen, most heart attacks occur among lower-risk people. In these sorts of cases—and Rose thinks most health-relevant matters are more like the driving and heart attack examples than the HIV/AIDS one—a population approach such as improving the roadways or reformulating processed foods makes more sense than an individual-level, high-risk intervention.

Rose's Principal Conclusions

Rose sums up his key arguments with four criticisms of the individual-level, risk factor approach:

1. It addresses only a small proportion of the total incidence of disease, injury, and premature death.
2. It is palliative, a band-aid approach, failing to address root causes.
3. It is behaviourally inadequate.
4. It involves attribution errors and mistakes about causality.

Fails to Address the Majority of Cases

We have already discussed the problem of addressing only a small proportion of total incidence of health-related problems. Because high risk is by definition a small minority and because cases arise within the much larger lower-risk population, a high-risk approach will always, unless the problem is highly concentrated in a small group within the population, fail to address the majority of cases.

Fails to Address Root Causes

The high-risk approach is palliative, a "band-aid solution," because it fails to prevent future cases from arising. If we address malaria incidence in Africa by supplying mosquito bed nets to prevent children from being bitten at night (based on children being at high risk of such bites), we may well protect some children, but the population will still be plagued with malaria. But if we drained the swamps and constructed better housing for the population, we might come close to eradicating the disease. Likewise, if we put all men with blood pressures over 160 on blood pressure–reducing medication, we would prevent in that small high-risk group some heart attacks. But the heart-attack rate would not be significantly changed in the population because new cases would continue to arise. If, alternatively, we were able somehow to get the population to exercise more and eat less-refined carbohydrates, we would lower the overall incidence of heart disease across the board.

Fails to Understand Human Behaviour

The risk factor approach is behaviourally inadequate because it fails to recognize that the individual is not the bearer of some risk but instead is a member of social group living in a context. What people do is shaped by their relationships with others and by group norms. It is not realistic, for example, to expect a woman who also shops and cooks for a spouse and children to completely change her diet. Moreover, people respond poorly to demands that they behave differently from their friends and family members. Why should I have to take pills or exercise more or give up smoking when the people around me are not required to?

Fails to Incorporate an Adequate Concept of Causality

Importantly, the risk factor approach erroneously attributes risk and implies causes when there are in fact none. The risks of high blood pressure or smoking or any other risk factor are calculated probabilities based on the incidence, the number of new cases, arising over a specified period of time, in a given population. The risks are probabilities appropriately applied to populations, not individuals. A population of smokers will have more deaths from lung cancer than a population of non-smokers, thus making smoking a risk factor for lung cancer. But this tells us very little about an individual smoker's risk of lung cancer. It is no doubt healthier if the smoker quits, but we have no way of knowing how much the person's odds of disease have been changed by quitting.

Confusing population probabilities with personal ones and risks with causes becomes important if we aim to treat high-risk individuals. Unless we know the proposed treatment to be completely acceptable to the person and reasonably benign, we could do more harm than good. In other words, there are important risks associated with managing risks. Rose pointed out that to gain 10 fewer heart attacks we would need to put 1000 high-risk middle-aged men on daily aspirin for one year. Even though aspirin is one of the safest drugs known, those 1000 person-years of aspirin taking would induce 21 extra strokes, 31 extra cases of peptic ulcer, and 731 cases of gastric bleeding—20 of them serious (Rose & Arthur, 2008, p. 147).

Rose was not opposed to reducing the burden of illness by treating people at high risk of disease. But he was opposed to putting all of our energy and resources into individual-level interventions and failing to see that there were more effective and often safer and cheaper alternatives. He wanted us to be clearer headed about what we were doing and what we might achieve. Along the way, he certainly made a significant contribution in distinguishing between individual-level and population-level approaches to human health.

The Impact of Recent Studies on Thinking About Health

Three research initiatives can be credited with substantially increasing interest in the differences in health across populations. They are the Whitehall Studies, the research conducted by the Working Group on Inequalities in Health, and Richard Wilkinson's studies on health inequalities in affluent countries.

The Whitehall Studies

The Whitehall Studies comprise two studies investigating the determinants of health and disease among British public servants—salaried government workers. The first study, Whitehall I, enrolled 18,000 male public servants in 1967. The second study, Whitehall II, enrolled 10,308 male and female public servants in 1985. Whitehall II is ongoing; wave 10 commenced January 2011. Dr Michael Marmot (now Sir Michael) of University College London heads the Whitehall research project.

The Whitehall Studies are **prospective cohort studies**. They are prospective because they begin at a point, 1985 in the case of the current study, and work forward in time. They involve cohorts, a defined group of people recruited into the study and then followed up as the study progresses. By having baseline data on members of the cohort (their state of health, biological measures, their health-relevant behaviour), changes in those variables can be monitored and the relationship between those variables and outcome measures, such as future state of health, can be inferred. Because the order in which things happen is known, probable pathways of causality can be worked out. In short, the approach is very powerful and yields rich results. However, on the down side, prospective cohort studies are expensive and time consuming.

Whitehall I demonstrated that employees in more highly paid, higher-status jobs enjoyed better health over a range of measures than workers in lower-status, lower-salary positions (Marmot, Rose, Shipley, & Hamilton, 1978). Since the study was primarily concerned with risk factors for coronary heart disease, it tracked a number of variables known to be associated with the incidence of heart disease: body mass index, activity level, smoking, and blood pressure. While the study showed that not only disease rates but also the various risk factors were more common the lower the employment grade, it also yielded a more surprising result. Risk factors accounted for only a small fraction of the differences in incidence of coronary heart disease. The lion's share of the differences in health was directly attributable to features associated with employment grade—salary, education level, and working conditions.

In other words, the study showed that workers in lower-status, lower-paid government jobs, such as junior clerks, smoked more, exercised less, were more likely to be overweight, and were more prone to high blood pressure than workers in higher-status jobs earning higher incomes. But the differences in risk factors could account for only a small portion, no more than 25 per cent, of the difference in incidence of heart disease between the various employment grades. And those differences were vast. Workers in the best-paying jobs were twice as likely to be healthy than those in the worst-paying jobs. Remember, all the workers in the study, regardless of their employment grade, were government workers, working indoors in safe and secure employment, with excellent health, unemployment, and pension benefits.

The other major surprise was the discovery that there was a distinct **gradient in health** (see Table 3.1). Not only were people in the top jobs doing better from a health point of view than people in the bottom jobs, but also every employment grade from top to bottom was associated with a change in health status. Senior clerks enjoy better health than junior clerks, and junior administrators enjoy better health than senior clerks, and senior administrators enjoy better health than junior administrators.

The health gradient, a different level of health associated with each social position, has been confirmed to exist in every affluent country in the world, albeit the steepness of the gradient, how big the differences are for equal-sized increments of education or income, varies from place to place for reasons we will explore later in the book.

Table 3.1 Selected Data from Whitehall I

Cause of Death	Senior Executives	Managerial/ Professional	Clerical
Lung cancer	0.35	0.73	1.47
Other cancer	1.26	1.70	2.16
Heart disease	2.16	3.58	4.90

Source: Adapted from Marmot et al., 1978.

In summary, Whitehall I showed that

- even within a privileged part of the workforce, large differences in health exist between employment grades, presumably due to differences in the employees' education, the nature of the work, and salary;
- risk factors such as smoking and inactivity are more common among lower-paid, lower-status workers than among higher-paid, higher-status workers;
- individual risk factors such as smoking or high blood pressure cannot account for the size of the differences in health between different employment grades; and
- a health gradient exists in which a different level of health is associated with each change in employment grade.

Whitehall II was able, since it recruited both women and men, to extend the results of Whitehall I to women. In Whitehall II, the researchers examined characteristics of jobs at each of the different employment grades and thus were able to show that part of the difference in health could be attributed to job factors. The most important factor is the degree of control the employee has over his or her work (Kuper & Marmot, 2003). Men and women in high-demand but low-control jobs suffer worse health than men and women in jobs where they can exercise more control over their work. Contrary to popular belief, it is not the senior manager who is likely to have a heart attack, but rather the junior clerk. We will explore these findings in more detail in Chapter 9.

A report from the Whitehall II study showed that a man aged 70 who, before retirement, occupied a high-paying, high-status job, had the same level of health as a 62-year-old man who worked in a low-status job (Clandola, Ferrie, Sacker, & Marmot, 2007). Income, education, and job characteristics resulted in an eight-year health gap. Differences between women of difference status are generally smaller but nevertheless significant.

The Whitehall Studies are of the utmost importance. For the first time, high-quality, reliable studies established that a hierarchy exists in health with people in more privileged positions—whether measured in terms of education, income, or job status—enjoying better health than those in less-privileged positions. For the first time it had been shown that conventional individual-level risk factors do not account for most of the variation in disease incidence. That variation has more to do with the conditions under which people live and work.

The *Black Report*

Shortly after Marmot and his colleagues released the reports on the first Whitehall Study, the Working Group on Inequalities in Health completed their project. The UK Labour government asked Sir Douglas Black, a prominent British physician, to convene the working group in 1977. Its task was to examine health inequalities in the United Kingdom and assess how effective publicly funded health and social services, in particular the National Health Service, were in reducing the gap in life expectancies between poor and rich in the United Kingdom.

By the time the report was complete, the Labour government had been defeated and replaced by a Conservative government. Understandably, the Conservative government was not sympathetic to expanding public services, nor was it inclined to reduce the social and economic gap in the UK. Black's report, then, was an unwelcome shock because it showed clearly that the gap in health between social classes was huge, and worse, that it was growing. The government chose not to publish the *Black Report* and it was not widely available until Penguin Books printed a paperback in 1982 (Townsend & Davidson, 1982).

Black's team of researchers found that the death rate of men in the lowest social class, social class V, was more than two times greater than the death rate of men in the highest social class, social class I. And just like Marmot and his team working on the Whitehall Studies, Black's team working on health inequalities found a distinct gradient. Men in social class V were less healthy than men in social class IV, and so on all the way to the top.

As already noted, Black's team also found that there had been no progress in closing the gaps in health. Data from 1911 onward show that the gap between professional (class I) men and unskilled (class V) men actually grew (see Table 3.2), in spite of all the welfare programs that were put in place between 1946 and 1970, and the establishment of the National Health Service in 1948 (Townsend & Davidson, 1982).

More recent data show that the situation with respect to gaps in life expectancy has not improved. In 1982, lower-class men lived four fewer years than men who were managers or professionals. The gap had grown to five years by 2002. For women, things are not much better. The difference in life expectancy between professional-class women and unskilled manual workers grew from 3.8 years in 1982 to 4.2 years in 2002 (Office for National Statistics, 2011a).

Richard Wilkinson

British economist Richard Wilkinson spent his career investigating what we now refer to as "health disparities." Specifically, he was interested in the relationship between socio-economic variables and mortality rates. Shortly after the publication of the *Black Report,* Wilkinson published findings from his study of **Organisation for Economic Co-operation and Development** (OECD) countries (a group of the 32 most affluent countries). He found that there was a strong correlation between life expectancy and the proportion of income received by the lower 50 per cent of the income distribution.

Table 3.2 Death Rates per 10,000 (Male), England and Wales, 1911–1981 (ages 15 to 65)

Year	Professional	Managerial	Skilled	Semi-Skilled	Unskilled
1911	88	94	96	93	142
1921	82	94	95	101	125
1931	90	94	97	102	111
1951	86	92	101	104	118
1961	75	81	100	103	143
1971	75	81	104	114	137
1981	66	76	103	116	166

Source: Adapted from Black, Morris, Smith, & Townsend, 1980.

Wilkinson argued in his early papers, and continued to advance the claim in subsequent work, that he had proved that more equal places, those with similar proportions of income flowing to the top and bottom half of the income distribution, were healthier places. Contrariwise, Wilkinson labelled unequal societies "unhealthy societies" (Wilkinson, 1996). In other words, in rich countries at least, Wilkinson contended that the degree of inequality in a society measured by the proportion of income received by the poorer half of society, influences human health and life expectancy (Wilkinson, 1986).

Wilkinson's findings have been challenged, based on concerns about measurement, the data he used, and his interpretation. One problem arises from the metric applied. Proportion of income flowing to each half of the income distribution is very easy to calculate but is a weak measure because it tells us nothing about how equally the income is shared within each half of the population. Other more sophisticated measures of income inequality such as the Gini coefficient, the Atkinson index, the Robin Hood index, and the Sen poverty measure yield different and often contradictory results. Another problem arises from the choice of years and countries to include in the analysis. Depending on which years' data and which countries a researcher uses, the results will be slightly different.

Nevertheless, Wilkinson's research made an important contribution to the growing realization that health and life expectancy are to a significant degree determined by social position. Wilkinson showed that differences in health, life expectancy, and causes of disease and disability, between places, times, and social groups were much larger than had been previously expected. Moreover, he established a link between life expectancy and social position. Others, such as American epidemiologists Kawachi and Subramanian, took note and conducted a host of studies that we will be examining in Chapter 4, on inequality.

The Gradient in Health

Pause and Reflect   Why a Socio-Economic Gradient in Health?

In every known affluent society, the better-off have superior health to the next best-off who in turn have better health than the less well-off all the way down to the bottom of the socio-economic ladder (Marmot, 2010; Wilkinson, 1996).
Why might this be so?

The gradient in health is usually expressed in terms of differences in income. However, similar associations exist between education and health. Figure 3.5 illustrates the gradient in health measured by education level in the United States.

The educational level of his or her parents largely determines whether an individual receives higher education. There are several reasons for this: first, the educated family is more likely to have income to support their child in continuing his or her studies; second, the educated family is more likely to value and promote the pursuit of education; and third, the child of an educated family, over his or her life, is more likely to have a home environment that stimulates learning, brain development, and pursuit of intellectual challenges.

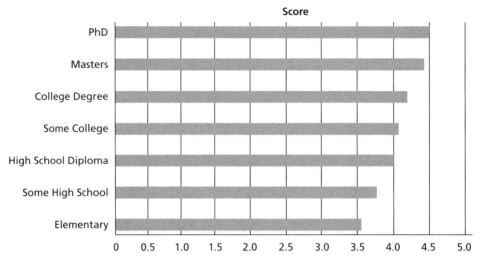

Figure 3.5 The Health Gradient and Education: Self-Reported Health by Educational Attainment, United States (5 = perfect health)
Source: Ross & Mirowsky, 1999.

Student loan, bursary, and preferential admission programs for disadvantaged university applicants make very little difference to the underlying inequality, as Figure 3.6 shows. In Canada, for example, programs to promote participation of less-privileged students in university education have done little to close the gap between children of privileged families and children from less-advantaged backgrounds (Turcotte, 2011a). Between 1986 and 2009, there was only a slight decline in the disparity, mostly attributable to the dramatic increase in the number of women attending Canadian universities.

Table 3.3 shows that health, as measured by the **Health Utilities Index** (1 = perfect health) varies by educational level, and Table 3.4 shows that health, also measured by the Health Utilities Index, varies by income, which is primarily determined by education. In

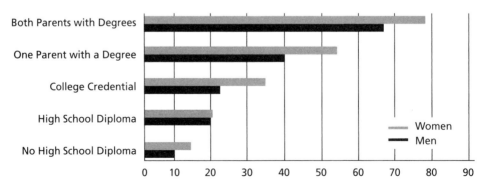

Figure 3.6 The Gradient in University Graduation by Educational Attainment of One or Both Parents (2009)—Per Cent Graduating
Source: Turcotte, 2011a.

Table 3.3 The Gradient: Education and Health Utility Scores
(1 = perfect health)

Educational Level	United States	Canada
<High school diploma	0.786	0.822
High school diploma	0.863	0.886
Some college	0.876	0.897
College degree	0.921	0.925

Table 3.4 The Gradient: Income and Health Utility Scores
(1 = perfect health)

Household income	United States	Canada
<$10,000	0.757	0.818
$10,000–$19,999	0.837	0.823
$20,000–$29,999	0.884	0.879
$30,000–$49,999	0.911	0.910
>$50,000	0.928	0.933

Source: Based on McGrail, van Doorslater, Ross, & Sanmartin, 2009.

both cases, there is a significant, consistent gradient, with health improving alongside increases in education and income.

The Building Blocks of Theory

It is one thing to note that human health is largely determined by social factors, but it is quite another to explain why this might be so. In this section, we will take a quick look at the competing theories regarding the gradient in human health and the persisting association between income level and health. We will return to and deepen our understanding of the strengths and weaknesses of these theoretical frameworks as we examine the various determinants of health in the chapters that follow.

Materialist Theories

The simplest explanation of inequalities in health rests on the hypothesis that it is the resources available to the individual that ultimately determine how well he or she does. This is a **materialist hypothesis** that links absolute level of resources at the individual level—my income, my level of education, and my ability to draw on resources from my social network—with health. Measuring the strength of association between individual resource variables and health status can test the hypothesis. When this is done, the hypothesis stands up well to evidence.

One question arises: If in the end everything depends on resources at the individual level, why do we find that more equal affluent societies have better health than less equal ones? The answer lies in the concept of diminishing marginal returns. Once my personal resource level reaches a certain point, say compares favourably with multi-billionaire Bill Gates, additional resources are not going to make much difference to my health and well-being. If some of my resources are transferred from me to a much poorer person, that increment will have much greater positive impact on the recipient compared to any harm done to me, the donor. It follows that evening out the income distribution should benefit less well-off people more than it harms well-off ones, at least in terms of their health. Thus we would expect to find, at the population level, better overall health in more-equal affluent societies like Japan than in less-equal affluent ones like the United States. And in fact we do.

However, by 2000, the materialist theory hit a speed bump. As we will see in Chapter 4, comparisons between the United States and Canada failed to show a consistent relationship between resources available at the individual level and health outcomes. Canadians were healthier than they ought to be, and income inequality in Canada did not have the same health effects as income inequality in the United States (Ross et al., 2000). This discovery led to the realization that not only individual income matters but communal and public resources may matter as well. If there is a decent, inexpensive recreation centre within walking distance, I do not need to install a home gym. If there is excellent, affordable public transit, I do not need to incur the expenses of buying and operating a car. If health care costs are insured by a tax-funded scheme, I do not have to pay for private health care insurance premiums. In short, public goods can substitute for private ones, and a society such as Canada providing a high level of public goods may at least partially mitigate the effects of income inequality.

Tax policies may also mitigate inequality. Progressive taxes that take a larger proportion of income from wealthier people than from less-wealthy ones have big effects on disposable (after-tax) income, and thus on the size of the difference in potential consumption patterns between income groups. Moreover, social programs are supported by tax revenues and tend, whether they are schools or health care or social welfare programs, to advantage the poorer population more than the rich. Thus, social programs also tend to be progressive, disproportionally helping the less well-off. The double effect of progressive taxes and public programs is very large.

Contextual features can matter as well. Public services, the quality of neighbourhoods, the nature of the transportation infrastructure, and community resources, such as the proximity of parks, good-quality shops, schools, and health care, are also important to the individuals living in the area (Dunn et al., 2005).

Factoring in the effects of public goods and contextual features gave rise to the **neo-materialist hypothesis**. This hypothesis, like the materialist one, focuses on the idea of resources available to the individual, but it is broadened to include a range of communal and public resources, as well as tax policy. As we will see, most theorizing about the determinants of health works within the neo-materialist paradigm and its explanatory force remains unsurpassed.

Psychosocial Theories

There is, however, an alternative to the materialist view and the neo-materialist variant, both of which construe relevant differences in terms of resources, capabilities, and opportunities available to individuals. Most closely associated with Wilkinson (1996), this alternate view argues that in affluent societies it is not income or education or other resources that matter but rather the status of the person who has those resources. In other words, income or education can be seen as markers of an individual's social position. Income and education are signifiers of rank or status within social hierarchies. From this perspective, the reason why we see poorer health in less equal places is that those places are more hierarchical. That is, bigger gaps exist between richer and poorer. Wilkinson contends it is the size of those gaps, not the income available to people, that matters.

If it is not resources and capacities that contribute to health, what could be causing the differences we observe in unequal societies? Wilkinson's answer is that unequal societies foster more competition and envy due to conflict over status. Steeply hierarchical social arrangements fail to generate co-operation and a sense of solidarity and thus are likely to have higher rates of anti-social behaviour and crime than more equal societies. The individual, especially the individual with low social status, feels less secure. All of these features will work their way into human biology through the elevated stress experienced by people lower down in the social hierarchy.

This alternative view is relative, as opposed to absolute, because its focus is on the position of individuals relative to others within their society. It is also a **psychosocial hypothesis** because it posits a mechanism—the feelings of stress that arise regarding an individual's position ultimately drive his or her health status.

At first glance, this appears to be quite a load to be carried by stress. But keep in mind that stress significantly impairs our capacity to cope with challenges. Moreover, chronic stress has been linked to smoking, excess alcohol consumption, overeating, depression, and breakdown of social relations. People under stress have a heightened sensitivity to pain and are susceptible to debilitating chronic pain syndromes. And there is evidence that stress can affect basic metabolic pathways, contributing to diabetes and impaired immune function. Chronic stress is also associated with coronary heart disease.

Wilkinson (1996) asserts that in poorer countries material differences are what matters. The big health problems in poorer societies, as we have seen, are infectious and parasitic diseases. But as we have also seen, once a society crosses the epidemiologic transition, becoming more affluent, the big problems facing it become the chronic diseases like cancer and heart disease. The transition, in Wilkinson's interpretation, represents a shift from material differences between people to social differences. In other words, material disadvantage lies behind infectious disease, but social disadvantage lies behind chronic disease. Wilkinson thus provides an elegant and coherent explanation of the epidemiologic transition.

We will be fleshing out these two families of theories, materialist and psychosocial, putting them to work and evaluating how satisfactory they are in the chapters that follow.

Theoretical Considerations

This chapter introduces the conceptual model underpinning the social determinants of health, as sketched out in Figure 3.7. Dark lines imply strong determining relationships; lighter lines imply weaker relationships. Perhaps the hardest part of the model to grasp is the interaction between biology, social status, and social interactions. Bear in mind epigenetics, the entangled nature of sex and gender and the social interactional influences

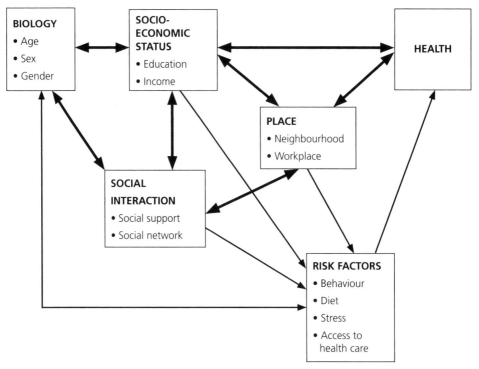

Figure 3.7 Conceptual Model of Determinants of Health

on our brain and cognitive development—all matters we will explore in some detail in Chapters 5 and 7.

Summary

Rose showed that focusing on risks in society, such as high blood pressure or abnormal blood lipid profiles and building disease-preventive strategies around these, is neither entirely coherent nor very effective. If we are serious about health, we need to find approaches that shift the baselines, improving conditions for the entire population.

Higher rates of disease among less well-off people are not due to poverty effects, although those play a role. In every known affluent society, there is a gradient: the richer you become, or the longer you attend school and college, the better your health and the longer you will live. Social and economic advantages confer health and life-expectancy advantages.

This chapter introduced some hypotheses about why income, education, and social position might matter so much to health. Those hypotheses aim to explain the gradient in health. Recall that there are three: materialist, neo-materialist, and psychosocial. The key difference is that materialist hypotheses construe the main driver of health differences to be individual resources or capacities, whereas psychosocial hypotheses construe differences in health to arise from differences in social status or rank.

Critical Thinking Questions

1. Canada and the United Kingdom have free universal health care and fairly extensive welfare programs to support their populations. Yet, since the introduction of universal health care (1948 in England; 1968–1971 in Canada), the gaps in health and life expectancy between richer and poorer people have gotten larger. How is that possible?

2. Preventive medicine—screening, early diagnosis, and putting people on medication to modify risk factors like blood pressure—is not making much progress in creating a healthier public. Why?

3. Why might the distribution of resources within a society have a decisive impact on its health?

4. Inequality has grown tremendously in the United States, especially over the past decade. Yet the incidence of coronary heart disease and many other chronic diseases such as colon cancer and dementia has declined dramatically. What problems do those data pose for Wilkinson's hypothesis?

Annotated Suggested Readings

The most comprehensive resource on social determinants of health is the World Health Organization's 2008 publication *Closing the Gap in a Generation: Health Equity Through Action on the Social Determinants of Health*. The full report is available free of charge at http://www.who.int/social_determinants/thecommission/finalreport/en.

Richard Wilkinson expressed his views most clearly in his 1996 book *Unhealthy Societies, the Afflictions of Inequality* (London: Routledge). He outlines the basis of his case for a psychosocial account of health inequalities and makes a series of policy recommendations for affluent countries.

A more recent, but specifically British, account of health inequalities can be found in a 2010 report by Sir Michael Marmot, the esteemed English epidemiologist. An electronic version of the report *Fair Societies, Healthy Lives* may be found at http://www.instituteofhealthequity.org/resources-reports/fair-society-healthy-lives-the-marmot-review.

Annotated Web Resources

"About Professor Sir Michael Marmot"
http://www.instituteofhealthequity.org/about-us/about-professor-sir-michael-marmot
Many valuable resources associated with the work of Sir Michael Marmot are available at the Institute of Health Equity's website.

"Science: from Cradle to Grave"
www.bbc.co.uk/iplayer/episode/b012wg2q/Science_From_Cradle_to_Grave
The BBC audio file "Science: from Cradle to Grave" discusses prospective cohort studies.

The Best of Ideas Podcast
www.vivele canada.ca/article/235929840-sick-people-or-sick-societies
The CBC podcast *The Best of Ideas* includes interviews with many of the top researchers in the population health/social epidemiology field. Specific recommended episodes on health are available at the link above (the full archive of the podcast is also available on the CBC website).

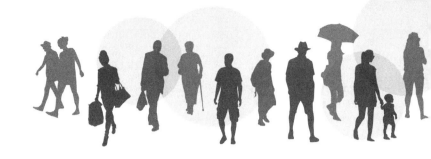

4 Income, Income Inequality, Wealth, and Health

Objectives

By the end of your study of this chapter, you should be able to
- appreciate the importance of income as a determinant of health;
- understand the strengths and weaknesses of the "inequality hypothesis";
- distinguish between the individual-level analysis (embedded in materialist hypothesis) and the collective-level analysis (embedded in the psychosocial hypothesis);
- appreciate the policy implications for taxation, income maintenance, and public services that flow from an analysis of inequality and health.

Synopsis

Chapter 4 discusses the profound effect income has on health and life expectancy. The chapter then reviews the emergence of theory relating to *income inequality* and the continuing controversies over the extent to which population-level income inequality affects human health. It then moves to an overview of the extent of inequality in liberal regime countries, some of the reasons for rising income inequality, the increasing concentration of wealth, and the importance of policies relating to taxation and public spending in mitigating health inequalities arising from the operation of market economies.

Income and Health

Income is the single most important determinant of health. Higher-income populations enjoy better health and live longer lives. This impact of income on health is not a poverty effect, an observed difference between deprived populations and privileged ones, but rather a curvilinear relationship, with each additional income increment yielding an additional health increment (albeit a shrinking one at very high incomes).

Income (and the related factor of education) has the effects we observe because of the kind of society in which we live. In modern market (capitalist) societies, goods, services, and labour are traded for money; hence, money is central to virtually every transaction, a feature that would not be true of subsistence agricultural societies. Income and education in our society are very closely related, although the association is less than perfect. Celebrities may be highly trained (but generally do not have advanced education), yet they have substantially higher incomes than university professors. Despite exceptions, income and education are covariates; *typically, income rises with education.*

The reasons for the relationship between income and health are explored throughout the book. Here we will observe only some generalizations about why the relationship exists and is so strong. In our society, income is the necessary means to a great many things: food, housing, transport, recreation, and health care, to name but a few. The quality of our diet, homes, and neighbourhood is a function of our income. Income is thus *the principal means to the resources necessary for a healthy life*. Income is also associated with status—our standing in our society. Status is a determinant of our influence over other people, how respectfully we are treated, and the size and supportiveness of our social network. Those variables all impact on our health (see Chapter 7).

Like income, education is associated with status. Additionally, education influences a number of health-relevant variables such as the amount of information we have, our capacity to acquire and utilize new information, and our ability to plan. These all affect our health-relevant behaviour (see Chapter 13). Education also determines our employment, which affects our health not only though the income attached to the kind of work we do, but also through the effects of working conditions on health (see Chapter 9).

Health increases as income increases and, at least partly independently, as education increases. But because income and education are so closely linked, studies often examine only income effects on health. Here we will do likewise, though we will also look at some data linking education to health.

The Gradient in Health

The association between disease and income is one of the strongest and most consistent correlations in population-health research. Everywhere we look, death rates are inversely related to area income. Moreover, not only deaths but also rates of disease and disability are sensitive to income levels. Morbidity incidence shows the same distinct-income gradient, with every population's health improving as its income rises.

While the health gradient is a universal feature of affluent societies, researchers have found some anomalies. The most important exceptions to the pattern of incidence of disease declining with rising income, in terms of frequency and contribution to premature death, are breast cancer and prostate cancer, both of which tend to be more common in affluent as opposed to poorer populations. And for unknown reasons, some rare diseases like cancer of the brain and Parkinson's disease are more common among relatively privileged as opposed to relatively deprived people. Disadvantaged people are not worse off across the board. For example, African Americans have lower rates of cancer (apart from prostate) and mental illness than white and Hispanic Americans. Nevertheless, the relationship between all-cause morbidity, all-cause disability, and overall mortality rates and income is stable. *Wherever we look, richer people are healthier and live longer disability-free lives.*

The Canadian mortality picture is shown in Table 4.1.

The US data shown in Table 4.2 paint a similar picture, this time for morbidity. Kennedy and colleagues show that the likelihood of reporting poor or fair health (as opposed to excellent or good health) is nearly 7.5 times greater for poorer than richer Americans. Canadian data, mortality rates rather than morbidity, also illustrate the same relationship between income and health (see Figure 4.1).

Table 4.1 The Gradient: Total Deaths and Infant Mortality Rates by Income Quintile, Canada, 1996

Income Quintile	Male Deaths	Female Deaths	Infant Mortality Rate
Quintile 1 (richest)	8,359	6,909	4.0
Quintile 2	9,327	7,449	4.7
Quintile 3	10,811	9,163	4.9
Quintile 4	12,495	10,852	5.0
Quintile 5 (poorest)	14,384	11,737	6.4

Source: Adapted from Wilkins, Berthelot, & Ng, 2002.

Table 4.2 Odds of Poor Health by Income Level, United States, 1996

Income	Likelihood of Reporting Poor Health (Odds)
<$10,000	7.43
$10,000–$14,999	5.32
$15,000–$19,999	3.62
$20,000–$24,999	2.71
$25,000–$35,000	1.98
>$35,000	1.00

Source: Adapted from Kennedy, Kawachi, Glass, & Prothrow-Stith, 1998.

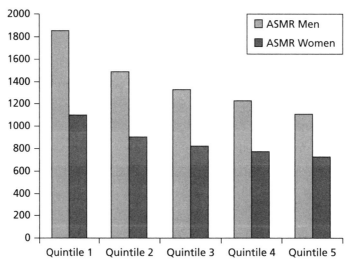

Figure 4.1 Age-Standardized Mortality Rate (ASMR) per 100,000 Person Years, by Sex, by Income Quintile, Canada, 1991–2006 (1 = lowest)

Source: Adapted from Statistics Canada (2015). https://www.statcan.gc.ca/pub/82-003-x/2013007/article/11852-eng.htm

Box 4.1	Case Study ○ The Gradient: Life Expectancy in and around Washington, DC

If you ride the metro from southeast downtown Washington DC out to Montgomery County in Maryland, for every mile you travel, residents live 1.5 years longer. Residents of Montgomery County live 20 years longer than the African Americans of southeast downtown Washington, DC (Marmot, 2006).

How might such results be explained?

Understanding the Complex Relationship Between Income and Health

One question aggregated nation-wide data fail to answer is whether the observed effect is a relationship between income and health or a relationship between the things income *is a marker of* and health. Higher population income typically signifies higher education levels, improved living conditions, improved housing, better diet, and safer, more rewarding work as well as a great many other things. Moreover, having a relatively affluent population is a precondition for stable government, development of infrastructure such as roads, collective garbage removal, safe water and sewage disposal, and social programs such as universal education, health care, and social services. This complex relationship among potentially relevant factors is the problem of **collinearity**. Several predictive variables are highly correlated with each other, making it difficult to ascertain the relative contribution of each to the outcome. One way of approaching this problem is the careful comparison of populations, internationally by country and domestically by province, state, county, municipality, and neighbourhood. The past 20 years have seen a plethora of just such studies, and thus our understanding of the relationship among the variables associated with income has become much deeper. That relationship is the heart of the materialist health hypothesis, discussed further in this chapter.

An important question arises when we consider health, populations, and incomes: Does inequality at the societal level affect health at the individual level? A brief history of the income inequality hypothesis best starts with the groundbreaking work of the American demographer Samuel H. Preston (1975).

The Inequality Hypothesis: Preston, Rodgers, Kaplan, and Wilkinson

Income is an individual-level variable, an attribute of a person or a person's household. As such, it exercises a profound effect on health, as we have already seen. A separate, though related, question is whether macro-level, contextual variables relating to income also affect health and mortality. The most obvious variable is *income distribution*—how equally income is distributed across individuals in a population. Average and median incomes for a population are themselves aggregate measures that apply to the population and not to any one person. But we often assume a measure like per capita income (total country income divided by the number of people) serves as a proxy for what each person receives. That might not be too misleading for very poor countries, with subsistence agricultural economies, but it would be wildly off the mark for affluent industrialized countries, which are characterized by a very wide income distribution from poor to rich.

Well over a quarter-century ago, Preston discovered that a country's gross domestic product (GDP) per capita correlates strongly with life expectancies in poorer countries but very weakly with life expectancies in richer ones. At some point around $10,000 per capita (in 2018 dollars), the relationship between income and life expectancy virtually disappears. Notice that this would also be a point, in terms of average income in a population, at which we would expect both the demographic and epidemiological transitions to have occurred.

Preston's findings have been replicated and the relationship he discovered between diminishing health returns from higher incomes above a certain threshold is now referred to as the "**Preston curve**." The Preston curve shows a *curvilinear relationship* between income and life expectancy (see Figure 4.2). Each new income increment in an already affluent place such as Canada has less effect on health and life expectancy than the same increment of wealth in a poorer one such as India.

Preston's finding is of great importance because it suggests that absolute income is the main consideration with regard to life expectancy only up until the population becomes relatively affluent. Preston (1975) drew the conclusion that total income and *average income* matter most in poorer places but the *distribution of available income* matters more in affluent ones. This makes intuitive sense. If we redistribute food in a situation where everyone is near starvation, we make that population of people worse off because now a proportion of them will die. But if we redistribute food in a situation

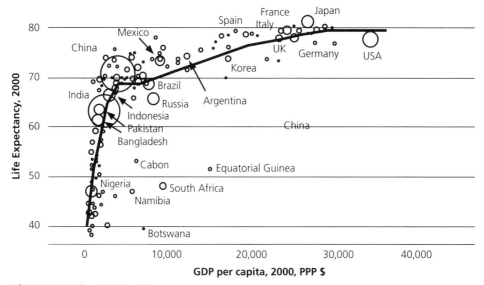

Figure 4.2 The Preston Curve

Circles have a diameter proportional to population size. GDP per capita is in purchasing power parity (PPP) dollars.

Source: World Health Organization, 2008.

where some people have plenty and some are near starvation, the health of the overall population improves.

It follows from Preston's analysis that overall life expectancy (and presumably overall health) would be improved by redistributing income from the wealthy to the less wealthy within rich countries and redistributing income from wealthy countries to poorer ones between countries. It also follows, as Preston himself pointed out, that countries like the United States have worse health and lower life expectancies than their average per capita GDP would warrant. In short, *affluent countries with significant income inequality have sub-optimal health outcomes.*

It is important to note the ethical implications of Preston's findings. Preston showed that income inequality in more affluent societies (and income inequalities between rich and poor countries) harm human health. It does not follow that such inequalities are morally wrong or unjust, but it does follow that they are wrong or unjust if the inequalities cannot be justified on some basis other than health—for example, if inequality is necessary in order to sustain a productive economy. If existing inequalities cannot be justified, those inequalities are arbitrary. If arbitrary, they are morally questionable or, in other words, not just inequalities, but also social injustices.

Later research by Rodgers (1979) shows a correlation between infant mortality rates—quite a robust measure of the overall health of a population—and country-level income inequality measures. Rodgers argued that the relationship between income and life expectancy at the country level was roughly linear. In broad-brush terms, the higher the country-level income the better the country's overall health would be. Rodgers believed the effect existed mostly because national income was such a strong determinant of other things important to health such as education, health care services, nutrition, and housing. But at the individual level, Rodgers found that more income does not lead in a linear way to better health, at least not after a certain level of wealth is achieved. Instead, the relationship between income and life expectancy at the individual level is **asymptotic** (Rodgers, 1979). Once a person had a sufficiently high income, more income would lead to only small marginal improvements. Like Preston's findings, Rodger's results strongly suggest that taking action to reduce inequalities in income through taxing the more affluent and providing better income support and public services for the less wealthy would improve the health of a population.

We already mentioned Wilkinson's (1986, 1996) work on life expectancies in countries belonging to the Organisation for Economic Co-operation and Development. Recall that Wilkinson showed that life expectancies are correlated with the share of income received by the poorer half of the income distribution. In short, Wilkinson showed that the more unequal the society, in the case of the rich nations, the worse the health of its population.

Kaplan is a distinguished professor of epidemiology at the University of Michigan. Kaplan and colleagues (Kaplan, Pamuk, Lynch, Cohen, & Balfour, 1996) undertook sophisticated multi-level research in the United States. The results show that the income share of the lower half of the income distribution is strongly associated with the state-level mortality rate. Even when Kaplan controlled for differences in the median incomes and differences between states with respect to their poverty rates, the results held up. Kaplan's study shows, in the United States at least, that the extent of income inequality is predictive of poor health, and the effect is not caused by there being more poor people in places with higher inequality (although that is likely to be true). In other words, both the proportion of poor people (a compositional variable) and the nature of the income distribution (a collective or population level variable) affect population health. Kennedy et al. (1998) added to Kaplan's findings by showing that people living in more unequal US states were 32 per cent more likely to report bad health (see Table 4.3). By the mid-1990s, good-quality research established that income inequality in affluent countries harms human health.

By 2009, some researchers were contending that not only health but also social problems in affluent countries were functions of the level of inequality (see Figure 4.3).

Table 4.3 Odds of Reporting Poor Health

Extent of State Income Inequality	Odds Ratio for Reporting Poor Health
High inequality (GINI > 0.355)	1.32
GINI 0.332—0.355	1.29
GINI 0.320—0.331	1.19
Lowest inequality (GINI < 0.320)	1.00

Source: Adapted from Kennedy et al., 1998.

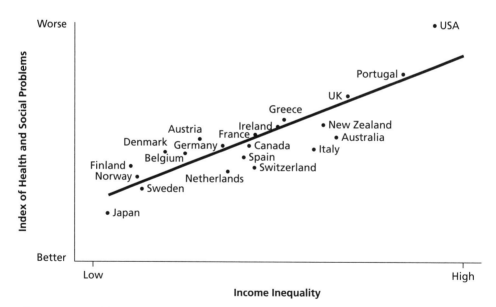

Figure 4.3 Health and Social Problems Worse in More Unequal Affluent Countries
Source: Wilkinson & Pickett, 2009.

Pause and Reflect   What Links Income to Health?

Through what mechanisms might a person's income affect his or her health? Through what mechanisms might the income distribution in the place where the individual lives affect his or her health?

Components of the Wilkinson Synthesis

The first person to develop an integrated theory around the findings respecting income inequality and health was Richard Wilkinson (1996). He drew from four sources:

1. Social capital theory as it had been developed by political scientist Robert Putnam (Putnam, 1993).
2. Sociologist Émile Durkheim's concept of "social facts," in particular the significance of norms of social interaction (Durkheim, 1897).
3. Criminology and the findings that crime rates and anti-social behaviour tend to reflect the extent of social inequality.
4. Primatology, notably the work of Sapolsky (1990) on stress responses of primates in troop hierarchies.

Social Capital Theory
Robert Putnam advanced an argument in his book *Making Democracy Work* (1993) that norms of reciprocity and mutual trust are essential for stable and accountable governance. The norms, such as seeking out social and economic exchanges with others, are generated, according to Putnam, through social transactions in the family and community, in particular via participation in economic life and voluntary associations. Social hierarchy, as opposed to day-to-day interactions among near equals, corrodes **social capital**. Hierarchies foster factionalism, discord, and anti-social behaviour, whereas more equal social conditions support constructive interaction within communities. Putnam claimed that southern Italy, with its high crime rate and fractured communities, illustrates low social capital, whereas northern Italy, with its well-functioning and integrated communities, illustrates high social capital (more on social capital in Chapter 7).

Sociology and Criminology
Émile Durkheim claimed that a degree of stability and predictability is essential to human well-being. He argued (1897) that breakdowns in stability and predictability, such as may occur during rapid social change, create stress that in turn drives suicide rates. Modern sociology and criminology have built on Durkheim's findings, exploring the relationships between social change, inequalities in society, breakdowns in social integration, and crime rates. In general, criminologists contend that more unequal places will exhibit more discord, more anti-social behaviour, and more crime. For example, criminologists predict that a highly unequal, hierarchical community such as New Orleans will have a higher crime rate than a more equal community such as San Diego.

Primatology
Primatologists have shown—among Rhesus monkeys, baboons, and chimpanzees, all of which live in social hierarchies—that dominant animals are healthier and have longer lives. Contrariwise, subordinate animals are more frequently ill and live shorter lives. The neurologist Robert Sapolsky (1990) showed those results do not stem from diet—an inability on the part of subordinate animals to compete successfully for food. Rather, the basal cortisol levels (normal levels of stress hormone) are different in dominant and subordinate animals. A chronically elevated stress response can be shown to affect things like

deposits in the arteries, linking biological outcomes with the animal's social position. The psychologist Stephen Suomi (2005) added to this line of research by showing that healthy dominant animals can be made sick and sick subordinates can be made healthier by manipulating the animals' positions in the troop hierarchy.

Wilkinson's Theoretical Synthesis

Wilkinson's argument runs along these lines. Income distribution is a marker of how unequal a society is. The size of income inequalities reflects how hierarchical the society is. In other words, income inequality measures the differences in social standing or social status. Because education and the nature of your job and the quality of your house and the safety of your neighbourhood are all reflected in your income, income serves as a reliable marker of your social standing. A big difference in income between two individuals suggests big differences in education, housing, neighbourhood, job, and capacity to influence social and political life. And big differences between individuals across society will diminish social capital, fuel envy and discontent, undermine social and political processes that could lead to fairer compromises, contribute to social breakdown and crime, and thus make life more difficult and stressful for everyone, but especially for the less well-off members of society (Wilkinson, 1996; Wilkinson & Pickett, 2009).

Stress will also be generated among the less well-off because they perceive their situation to be that of inferiors. They will feel shame and they will be driven to be more competitive. All of this will work its way through our biological stress mechanism—the hypothalamic-pituitary-adrenal system (HPA axis)—affecting mental and physical well-being and life expectancy.

It is important to recognize that stress per se is not a risk to human health. When we are startled or frightened, our HPA axis is activated. Our blood cortisol levels spike, an evolved response to danger. Our heart rate rises, our peripheral arteries constrict, making more blood available to muscles, and glucose is mobilized for energy, all in preparation for flight (running away) or fight (confronting the perceived danger).

When manifested as a temporary response, stress is a motivator and feeling under pressure can get us into action and improve our performance. We even seek out stress in the form of thrills and competitive sports. Intermittent stress, at levels with which we can cope, enhances our productivity and sense of well-being. This is sometimes referred to as eustress (good stress) or simply as arousal.

Problems arise when stress and the resulting elevated level of cortisol become chronic. People perceiving themselves to be constantly under assault or constantly on their guard or not in control of their situation will experience this chronic elevation of their blood cortisol levels. Under such circumstances, the normal cortisol response becomes blunted. Instead of their blood cortisol spiking to high levels and then rapidly falling back to its normal low level, people under chronic stress will exhibit a small rise from a high baseline, "basal" level, to a slightly higher level, then a slow decline back to that elevated baseline. That abnormal response is the hallmark of an elevated basal cortisol level, a condition that causes damage to blood vessels and adversely affects sugar metabolism.

Chronic elevated basal cortisol levels are associated with insulin tolerance and type-2 diabetes, plaque buildup in arteries, coronary heart disease, and kidney disease. Thus, a robust biological model exists to link high levels of ongoing stress with some important health outcomes, notably diabetes and heart disease.

Emotions, Mind, and Body

Our reaction to emotional stress is biologically complex. At least two fundamental body systems are involved. The brain and the range of powerful hormones that it controls comprise the neuroendocrine system. The second major system affected by stress is the immune system.

Two sub-systems, the HPA axis and the sympathetic nervous system, make up the neuroendocrine system. The HPA axis involves both direct and feedback effects among the hypothalamus, the pituitary gland, and the adrenal cortex. Fear and anxiety trigger the release of hormones from the brain's hypothalamus, leading to the release of glucocorticoids from the adrenal glands (see Figure 4.4). Chronic exposure to one glucocorticoid (cortisol) affects ageing, promotes changes in brain structure, can damage the cardiovascular system, and depresses the immune system.

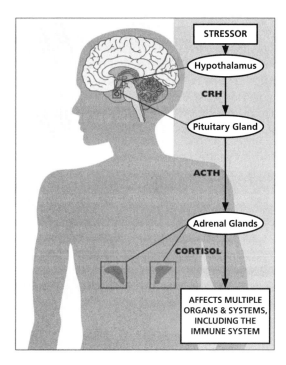

Figure 4.4 The Science of Stress

Source: Robert Wood Johnson Foundation, 2011. Reproduced with permission of the Robert Wood Johnson Foundation, Princeton, NJ.

The adrenal glands are also stimulated through the sympathetic nervous system to release catecholamines, which include adrenaline and noradrenaline. Fear and anxiety, through the action of these hormones (which are also neurotransmitters), raise heart rate and blood pressure, cause the liver to release stored energy, and direct blood away from the body's periphery to the brain, vital organs, and major muscle groups. The reaction is essential to the "fight or flight" response to physical danger, but is itself a threat to health if repeatedly, regularly engaged.

Stress also directly affects the immune system. Chronic stress is linked to chronic inflammation, which in turn is implicated in heart disease and diabetes. Moreover, chronic stress reduces the body's capacity to resist infection or overcome the toxic effects of negative environmental exposures.

Pause and Reflect   Might Rich Neighbours Make You Sick?

How and why might it matter to your health and well-being if your neighbours are substantially richer than you are?

Wilkinson, in sum, argues (1996; Wilkinson & Pickett, 2005, 2009) that rising social inequality means a more hierarchical social structure which in turn damages social capital, undermining positive social interaction. Low levels of social capital at the macro, societal level induce high levels of stress at the individual level. Stress provides the biological mechanism for damage to health. Stress also induces health-damaging behaviours ranging from overeating, to drug and alcohol use, to smoking. Thus, for Wilkinson, *unequal societies are unhealthy societies.*

The Inequality Hypothesis Under Assault

In 1996, the prestigious *British Medical Journal* declared that the relationship between income inequality and health was the "Big Idea" of our age. However, matters did not rest there. In 1998, Gravelle argued that the correlation between income inequality (at the population level) and poorer health was a statistical artifact arising from the fact that more income had a bigger effect on less well-off people than on more affluent ones (Gravelle, 1998). Critics accused Wilkinson of cherry-picking the OECD data. They claimed he used data that fit best with his hypothesis and ignored data that called it into question (Lynch et al., 2004a). Then, in 2000, Nancy Ross and colleagues showed that there was no population-level income inequality effect in Canada (Ross et al., 2000). Later, Shibuya, Hashimoto, & Yano (2002) showed there was no income inequality effect in Japan (beyond differences in individual and household incomes), followed by Blakely, Atkinson, and O'Dea (2003), who showed there was no population-level inequality effect in New Zealand. Deaton and Lubotsky (2003) called into question the inequality effect in the United States by showing that the varying proportions of the population made up by racial minorities confound American data (i.e., the results of earlier studies might have arisen from compositional effects). McLeod and colleagues (McLeod, Lavis, Mustard, & Stoddart, 2003) established that income differences at the household level, not income inequality at the societal level, account for most of the differences in health status. Finally, it was discovered that the relationship between the amount of inequality in a place and the size of differences in health status appears to exist at some high levels of data aggregation (country level or state level in the United States), but disappears at some lower levels (municipal level or neighbourhood level). That means you might be able to show a relationship between health and inequality comparing the more unequal Louisiana with the more equal Washington State but not by comparing two cities in Louisiana. In other words, the statistical association between the amount of inequality in society and health appears unstable, calling into question whether the relationship actually exists.

It is important to understand what is at stake in this dispute. Everyone agrees that *people with more resources are healthier*. That statistical association is robust. The dispute is about whether societies that are more unequal, such as the United States, will be more unhealthy than countries like Sweden or Japan (which are more equal) because income inequality harms health *or* simply because individuals with more resources do better than those with fewer resources (e.g., the US has a larger number of disadvantaged people). If it is only a matter of the resources each individual has, the **materialist hypothesis**, then it is the composition of a population that matters, the mix of richer and poorer people. It would make sense to disaggregate down to the individual level and measure each person's resources, safely ignoring any possible population-level effects.

But if inequality, the relative position of people in an income distribution, itself matters, then it should be possible, in theory at least, to show an independent effect of income inequality over and above the effects that arise from the features of individuals within the population. Some theorists (Wilkinson, for example) claim a big effect, in fact the largest effect, is attributable to the degree of social equality in a society. Others, Lynch and colleagues (2004a) for example, argue that the observed association with income inequality can be accounted for by diminishing marginal returns at the individual level. To the extent that Lynch is right and Wilkinson wrong, what ultimately matters is the concentration of lower- and higher-income earners in a given area (the "population composition") and not the collective variable "social equality."

Understandably, Lynch takes a dim view of Wilkinson's underlying psychosocial theory because Lynch denies at the outset that relative position in society matters (Lynch et al., 2004a). Other researchers with a materialist orientation attack Wilkinson's position on several grounds. The major objections are outlined in the following section.

Weaknesses in Wilkinson's Synthesis

The Problem of Scale

From our best data, inequality appears to matter only at high levels of aggregation such as the country or state level. If it is true that people compare their position to that of others and this comparison underlies the stress response that in turn affects health, one would expect to find the strongest relationship at the local level. But it is precisely here, at the local level, that the relationship breaks down. Hence Wilkinson's theory relies on interpersonal comparisons that are contrary to findings in psychology where it is well established that people compare themselves to those they interact with on a regular basis—i.e., locally.

The Problem of Inconsistent Correlation

If inequality matters, as societies become more unequal, health ought to get worse. Wilkinson claims that is true, citing the infant mortality rates in the United Kingdom and United States between the 1980s and 1990s. (Progress on reducing those rates stalled as inequality grew in both countries over that period.) Deaton (2003), however, attacks Wilkinson's claim, pointing to the fact that the period of flat development cited by Wilkinson followed a surge in the earlier period. Moreover, Deaton points out, life expectancies, at least for those over 45, continued to lengthen alongside growing inequality. Lynch and colleagues (2004b) show that the income gap in the United States grew, contracted, then grew again without evidence of a consistent relationship with mortality. In contrast, McGrail and colleagues (2009) find growth in health inequality comparable to growth in income inequality within the United States (from a gap of 2.8 years between highest and lowest income decile in the 1980s to 4.5 years by the end of the 1990s), but they find no evidence of a similar income inequality/health inequality relationship outside of the United States. In short, the relationship Wilkinson claims to exist universally appears to be rather hit and miss.

The Problem with Animal Models

Others argue that using animal models, particularly hierarchies of baboons and chimpanzees, is misleading because these animals are especially nasty and competitive (Abbott et al., 2003). There is no reason to think that humans are as combative as baboons. It is therefore highly unlikely that humans would suffer such dramatic consequences from living in status hierarchies. The association between hormones and status in primate hierarchies has also been questioned. Gesquiere and colleagues (2011) confirmed that higher-ranking baboons have higher levels of testosterone and lower levels of glucocorticoids than lower ranking animals. But this finding does not apply to the top, alpha males. The top animals have higher levels of stress hormones than subordinates, the exact opposite of what is predicted by the psychosocial hypothesis. Sapolsky himself (2017), the theorist upon whom Wilkinson based his hypotheses about stress, now holds that position in the social hierarchy is not the central determinant of the health of primates. The amount of support an animal garners from others is more important to its health and well-being than its place in troop hierarchy.

The Problem of Ideological Bias

An entirely different line of attack is to label psychosocial theorizing "ideological" (Navarro, 2002). Ultimately, Navarro points out, psychosocial theory relies on how individuals react to their circumstances, in other words, their emotional responses. It follows that if we can get people to be more accepting of their inferior positions, the bad health effects can be reduced or even eliminated. Navarro thinks psychosocial theory is politically dangerous because it opens the door to manipulating how people think about their circumstances rather than undertaking necessary social reforms.

The Confounding of Status with Income

John Lavis and colleagues (Lavis, McLeod, Mustard, & Stoddart, 2003) devised an ingenious study of possible status effects on health. Noting that status differences are highly significant in the British peerage system, yet aristocratic standing aligns poorly with income and wealth, the researchers worked out the correlations between aristocratic standing and life expectancy. It turns out that once income is detached from social standing, the relationship with life expectancy breaks down. In short, Lavis et al. establish that personal resources, not social status in a hierarchy, drive health outcomes.

While the dispute over resources available to individuals versus relative social standing sounds trivial, a lot is at stake. Conservative-minded governments often reach for strategies to make people feel included while avoiding real change in their material circumstances. In the United Kingdom, a few years ago, Prime Minister Cameron's Conservative coalition government floated the idea of a "Big Society," encouraging families and communities to pull together and reach out for common understandings. At the same time the government was cutting funding for programs and services that redistributed resources from richer to poorer citizens. President George W. Bush played a similar hand in the United States when his government sponsored more "civic-mindedness" while cutting programs serving minorities and other less-affluent Americans.

Is Wilkinson Wrong?

In spite of all the recent criticism, Wilkinson discovered an important relationship. A seminal study by Subramanian and Kawachi (2003) shows that income inequality between US states matters for human health, even after controlling for population composition, including race. Since then, a large number of American studies show that relevant metropolitan, state level, and regional health disparities are associated with population-level inequality. Some of those high-quality studies control for median income, household income, and poverty levels as well as race. It now looks like inequality, and not just racial inequality, really matters in the United States, but apparently not elsewhere. The findings in the US may be explicable in terms of social relations theory, discussed later in this chapter. Combined with neo-materialist concepts, the health impact of inequality can be explained. Lynch, the most hard-core materialist, has moved in recent years to this more synthetic position.

What Are We to Make of the Literature on Inequality and Health?

A high-quality multi-level Canadian study by Hou and Myles (2005) shed some light on what had become an increasingly confused field. They show, contrary to psychosocial theory, that poorer people living among richer people gain "positive externalities"—they actually benefit from inequality at the local level. There are several reasons why this might be: (a) people may model their behaviour on the health-enhancing behaviours of their better-off neighbours; (b) the neighbourhood may benefit from having a mix of people; and (c) having more affluent neighbours may mean better municipal services and higher-quality schools. Hou and Myles also found a strong association between household income and health but no association between neighbourhood inequality and health.

In yet another high-quality study, Dunn, Veenstra, and Ross (2006) show that neo-material explanations of variations in health status in Canada (such as the availability and configuration of public services and other neighbourhood characteristics) are much more strongly predictive of health than psychosocial explanations. Presumably those resources compensate for the lack of health-relevant resources at the individual level.

What are we to make of all of this? First, the evidence is incontrovertible regarding income and health. The more affluent a population is, the better its health. Everywhere, richer individuals enjoy better health than poorer ones. An individual's economic position, measured by income, is a close correlate, and arguably is the principal determinant, of other critical variables, not only education, but also access to other resources crucial to good health.

Second, diminishing marginal returns have been demonstrated consistently at both the individual and societal levels. Once an individual reaches a certain income threshold, additional increments of income provide smaller and smaller health benefits. Intuitively, that finding is pretty obvious. An extra $10,000 for a homeless woman would affect her life much more than an extra $10,000 would affect the life of a millionaire. Likewise, at the societal level, as we saw with the Preston curve, once a society reaches an income threshold measured by per capita income, additional increments of income provide smaller and smaller health benefits. For those reasons, it follows, as Preston argued over 25 years ago, that greater equality in affluent societies and greater equality between affluent and poorer societies would yield greater health at the population level. The transfer of resources from richer to poorer would drive death rates down and life expectancies up.

This remains an individual-level argument. It is about weighing the impact of one person losing some of their resources against the gain of another person receiving some resources. It is not about how hierarchical a society is and does not imply that social hierarchies harm health. It is also, as we have seen from the disputes about inequality, an argument that can carry most of the weight regarding the differences we see in the health status of different populations. But as we have also seen, other social dimensions of inequality, inequality at the population level, may have health effects in certain contexts, notably the United States. The difference across societies requires an explanation, one that probably lies in correlates of social and income inequality, such as quality of and access to public goods and services, neighbourhood characteristics, social solidarity and support, education and other important sources of health-enhancing support to individuals.

Third, analysis of differences between modern, affluent states has drawn attention to the willingness of populations to pay taxes for public services. In general, countries with high levels of income inequality have tax-resistant populations, whereas countries where income is distributed more evenly are able to support more public programs and services from taxes because of greater willingness on the part of the population to pay the taxes needed to support them (Esping-Andersen, 1990). More equal societies tend to move toward greater equality in two ways. First, progressive income taxes take a bigger bite out of higher incomes than lower ones. Second, the effects of using those tax dollars to provide free or highly subsidized education, health care, recreation, and so on, are redistributive because those public services are more heavily used by the less well-off than by the affluent. In other words, in more-equal countries, the healthy and wealthy contribute to programs and services that are used by those who are less healthy and less wealthy.

The effect of this is an increase in overall population health, whereas exactly the contrary effect will be found in tax-resistant countries because income and wealth become increasingly concentrated, thereby boosting tax resistance and increasing political pressure to cut what public programs do exist.

The trend in unequal societies is toward further disadvantaging the less healthy and less wealthy, whereas the tendency in more equal ones is to extend support to the less well-off. These and related findings are incorporated into the neo-materialist understanding of health inequalities in affluent societies, and they go a considerable distance toward explaining the differences we see in the health of different wealthy countries.

Finally, an important study may explain the reasons why inequality effects are found sometimes but not universally. Zheng (2012) argues that inequality at the national level has a very large detrimental effect on individual mortality risk but that this effect only manifests itself over time. Cross-sectional studies looking at inequality and health at a single point in time fail to take into account latency—the fact that it takes upwards of five years for the unequal conditions to work their way into human biology. Zheng demonstrates distinct time lags, with health effects appearing in the data five years following rises in national-level inequality and peaking seven years later. If this line of evidence holds up, the importance is difficult to underestimate. The findings mean that countries experiencing rapidly increasing inequality, notably the United States, are creating a legacy of serious ill health and premature mortality for their populations.

The Importance of Keeping Materialist Arguments Separate from Ones About Hierarchy and Control

Many analysts—Marmot is a notable one—tend to run together arguments about income, education, rank, and the degree of control one has over one's life. From a policy point of view, it is important to separate them out. Progressive income taxes reduce the income of richer people and increase resources for poorer people, but they do not change rank order and would be unlikely to change social status. A materialist theory would lend support to progressive tax policies because the theory would predict improved health results. A psychosocial theory would not, because progressive taxation leaves status untouched. Yet the evidence is strong that progressive taxes and public programs do improve population health, suggesting the materialist view is right and the psychosocial one is wrong. Likewise, a tax on wealth would certainly reduce differences in power between rich and poor, but it probably would not affect how much control a poorer person felt over his or her life. Wealth taxes might impact on status and they would create pools of money for redistribution through public programs. Therefore, both psychosocial and materialist theory would support wealth taxes, but a theory of health based on ideas of personal control would not.

Wilkinson and Pickett (2009) tend to run together resources and capabilities such as income and education with status differentials, whereas it would be more helpful to separate them out so that the influence on health of differences in resources (materialist) can be tested against the influence on health of differences in status (psychosocial).

When we take the precaution of separating out possible factors, the evidence to date suggests materialist explanations have more force than psychosocial ones. Most of the differences we see associated with inequality stem from diminishing marginal returns. That does not mean, however, that there are no aspects of life to which the psychosocial model properly applies. Similarly, the idea of personal control may well have force in certain health-relevant contexts. The world of work appears to be one of those places where both psychosocial factors and personal control matter, as we shall see in Chapter 10.

Other Explanations for the Correlation Between Social Inequality and Health in the United States

One psychosocial and three neo-materialist hypotheses have been proposed to account for the enormous differences observed in the health of different populations in the United States. They all relate to inequality in income, and they all see the neighbourhood as being the key intermediate variable. Income differences drive differences in terms of where people live and work, and those differences affect health.

Social relations theory proposes that income differences segregate (spatially and culturally) the less well-off from the more affluent, with the degree of segregation depending on how unequal incomes become. Social distance between groups increases as differences in income-related status grow; people with very different incomes will live in different types of home, own different things, and cultivate different interests, until they have virtually nothing in common and no basis for common understanding and co-operation. Fellow feeling diminishes, and hostility and stress increase. This theory is psychosocial.

Social isolation theory postulates that once people become much more affluent than those around them, they will relocate to create a privileged enclave for themselves. Resources such as good schools migrate with them. Less well-off people are concentrated in areas of decline and as the area becomes less and less supportive of its population, all those with the means to leave will do so, creating a blighted neighbourhood and a sub-culture of poverty. This theory is neo-materialist.

Health-enhancing goods theory is similar. An area in decline because of departure of the more affluent will see a fall in property values relative to other areas and hence a relative decline in property tax—the major source of funding for most community-level services. Contrariwise, areas experienced gentrification or attractive affluent suburbs will see rising property values, higher tax revenues, and hence greater capability to deliver services important to people's health such as policing, parks, recreation facilities, etc. This theory is also neo-materialist.

Opportunity structure theory looks at the range of possibilities and constraints a neighbourhood presents to its residents. The theory is central to most thinking about health and neighbourhoods and is discussed in Chapter 10. This theory is also neo-materialist.

These four theories are not mutually exclusive. Each of them captures an important dimension of inequality that may be relevant to health.

Income and Income Distribution

Available income shapes a person's opportunities, sense of his or her capabilities, living conditions, diet, health-relevant behaviour, and much else. In addition to earnings from employment, available income is determined by personal savings and investments such as annuities and private pensions; transfers from government such as income assistance, public pensions, disability allowances, food stamps, and unemployment insurance payments; and public services for which the individual would otherwise have to pay out of pocket, such as public health care, insurance, and public school education.

The amount of disposable income (spending money) a person or household has depends on taxes and transfers. Governments not only tax their citizens but also transfer substantial amounts of cash to them in the form of tax credits, allowances, pensions, and other payments.

Pause and Reflect   Are Fair Taxes Required for a Healthy Society?

US jurist Oliver Wendell Holmes (1841–1935) argued that taxes are the price we pay for civilized society. Was he right? How might taxation affect the health and well-being of people in our society?

Incomes, to be comparable, must be adjusted for household size. There are considerable economies of scale associated with sharing the costs of accommodation, utilities, and transportation. In general, the smaller the size of a household, the more expensive it is to support each person in it, hence the lower the value of any given level of disposable income. One feature of advanced countries such as Canada, the United States, Australia, and the United Kingdom is that household sizes have been shrinking and more people are living alone. This places more people at risk of low income, food insecurity, and substandard housing.

Countries differ not only in terms of how high their average taxes are but also in terms of how progressive their taxes are. Advanced countries rely most heavily on income taxes to raise government revenues. Income taxes may be proportional, in other words, take the same percentage of everyone's income ("flat tax") or, alternatively, they may be engineered to take a bigger proportion of a higher income than of a lower one ("progressive"). In Canada, the United Kingdom, Australia, and the United States, income taxes are progressive and the tax systems actually give cash to, as opposed to taking money away from, low-income individuals. Table 4.4 shows income through employment (earned or market income), government transfers, and income taxes, by family type. Below a family market income of $65,000, every family type ends up with more disposable income than it earns. That means, of course, that families above the median incomes shown here are contributing more by way of taxes, thereby supporting the income transfer to the less well-off. (Note: Disposable income in the chart does not equal earned income plus transfers minus taxes because of various other factors incorporated in Statistics Canada's analysis.)

Table 4.4 Median Income by Family Type, Canada, 2010

Family Type	Market (Earned) Income	Government Transfers (tax credits, pensions)	Income Tax Paid	After-Tax (Disposable) Income
Family, two persons or more	64,900	6,500	8,200	65,500
Family, over 65	23,700	25,300	1,500	46,800
Family, female lone-support	28,000	9,500	0	38,700

Source: Statistics Canada, June 18, 2012.

Progressive tax systems use brackets: one tax rate for income up to a certain level, then a higher tax rate for income beyond that level up to a certain higher level, and so on all the way up to the top marginal income bracket, beyond which all further income is taxed at the same top rate. The Nordic countries (social democratic regimes) of Europe, committed to achieving greater social equality, have steeply progressive tax systems with top marginal rates over 60 per cent. The world of liberal regimes has a much flatter tax system, with top rates hovering around 47 per cent. An important trend has been the move to increasingly flatter rates (less progressivity) in Canada and the United States, a trend that contributed to the rapid rise of post–tax income inequality in those countries (recently partially reversed in Canada but worsened in the US by the 2017 Republican tax reform). Oddly, Canadians have consistently signalled their willingness to pay more in taxes to create a more equal society (Galloway, 2012), but until recently governments ignored them, choosing instead to follow the US lead by continuing to cut taxes for the wealthy up until the modest taxation changes made by the federal Liberal government in 2017.

From the mid-1970s to the present there has been a sharp increase in inequality across the developed countries of the Organisation for Economic Co-operation and Development, with the exception of a decrease in Australia (Organisation for Economic Co-operation and Development, 2008). Canada's situation is now stable, with a GINI coefficient hovering around 0.32, placing Canada twelfth among its 17 peer countries (Conference Board of Canada, 2013).

From the mid-1980s until the mid-1990s, government expenditures through transfers and social programs dampened the rise in poverty. But cuts in taxes on wealthier citizens and reductions in programs benefiting mostly poorer ones contributed to rising inequality and to a growing number of poor people, particularly between 1990 and 2004. In general, countries with wider income distributions (greater inequality), such as the United States, have more poor people. Top marginal tax rates for 1979 and 2017 are shown in Table 4.5.

Table 4.5 Falling Tax Rates for the Wealthy

Country	1979 Top Marginal Tax Rate	2017 Top Marginal Tax Rate
Australia	62	45
Canada	58	47.7 (BC)
United Kingdom	87	60
United States	70	39.6

Incomes of rich households have grown enormously in the United States and Canada (OECD, 2008; Yalnizyan, 2010), but incomes of the bottom 20 per cent of income earners have actually shrunk. In the United States, the top income quintile (20 per cent) earned 10 times more than the lowest income quintile in 1969. That grew to 14 times more by 2009 (Robert Wood Johnson Foundation, 2011).

> The gap between the families with the lowest and highest incomes, an indication of income inequality, widened during the past decade. The gap between the top and bottom quintiles started at $83,800 in 1980, and fluctuated between $79,500 and $84,500 until 1996. By 2005, the gap had reached $105,400. (Statistics Canada, 2005)

In Canada and the United States, from the Second World War into the 1970s, the proportion of total income going to the richest people shrivelled. But over the past 30 years, the trend has been reversed. In Canada, the very rich (0.1 per cent at the top of the income distribution) saw their share of income triple; the super-rich (0.01 per cent at the top) saw their share increase by more than fivefold (Yalnizyan, 2010).

Part of the trend toward growing inequality is attributable to tax cuts for the wealthy, but part of it is also due to changes in earned incomes. Incomes for males, in particular, have declined for people with lower incomes and less education, whereas the pay of senior executives in the form of salaries and bonuses has skyrocketed: "In 2005 the share of the top 1 per cent in pre-tax income varied from 5.6 per cent in the Netherlands and 6.5 per cent in Denmark and Sweden to 12.7 per cent in Canada, 14.3 per cent in the UK and 17.4 per cent in the US" (Wolf, 2011). The richest Canadians are now paying themselves 189 times the average Canadian wage. CEOs of Canadian companies have been rewarded with 27 per cent raises year-over-year in compensation versus 1 to 2 per cent increases for average Canadian workers (Scoffield, 2012). We will look at the growing gulf between workers and executives in Chapter 9, on employment.

In the past, there was little concern about income distribution because it was assumed that everyone had a reasonable opportunity of rising up the income ranks. Specifically, it was believed in Canada, and it still is in the United States, that our societies have equality of opportunity—that children from less well-off families have fair opportunity to become more affluent adults if they are motivated and work hard. However, recent evidence (see Figure 4.5) does not support this. The primary, indeed the only, significant determinant of a child's income in adulthood is the income of his or her family of origin.

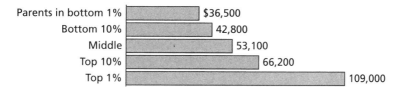

Figure 4.5: How Much a Canadian Child Would Earn in Adulthood, Based on His or Her Parents' Position on the Income Ladder

Source: https://www.theglobeandmail.com/news/national/a-tale-of-two-canadas-where-you-grow-up-affects-your-adult-income/article35444594/; note that this figure was compiled from data at this source: https://milescorak.com/equality-of-opportunity/

The mal-distribution of income and the growing debt of less well-off Canadians, Americans, Britons, and Australians, are related problems seriously impacting the resources and opportunities available to people. They are problems that have grown much worse since the 2008 economic crisis. In Canada, the debt-to-disposable-income ratio has sky-rocketed to 152 per cent and is currently growing at 2 per cent per quarter (Statistics Canada, 2012). Once rates reached 160 per cent in the UK and the US, bankruptcies and foreclosures became commonplace.

Box 4.2   Case Study ○ Canada's Recent Report Card

The prestigious think tank the Conference Board issued a report in February 2013 that as-signed Canada a rank of seventh and the United States a rank of seventeenth out of seven-teen affluent peer countries. The top countries are Denmark, Norway, Sweden, Finland, the Netherlands, and Austria. The UK placed fourteenth. All ratings were based on sixteen social indicators.

Canada earned a grade of A on life satisfaction and acceptance of diversity, but only a C on child poverty and closing the gender income gap. Canada and the US received a D on working-age poverty. Canada scored a C on income inequality and the US scored a D.

The Conference Board noted that Canada's reputation as a fair, kind, and gentle nation is misplaced—a "myth." Poverty rates for working adults and child poverty are serious prob-lems and are areas in which Canada is doing worse than other developed countries except the US. Gender inequity and income inequality are also serious, unresolved problems in Canada. The Board noted that Canadians fail to see how poorly they do with respect to equity and dealing with poverty because the point of reference is the United States rather the rest of the world.

Source: Adapted from How Canada Performs: Conference Board, February 04, 2013, www.conferenceboard.ca/hcp/details/society.aspx?pf=true.

Wealth

Wealth is not income, though income is the principal means, apart from inheritance, to build wealth. Wealth is accumulated assets such as real property, investments, and sav-ings. It is a better measure of power and privilege than income, and is more closely aligned with status. Wealth is even more unequally distributed than income, and the inequality is getting worse faster for wealth than for income, mostly because of ballooning values of assets such as real estate (see Figure 4.6). Canada's poorest have no wealth; in fact, they have negative wealth—debt. In the United States, one of the world's most unequal coun-tries, less than 1 per cent of the population holds well over 50 per cent of the total assets of the country.

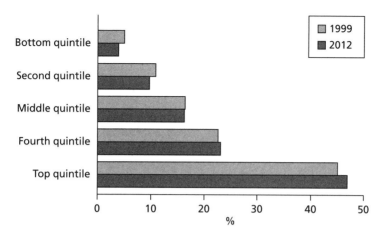

Figure 4.6 Share of Wealth (or Net Worth) Held by Each Income Quintile, 1999 and 2012

Source: Statistics Canada, 2015. http://www.statcan.gc.ca/daily-quotidien/150603/cg-b001-eng.htm

Public Programs and Services

Not only taxes but also government programs may be more or less progressive. Programs that target the poor or disadvantaged disproportionately benefit the less well-off, narrowing the gap between them and more wealthy people. This is especially obvious with programs that involve cash, such as the child tax credit schemes in Canada and the United States, which provide, through the income tax system, cash payments to lower-income families. But progressivity may also be true of other health and social programs. Poorer people have worse health and greater needs for health care services than more affluent ones (Humphries & van Doorslaer, 2000; Hernandez-Quevedo, Jones, Lopez-Nicolas, & Rice, 2006). Public health care insurance programs, therefore, transfer resources disproportionately to the less well-off.

Kim McGrail (2007) showed that poorer people made greater use of doctors and hospitals under Canada's public health care insurance plan. Overall, health care service provision in Canada is highly redistributive from the healthy rich to the unhealthy poor. Moreover, since illness is concentrated among the elderly, and the elderly pay less in taxes, they especially benefit—both as disproportionately heavy users of health care and from contributing less to the cost.

Programs like comprehensive public health care have a powerful equalizing effect. They also mitigate the negative impact out-of-pocket payments have on low and medium income earners. Those impacts extend directly to negative health outcomes. For example, in the United States, children with gaps in health insurance coverage (an estimated 15 to 20 per cent of children) "commonly do not seek medical care . . . and do not get prescriptions filled" (Olson, Tang, & Newacheck, 2005).

Among the **liberal regimes**, the distribution of benefits through public programs is most progressive in Australia and least progressive in the United States. Together, the effect of progressive taxes, progressive transfers, and progressive programs is significant. The OECD (2008) estimates the reductions in inequality achieved by the combination of taxes and programs to be less than 20 per cent in the United States, about 25 per cent in Canada, slightly less than 30 per cent in the United Kingdom, and over 30 per cent in Australia. (The **social democratic regimes** of the Nordic countries achieve inequality mitigation of about 40 per cent.)

Many programs and benefits provided by liberal regime governments are not progressive. For example, most cash benefits received from public programs are not truly redistributive because the person benefiting contributed toward the cost at some earlier point. Pensions based on employee contributions are like this, more akin to compulsory savings accounts than publicly bestowed benefits. Countries differ a great deal in terms of the mix of benefits they provide. Some are mostly of the prepaid sort; others are more redistributive—that is, the person paying and the person receiving the benefit are different. In the case of Australia, a moderately redistributive country with progressive taxation and progressive programs, about 40 per cent of benefits people receive are financed by taxes paid at another stage of their life whereas roughly 60 per cent of benefits are true redistributions. In the United Kingdom, the situation is reversed. Only 40 per cent of benefits are financed by redistribution and 60 per cent are of the prepaid sort (OECD, 2008).

Another useful measure of how a country approaches inequality is the share of public spending paid to people in the lowest income quintile, the bottom 20 per cent of the income distribution. The most recent OECD figures are as follows: Australia at 41.5 per cent, the United Kingdom at 31.4 per cent, Canada at 25.7 per cent, and the United States at 24.8 per cent. The numbers show a vast underlying difference in targeting of resources. Australia focuses on moving resources to those in greatest need, whereas Canada and the United States do not. It is worth noting that Australia has also been pulling ahead of Canada, becoming one of the healthiest places in the world. Contrariwise, in the United States health improvements stalled and are now in decline.

Standard Measures of Inequality

The GINI **coefficient** is the most commonly used measure of income inequality. A score of 0 would mean income is perfectly evenly distributed among everyone in the society. A score of 1 would mean a single person has all the income in that society. Current GINI scores range from a very equal Sweden (0.23) to a moderately equal Australia (0.30) to unequal Canada and United Kingdom (0.32 and 0.34 respectively) to a very unequal United States (0.45). The OECD average is currently 0.31 (OECD, 2011). Inequality has risen sharply in recent years, especially in the United States where the GINI now stands at 0.48, comparable to Mozambique or El Salvador (US Census Bureau, 2015). Again it is worth noting that, in terms of health, Sweden trumps Australia, Australia trumps Canada, Canada trumps the United Kingdom, and the United Kingdom trumps the United States. The liberal regime countries' GINIs and life expectancies are shown in Table 4.6.

Within Canada, inequality rose dramatically, especially in large urban areas. In Vancouver, Toronto, and Montreal the bottom 90 per cent of the income distribution made less in 2012 than they did in 1982, whereas the top 10 per cent made approximately $200,000 more. Calgary is the most unequal city in Canada; the bottom 90 per cent in Calgary make almost no more today than 30 years ago, whereas the top 1 per cent have seen their incomes rise by an average of nearly $600,000 (Canadian Centre for Policy Alternatives, 2013). The Canadian situation now appears to have stabilized.

Table 4.6 Income Inequality and Life Expectancy in Liberal Regime Countries

Country	GINI	Life Expectancy
Australia	0.305	81.2
Canada	0.32	80.7
United Kingdom	0.34	80.1
United States	0.45	78.2

Source: Adapted from OECD, 2011.

Poverty and Its Mitigation

Poverty

In 2009, nearly 15 per cent of the United States population, approximately 43 million people, fell below official poverty thresholds. Poverty is concentrated in the south, with all southern states, except California and Florida, reporting poverty rates in excess of 16 per cent of their population (US Census Bureau, 2015). Using a different measure, the LICO (low income cut-off), Statistics Canada estimates that roughly 14 per cent of the Canadian population is low income. As in the United States, poverty varies by region. Atlantic Canada has proportionally more people in poverty, and the western provinces proportionally fewer. The economic boom that kicked off in 2010 brought median incomes in Canada up 10 per cent over 2005 levels by 2016 (to $70,336), but that was mostly due to skyrocketing middle and upper-middle incomes in Alberta and Saskatchewan, which saw median income soar by nearly 25 per cent in Alberta and an astounding 40 per cent in Saskatchewan, despite the downturn in oil and gas prices (Statistics Canada, 2017b). Poverty rates did not improve and remained at 14 per cent of the population.

Thirty-one per cent of the US population experienced an episode of poverty lasting two or more months between 2004 and 2007, and about one-quarter of Americans had a two-month or longer spell of poverty in 2016 (US Census Bureau, 2017). Americans in minority groups have seen their average household income drop by nearly 15 per cent between the boom of 1999 and the recession of 2008. Canada is experiencing a similar trend, with unemployment, falling income, and poverty disproportionately affecting youth, recent immigrants, and people residing in central Canada, the region most affected by the economic downturn.

As one would expect with countries as unequal as Canada, the United Kingdom, the United States, and Australia, child poverty is a significant social problem. The OECD estimates child poverty rates to be 10 per cent in the United Kingdom, 12 per cent in Australia, 17 per cent in Canada, and 21 per cent in the United States. Those rates compare with Sweden at 4 per cent (OECD, 2008). In Canada, the problem is especially acute among Indigenous people. More than 40 per cent of Indigenous children are living in poverty (Canadian Centre for Policy Alternatives, 2018). Because of prevailing income support, child care, and employment policies in liberal regime countries, child poverty is concentrated in female sole-support households. Less than 10 per cent of children in Canada living in two-parent households are poor, but nearly one-half of those living in female lone-parent households are in poverty (Statistics Canada, 2017a). European countries with integrated approaches to income support, employment, and child care do not show those vast inequalities.

Box 4.3	Case Study ○ Disposable Income and Health

In the United Kingdom, it is estimated that a single man aged 21 requires approximately $210 per week to meet basic health requirements. If working full time at minimum wage, he would have a budget deficit of over $35 per week. A 21-year-old man would have to work over 50 hours per week at minimum wage to meet his basic health requirements (Morris, 2000).

How do you think that situation compares with Canada and the United States? What are the likely health implications?

Low household income translates into inability to maintain a healthy diet. Table 4.7 displays estimated proportions of the population of select countries unable to afford healthy eating. This is an aspect of the serious health problem of food insecurity, explored at length in Chapter 11.

Over the past 30 years, low income and poverty have grown worse for families of young children, young single adults, and people with limited education and job skills. But older adults, those in the 55- to 85-year-old cohort, have been doing better. Older adults have been beneficiaries of changes in tax codes, and they benefit disproportionately from programs such as Medicare in the United States, Canada, and Australia, and continue to receive public pensions/social security because governments have been loath to cut benefits to senior citizens. Poverty levels among older adults, in spite of the meagre public pensions provided in liberal regime countries compared to other advanced nations, have shrunk, although there are still pockets of older people, especially in the United States and the United Kingdom, who are vulnerable to **fuel** and **food insecurity**.

It is evident that too many people are living in poverty in Canada, the US, the UK, and Australia, and that this is seriously harming their health and shortening their lives. It is also evident that child poverty is a serious social problem in all four countries, and one worthy of special attention because of the importance of a good start in life. Further, the growing social and economic inequality in Canada and the United States is a negative trend that will compromise the health of present and future generations.

Table 4.7   Per Cent of Population Unable to Afford a Healthy Diet, Liberal Regime Countries, 2008

Country	Unable to Afford a Healthy Diet	Food Choices Constrained by Income
Australia	\<no data\>	3.0%
Canada	8%	\<no data\>
United Kingdom	8%	6.1%
United States	11%	16.4%

Source: Adapted from OECD, 2008.

Poverty Mitigation: Social Assistance or Welfare

As liberal regimes, Canada, the United Kingdom, the United States, and Australia have a common policy orientation referred to as residualism. **Residualism** is the view that a government ought to not be involved in matters associated with individuals or households unless there is no other party—such as a voluntary, non-government organization like a charity—willing or capable of addressing the need. In order words, residualism implies that (a) government intervention in support of individuals and families ought only occur as a last resort, and (b) the intervention should be as limited as possible. Government's role is to provide a safety net, not to support or facilitate health and human development.

Residualism arises from underlying liberal values of individualism, personal liberty, respect for private property, non-interference, and personal responsibility for one's own life. Those are all values characteristic of the United Kingdom and the countries most like it—the United States, Australia, New Zealand, and Canada (Esping-Anderson, 1990). In keeping with the residualist policy orientation, these liberal regimes target assistance programs at only the neediest of their citizens, keeping the level of assistance as low as possible. They also design assistance programs so that they will not undermine personal responsibility for one's own life and livelihood or provide perverse incentives (such as quitting a low-paying job in order to secure welfare benefits). Residualism is a policy analogue to high-risk interventions in health care, and it targets only extreme cases and those in greatest need.

To a greater or lesser extent (the United States being at one end on the spectrum and Australia at the other), these liberal regime countries operate on the principle of "less eligibility," first expressed by King Edward III in medieval England. Under no circumstances should anyone not in gainful employment be eligible for benefits equal to someone who is working. As King Edward saw it, not only would providing superior benefits be unfair to those working, but it would also undermine incentives to seek work, and would encourage idleness and foster social problems associated with lack of discipline and too much free time. In more modern phrasing, generous benefits would create and reinforce a welfare culture as well as undermine economic productivity. While plausible, the approach is plainly ideological. No amount of research has been able to show that Germans or Swedes have been made lazy or their countries' economies harmed by generous income support and other broad-based universal policies.

Programs of income support for the poor are referred to in Canada and the United States as "welfare programs," and beneficiaries are referred to as "welfare recipients." Elsewhere, notably in social democratic countries, income support programs are called "benefits" and people receiving them are "on benefits," a far less pejorative expression. Across the liberal world, since the mid-1990s, efforts have been made by governments to narrow the range of beneficiaries, tighten eligibility requirements, couple requirements to seek and obtain work with continuing eligibility and generally end "abuses." This term refers to people collecting benefits when they could be earning money through employment. A relatively recent example is the Canadian Conservative government's 2012 measures to curtail access to unemployment insurance, a policy aimed at forcing unemployed Canadians to take low-paid, insecure jobs.

Everywhere in the liberal world it is a duty of would-be beneficiaries to establish that they cannot support themselves and their dependents. This is accomplished through some form of needs testing, a process that can be experienced by clients as demeaning and stigmatizing. Employable recipients are required to participate in training and job seeking. The onus falls on the disabled and unhealthy to demonstrate the grounds for their exclusion from work seeking, a process that has recently become controversial in the United Kingdom because people with low intelligence or severe emotional and mental disorders often fail to understand what is required of them to maintain their benefits.

Benefits are deliberately set very low to incentivize job seeking. For example, in British Columbia, Canada, a single person deemed employable receives $235 in support and $375 toward housing per month for a monthly total of $610/month. The average rent for a one-bedroom apartment, away from the city centre, in Vancouver, BC, is $950 (Cost of Living Vancouver, 2013). Without spending anything on food, clothing, or transportation, the single welfare recipient faces a monthly budget shortfall of approximately $300. A sole-support mother with two children receives a total of $1724, made up of support, housing, and child support benefits. A two-bedroom apartment in Vancouver costs, on average, $1319 (Canadian Mortgage and Housing Corporation, 2011), and food costs for one adult and two children come to $659 (Cost of Eating, 2010). Without spending anything on other essentials like utilities and transportation, a sole-support parent with two children is short $254 per month of the disposable income minimally required for healthy living. Thus, it is next to impossible to live on welfare, except, possibly, on the streets. It is certainly next to impossible to secure the resources needed for a healthy life. And, as noted, that is deliberate public policy because the overriding goal is to force people to accept and keep low-paying jobs.

In 1997, the then Liberal federal government announced the Canada National Child Benefit, an effort to move children and families out of poverty and the stigma of welfare. A federal–provincial agreement in Canada launched the initiative, a supplement to the Canada Child Tax Credit. The benefit provides additional cash to low-income families through the income tax system. Similar arrangements are in place in the United States, the United Kingdom, and Australia. Canada and Australia have moved the furthest in terms of shifting support for families and children out of social welfare and into the tax system, where payments are income-based, as opposed to needs-tested—an arguably fairer and less stigmatizing arrangement for recipients. Recent changes in the federal government (2015) and the provincial governments in Alberta (2015) and BC (2018) have brought more tax credits, more progressivity to the tax system, increases in welfare benefits, and mandated rises in the minimum wage. However, political battles in Washington over taxes and government spending have taken the US in the opposite direction, threatening even bigger increases in inequality.

One problem with which all liberal countries have struggled since the 1980s is welfare traps. Reducing claimants' payments as their earned income rises obviously works as a disincentive to paid employment. Consequently, all systems have worked out ways to allow income support recipients to benefit financially from employment. The United States introduced an Earned Income Tax Credit to provide additional income and an incentive to low-wage earners to stay in paid employment. The amount of support, however, remains small ($2500 to $5000 credit). Moreover, none of these measures does much to mitigate the effects of poverty (but they have pushed many people off welfare and into low-paid work, which is the primary objective).

In general, the United States and Canada have not performed very well in terms of poverty mitigation through income supports, though Canada has improved its record considerably since 2015. Australia and the United Kingdom, until recently, did better.

Social democratic countries, with a different ideological policy orientation, have been much more proactive, with measures ranging from family allowances, special payments for sole-support parents, publicly funded child care for working parents, parental leave schemes, and a raft of other measures. In consequence, affluent social democratic and even conservative countries have lower rates of poverty than Canada and the US. They have, in consequence, performed better on population health measures.

Health-oriented policy remedies are straightforward. Canada, the United States, and the United Kingdom could restore more fairness to their taxation systems, not only making them more progressive, but also removing some of the patently unjust tax breaks that have been written into the tax codes. For example, Canada ended wealth taxes (on inheritance and gifts) and does not levy taxes on capital gains made on sale of personal primary residences. Those deliberate loopholes serve to concentrate wealth and income among the higher-income earners. Likewise, many tax deductions in Canada, the United States, and the United Kingdom, while technically open to all taxpayers, are meaningful, in reality, for affluent people only. Population health improvements require more progressive public programs that in turn require more progressive taxation to do the work of reducing inequalities and improving public health. Fortunately, this now seems to be recognized in Canada, although reforms have been modest.

In Canada and the United States, tax credits, such as the child tax credit system, could be bolstered to provide greater financial support to young families and especially sole-support parents. Existing social and health programs can be **targeted** to support the least well-off. But we must be mindful of the fact that it is often better to make programs universal, with benefits flowing to all citizens—first, because the more affluent will be less resistant to paying taxes in support of those programs and, second, because service standards and program quality will be higher in a universal program than in one targeting the poor or disadvantaged. Fortunately, Canadian federal, provincial, and municipal governments now seem to be taking this into account in the design of current programs.

Lower Taxes or More Public Spending?

Canada, the United States, and the United Kingdom have pursued low-tax policies since the mid-1990s. The belief undergirding low-tax policies is that people, if left to dispose of their money as they see fit, will make better use of it than government bureaucrats. Government tends to be inefficient and wasteful, is the argument. Individuals are more prudent. Ingenuity and the quest for a return on investment will foster innovation and growth in the economy and, ultimately, our individual and collective prosperity depend on economic growth. The best things government can do are (a) to take their hands out of our pockets so we can decide how we want to spend our money, and (b) to stop blocking innovation and flexibility. This drive to make government's footprint smaller is referred to as **neo-liberalism** (sometimes, confusingly, "neo-conservatism"). Taxation, government spending, and regulation of economic activity must all be cut back in the interests of freedom and economic growth.

There are several problems with this ideological perspective. First, much economic development over the centuries was actually government-led. China today, with its 7 to 10 per cent annual growth rate, provides a contemporary example of government-led economic activity. Even in the case of liberal countries, Canada could not have developed without government investment in railways, nor could the US have enjoyed the post-war boom without federal spending on interstate highways, electrical power generation, and university-based research. Second, private economic activity is nested inside a whole array of public laws and regulations without which it could not take place. Public laws and infrastructure are not impediments to economic activity, but rather its prerequisites. That became painfully obvious when governments had to bail out financial institutions in the aftermath of the 2008 economic collapse. Third, the combination of low taxation, easy credit, and self-regulation by individuals and companies, both in the past and now in our present, lead to rampant inequality, speculation, economic bubbles, and, ultimately, to bust and protracted recession. The near economic collapse of the United States, United Kingdom, and southern Europe are reminders of the folly of deregulation and cheap credit. Fourth, and of great importance from a public policy perspective, neo-liberalism wrongly devalues government's impact on lower- and middle-income earners. In a study of the economic value of public services to Canadians, Mackenzie and Shillington (2009) show that fully 80 per cent of Canadians would have been further ahead if the 1 per cent reduction in the federal goods and services tax had not occurred and the funds instead were pumped into public programs. Mackenzie and Shillington also show that the average Canadian receives, through a mix of tax credits, transfer payments, and public services, $17,000 per annum in benefits. Obviously someone comes out ahead from cuts in taxes and programs and services, but that someone is a high-income earner, not the average citizen. Contrary to what neo-liberals claim, what is at stake is not economic growth, but fairness, social equality, and the health and welfare of the overall population.

Neither tax reduction nor government program cuts are neutral. The former, tax cuts, advantage the richer without helping the poorer. The latter, program cuts, have little or no effect on the richer but substantially harm the poorer. In the United Kingdom, a study estimates that of the total interim program cuts the Conservative coalition government introduced in 2010, just over 8 billion pounds ($13 billion) fell differentially on citizens by gender and income. Nearly 72 per cent ($9.3 billion) of the cut is borne by lower-income women, mostly because of the concentration of low income and poverty among single-mother households (Fawcett Society, 2011). More recently, the US government's own analysis shows that the 2017/18 Congressional tax reform will end up, by 2025, costing people in the two lowest income quintiles more while providing substantial tax savings to people in the upper income quintiles, in particular those with incomes exceeding $912,000 (*Washington Post*, 2018).

There are good reasons to believe, as the Nobel Prize–winning economist Amartya Sen argues, that freedom is only meaningful in terms of human capabilities. Moreover, justice demands a fair distribution of those capabilities (Sen, 1999; 2009). Because the major determinants of human capabilities are income and education, freedom and justice require an active government, robust income distribution policies, and government-backed gender equity, all of which, in turn, require progressive taxation and substantial resource transfers to the less well-off. Countries where all of these are in place (most of the developed world), not only outperform the United States in terms of the health and welfare of their citizens, but also show more steady economic growth and greater resilience to recession. Paradoxically, even in the United States, economic prosperity turns on government-delivered welfare programs, in particular public education and public expenditure on infrastructure (Garfinkel, Rainwater, & Smeeding, 2010), rather than private-sector economic growth.

Theoretical Considerations

This chapter links individual-level considerations, such as income available to a person or a household, to health outcomes through a family of hypotheses broadly called "materialist." Essentially, the pathway is opportunities for healthy living—opportunities created by favourable circumstances including income, education, social network, and access to public goods and services. Health systematically differs between groups of people because their access to critical resources—healthy food, supportive relationships, good-quality housing, and parks and recreation—systematically varies in accordance with socio-economic position. One variant within the family is the absolute materialist hypothesis that emphasizes resources directly available to me as an individual; the other variant, neo-materialism, emphasizes resources available to individuals collectively through social programs, public assets, and the like. Leading theorists in this genre include Lynch (materialism) and Ross (neo-materialism).

Neo-materialist analysis is inherently multi-level because social structures, processes, and public goods (all collective features) may provide key health-relevant resources to individuals. Thus, theory in this genre considers jointly collective- and individual-level resource-relevant features. The model is illustrated in Figure 4.7.

An alternative to materialist thinking is psychosocial theorizing. The pathway from society to our biology is our perception, particularly our perceptions of our status and personal security. A sense of lack of respect or fearfulness can prime our stress response,

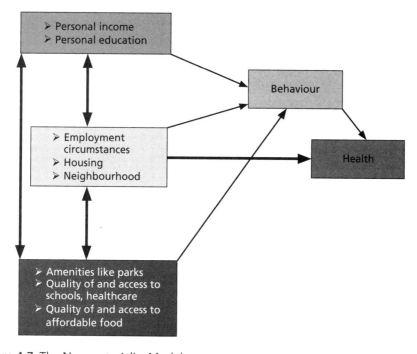

Figure 4.7 The Neo-materialist Model

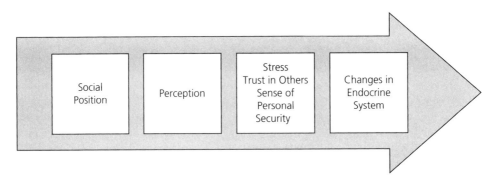

Figure 4.8 The Psychosocial Model

leading to chronic strain and elevated levels of cortisol, which in turn damage our emotional, mental, and physical health. The resources available to us as individuals, at least in affluent societies like Canada, matter much less, in this view, than our social position. More highly segmented and more hierarchical social formations will, it is hypothesized, drive poor health outcomes at the individual level. The model is illustrated in Figure 4.8.

Like neo-materialism, most psychosocial analysis is multi-level, as illustrated in Figure 4.9. Psychosocial theorists interested in social hierarchy and social capital regard relationships and community attributes—collective features—to be the central explanatory factors of individual health differences in affluent societies. The literature emerging from this theoretical perspective relies of concepts of inequality, community integration, and cultural inclusion, all social, not individual, attributes. Leading theorists in this genre include Wilkinson and Kawachi.

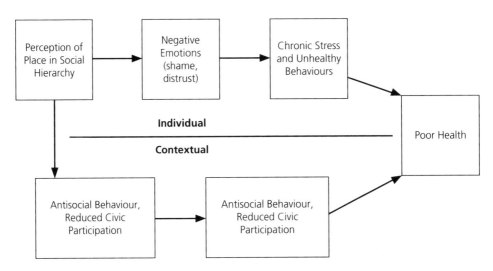

Figure 4.9 Psychosocial Income Inequality Pathways to Poor Health
Source: Used with permission from Maddison Spenrath.

The key theoretical issue at dispute is whether the contextual, societal level of inequality (neighbourhood, regional, or country-wide) affects human health—and if so, how? While results are mixed, it would appear society-level inequality does affect human health, but less so than the distributional effects at the individual and household levels. This is an alternative way of saying that effects seem to be mostly of a compositional nature—the attributes of individuals and households within a population—rather than of a collective nature—the consequences of the attributes of social formations per se.

Summary

Differences in health status have mostly to do with differences in the resources available to, and the related capacities of, individuals. The single most powerful measure of resources and capabilities is income.

More equal affluent societies, such as Australia, have a better health profile than less equal ones such as the United States. Important measures like life expectancy and infant mortality track closely with the amount of inequality. This has mostly to do with the composition of society, the mix of richer and poorer people. But social and economic inequality at the level of the country or the community can have direct effects on individual health, especially in the United States. Those effects may be delayed by five to seven years.

Inequality grew in Canada and the United States in the post-1980 period. Corporate compensation policies (bonuses and stock options for executives) and reduced taxes for the wealthy broadened the gap between the rich and the rest. Recession and rising unemployment have hit poorer Canadians and Americans much harder than richer ones. For example, real incomes for most American households declined over 5 per cent between 1999 and 2010 for white Americans and a stunning 14.6 per cent for black Americans (US Census Bureau, 2017). The GINI coefficient in the United States has soared to 0.47, making the United States as unequal as countries such as El Salvador, Rwanda, and Mozambique. The average American family has seen a 40 per cent drop in their wealth since 2007 (i.e., has lost all economic gains made over the preceding 18 years). And for the first time in a developed rich country, life expectancies in the United States are falling. For a time, Canada tracked closely with the US on inequality and changes to taxation and public policy, but that has changed since 2015 as a result of different political leadership federally and in a number of provinces. Meanwhile, recent US policy is creating even greater inequality and social division.

Materialist theories of health lend support to progressive income taxes and redistributive public programs. International data support the contention that overall population health would be improved by fairer taxation and more robust income redistribution.

Materialist theories of health also lend support to transferring some resources from richer countries to poorer ones. Countries like Canada could commit larger portions of their GDP to foreign aid and debt relief for poor countries. Global population health could be improved in consequence.

Psychosocial theories, at least at the population level, do not square well with the available evidence. But status hierarchies may be important at lower levels of analysis—for example, in the workplace. Characteristics of the organization we work for may well influence stress levels and hence health, as we shall see in Chapter 10.

The international evidence from population-health studies shows income policy must extend beyond mitigation of severe poverty to include a fairer distribution of post-tax/post-transfer disposable income. If improving health is the goal, advanced countries such as Canada should halt the trend toward higher consumption taxes (which are regressive) and restore a greater degree of progressivity to income taxes, a process that now seems to be underway.

Entitlements to income transfers through tax credits are preferable to means-tested benefits. Again, Canada seems to be back on track with targeted tax credits.

Special measures are required in all liberal countries to address child poverty. The importance of addressing child poverty in terms of health over the life course will be explored in Chapter 5.

Government spending is income to someone—businesses supplying goods or services to government, public sector workers, or beneficiaries of government cash transfers such as pensioners. Government spending is not a drain on the economy but a rather a central part of it, and needs to be managed as such. If improved health is the goal, spending, like taxation, ought to be progressive, aiming to reduce rather than compound social and economic disadvantages.

How a society organizes its taxation system, programs, and services has a dramatic effect on the incomes of households, the extent of inequality, and the numbers of children and adults in poverty. Public policy from tax laws to social programs is the primary determinant of resource allocation, which in turn is the primary determinant of the health of the population.

Critical Thinking Questions

1.   What factor or factors explain the Preston curve? How might the trends illustrated by that curve relate to the demographic and epidemiologic transitions?

2.   How might the materialist theoretical orientation influence thinking about taxation and social programs? Alternatively, how might the psychosocial orientation influence policy considerations? Where would the two theories lead to similar conclusions? Where would they yield different assessments of the outcomes of policies?

3.   Based on your current understanding, and the ideas presented in this chapter, do the reduced-health prospects of Canadian Indigenous people arise mostly from racism and social exclusion or from poverty and its correlates? Suggest how researchers might answer the question "Which is more important?"

Annotated Suggested Readings

The Spirit Level is a readable, comprehensive discussion of social hierarchy and the ideas associated with psychosocial theorizing. (Richard Wilkinson and Kate Pickett, *The Spirit Level: Why Equality is Better for Everyone*, New York: Penguin, 2010).

An excellent, although now slightly dated, meta-analysis of literature regarding inequality and
    health can be found in the paper by Lynch and colleagues, Lynch J., G. Davey Smith, S. Harper,
    M. Hillemeier, N. Ross, G. Kaplan, M. Wolfson (2004), "Is Income Inequality a Determinant of
    Population Health? Part 1. A Systematic Review." *Milbank Quarterly*, volume 82, no. 1, pp. 5–99.
A more recent paper does a superb job of analyzing US and Canadian findings regarding inequality
    and health. McGrail K., E. van Doorslater, N. Ross, and C. Sanmartin (2009), "Income Related
    Health Inequalities in Canada and the United States: A Decomposition Analysis," *American
    Journal of Public Health* (October), volume 99, no. 10, pp. 1856–63.

Annotated Web Resources

"How Economic Inequality Harms Societies"
www.youtube.com/watch?v=cZ7LzE3u7Bw&
    feature=related
Richard Wilkinson discusses his research on
inequality and health in a 17-minute TED Talk.

Gapminder
www.gapminder.org/world
Gapminder is a useful tool illustrating the
relationship between a country's average per
capita GDP and its life expectancy. This link
leads directly to an animation illustrating the
change in this relationship from 1800 to present
day. Notice the flattening of the curve. Small
amounts of extra income make for very large
increases in life expectancy in poorer countries
but make little or no difference in rich ones.

This is the Preston curve. Notice too how the
United States is very rich but life expectancies
are far from world class. Some relatively poor
countries such as Costa Rica and Cuba have
life expectancies that rival those of the United
States, presumably because they do a better
job of getting what resources are available to all
of their citizens through mechanisms like education, health care, housing, and social services.

Unnatural Causes
www.unnaturalcauses.org
The Unnatural Causes website ("Unnatural Causes:
Is inequality making us sick?") has a number of
valuable resources and interesting video clips. The
content is American, but the theory and evidence
are of broader application to the liberal world.

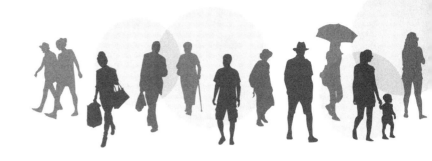

5 Childhood and the Transition to Adulthood

Objectives

By the end of your study of this chapter, you should be able to
- understand why and how fetal and early childhood development affects health over the life course;
- appreciate how programs and services targeting mothers and young children can alter health outcomes;
- describe and analyze factors affecting the health of older children and youth.

Synopsis

Chapter 5 outlines a life-course approach to human health, emphasizing the importance of fetal and early childhood development on subsequent health and well-being. Policies and programs that have been shown to impact on lifelong health are summarized.

Early Childhood

"Experiences in early childhood (defined as prenatal development to 8 years of age) . . . lay critical foundations for the entire life course." (Commission on Social Determinants of Health, 2008)

Pause and Reflect   Factors Affecting the Health of the Very Young

What factors influence the health of a newborn? An infant? A child aged one to four years? How might those factors play out over the life of the person?

The health of the newborn depends on a host of factors, including the health of the mother when she conceived, her activity level and diet during pregnancy, her age, the age of the father who provided the sperm, and her health-related behaviour such as smoking.

Many of those factors in turn depend on the mother's education and income level, how well supported she is by family and friends, and her access to services such as child care and health care. All of those determinants vary depending on where the mother happens to be on the socio-economic ladder and how supportive her particular society happens to be of women and children.

Once born, the quality of an infant's life depends on resources available to its mother. Is she well or poorly fed? Is she well or poorly housed? Does she have sufficient income to support herself and her baby? Does she have enough time to spend with the child to nurture it adequately? Does she have a deep enough understanding of what the child's needs are and how they are best met? Does she have a supportive partner? Are other caregivers available to provide her with some rest and relief? Can she afford and does she appreciate the significance of toys? How large is her vocabulary and how complex is her use of language? Is she literate enough to be comfortable reading aloud to her child? Does she interact verbally a lot or only a little with her child? All of those factors vary systematically with a mother's position in society, with more affluent women having ready access to most of the resources and less-affluent women having access to few or none.

Development in utero (mostly functions of the health status of the mother before conceiving and her diet and exercise during her pregnancy), combined with early childhood experiences, strongly influence the health and well-being of the child, not only at birth but also over his or her entire life. Conditions before birth and the kind and amount of social stimulation, support, nurturing, and exposure to language in the months and years immediately following it are particularly important for future cognitive, social, and emotional development. Partly, this is a function of neurology. Brain development in utero and in response to early childhood experiences determines neural pathways and the shape and structure of the brain, which in turn influence future intellectual, social, and emotional capabilities (Sapolsky, 2017; Mustard, 2007).

In general, fetal and early childhood experiences form the foundations for future learning, coping skills, resistance to health problems, and overall well-being. Consequently, the life course for disadvantaged children is different from that of more advantaged ones. Children from disadvantaged backgrounds are more likely to do poorly in school, end up in poorly paying, unstable employment, have children of their own early in life, become sole-support parents, and raise their own children under sub-optimal conditions. They are also more likely to develop diabetes and heart disease and to suffer from mental health problems. In this chapter, we will examine some of the reasons for these large differences in health and well-being.

> Research has shown that by age three, development is influenced by factors flowing from multiple levels of social organization. Not surprisingly, the environment of stimulation, support, and nurturance that families provide for their children matters significantly for early development. These qualities, in turn, are influenced by the income and other material resources that families can devote to child raising. . . . Familial dynamics in turn unfold within broader social networks. There is growing recognition that the "geography of opportunity" varies significantly. Children who grow up in affluent neighbourhoods, safe communities or areas that mobilize local resources to cater to the needs and desires of young families are less likely to be vulnerable in their development

than are children from similar family backgrounds living in poor, unsafe, and/or non-cohesive neighbourhoods. Development is also influenced by provincial and national government policy and political culture, especially policy that mediates access to quality early development, learning and care settings. (Kershaw, Irwin, Trafford, & Hertzman, 2005)

Programming, Latency, and Early Childhood Development

Programming and **latency** are concepts employed in life-course analysis. Both refer to how earlier events in human development can determine outcomes later in life. "Programming" is a term borrowed from computer systems: instructions are laid down for how future events will unfold; the parameters for outcomes are encrypted into our biology through early exposures or events. "Latency" is a closely allied concept referring to the capacity for an early exposure or event to influence later developments, even though no change is detectible for years, even decades. Early life experience may modify some outcome later in life irrespective of what occurs over the intervening years; the potential for that impact is invisible, covert.

It's helpful to look at an example of how each term is used. An epigenetic effect of poor maternal nutrition might not be evident in the infant or young child, but it may predispose that child to obesity in adulthood through its effects on regulation of genes affecting metabolism. The child has been *programmed* for obesity. A low-birth-weight baby may subsequently grow to be of normal weight for age, but in middle age, he or she has an elevated risk of heart attack. The child's high risk of adult heart attack is *latent*.

We will look at several types of programming and latency explored in the recent research literature. The **Barker hypothesis** is the earliest example. Barker (1998) postulates that "the fetus responds to under-nutrition with permanent changes in physiology, metabolism, and structure." Low-birth-weight babies, typically under-nourished during gestation, consequently are susceptible to adverse health outcomes. Barker was particularly interested in heart disease, and showed that low-birth-weight infants, irrespective of their weight or general health over their lives, are more likely to have a heart attack in middle age than babies born with normal weights for gestational age. Case studies and **birth cohort** studies have confirmed that babies born with low weights for gestational age are at higher risk than normal weight babies, in middle age, of developing heart disease, diabetes, respiratory disease, and mental health problems.

The incidence of low-birth-weight births has a distinct social and economic gradient. Poorer mothers, very young mothers, and Indigenous mothers are more likely than more affluent and more highly educated women to have a low-birth-weight baby. In general, the higher the income and education of the mother, the lower the probability of low birth weight. This is not surprising because more affluent and educated mothers will be healthier and better nourished before and during their pregnancies. They are also less likely to smoke—a risk factor for low birth weight.

Low birth weight, being small for gestational age, and failure to thrive have been linked to poor cardiovascular and respiratory health, schizophrenia, lower cognitive function, susceptibility to stress, lower educational attainment, lower adult income, and increased likelihood of smoking in adulthood. In short, a challenging start to life creates a series of health challenges, many of which do not manifest until adulthood. Figure 5.1 shows the relationships among household circumstances at birth, birth weight, and subsequent performance in school.

People who were small at age seven are three times more likely than normal-sized children to be unemployed at age 30. Income is also strongly correlated with adult height. In Canada, the United States, and the United Kingdom, employers pay taller men and women more than shorter ones. Height in adulthood is strongly correlated with size in infancy and early childhood, both of which are strongly correlated with parental income (Marmot, 2010). Thus, adult earnings are shaped by parents' earnings through biology, as well as by social vectors such as family level of education, family housing situation, and the like. The evidence strongly suggests that social and economic deprivation are transmitted inter-generationally through means such as low birth weight, failure to thrive in infancy, and dietary challenges in preschool years of life.

Over-nourished mothers also have adverse health impacts on their offspring. Autism and other neurodevelopmental disorders have been linked to maternal obesity. A child born of an obese mother is 67 per cent more likely than a child born of a non-obese mother to develop autism or learning disabilities (Krakowiak et al., 2012). Excessive weight gain during pregnancy amplifies the child's lifetime risk of obesity and chronic disease. Once again, there is a gradient due to the higher prevalence of obesity among lower-income women.

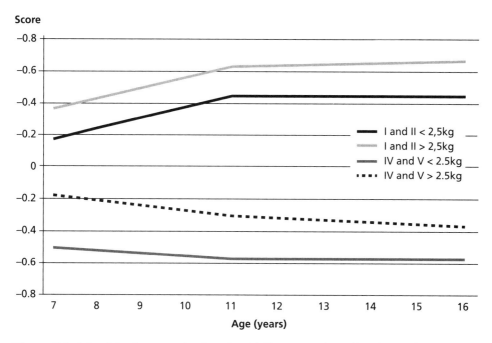

Figure 5.1 School Performance by Age, Social Class at Birth, and Birth Weight (England)

Maths score from ages 7–16 years by birth weight and social class at birth, 1958 National Child Development Study

Source: Marmot, 2010. Reproduced from Jefferis et al., 2002. Birth weight, childhood socioeconomic environment, and cognitive development in the 1958 British birth cohort study. With permission from BMJ Publishing Group Ltd.

Epigenetic Effects

Epigenetic effects may arise from environmental conditions in the womb, including nutrition, oxygen level, and maternal stress hormones, as well as from living conditions shortly after birth. The effects influence health and development over the entire life course by programming gene expression. Epigenetic markers are laid down in the genome, and those markers have **phenotypic** consequences for body size, likelihood of obesity, type 2 diabetes, and heart disease (Relton et al., 2012).

DNA methylation, one of the processes affecting gene expression, has been demonstrated in the offspring of mothers who, during pregnancy, were under extreme stress, or who were deficient in folate, or who drank alcohol, or who were undernourished. DNA methylation also occurs *after* birth in children who are under stress. The degree of methylation is partly a function of the quality of maternal care; a highly nurturing mother reduces the extent of DNA methylation in her offspring (Park & Kobor, 2014). However, a non-nurturing mother will increase DNA methylation. "Mothering style [in non-human primates] has epigenetic effects on more than a *thousand* frontcortical [brain] genes" (emphasis in original, Sapolsky, 2017).

A mother's diet during pregnancy can also affect the extent of DNA methylation; there are seasonal variations in the extent of DNA methylation in infants born in the Gambia, reflecting seasonal dietary factors (Dominguez-Salas et al., 2014). Extreme levels of stress can induce intergenerational epigenetic effects. Famines and wars can produce measurable epigenetic markers in children and grandchildren. Similarly, exposure to toxins such as cigarette smoke can induce effects in children and grandchildren. Somewhat surprisingly, men's exposures can affect their offspring in the same way as women's exposures. Methylation of DNA in sperm is incorporated into children and grandchildren.

Hormonal responses induced in the fetus or young child by stressful experiences have epigenetic effects. Cognitive ability, emotional control, mental health, and personality all may be affected in adulthood.

Box 5.1   Case Study ○ The Effects of the Seasons on Life Expectancy

In an interesting study, Doblhammer and Vaupel (2001) show that the month in which a person is born is predictive of life expectancy. In the northern hemisphere, being born in October or November confers an advantage over being born in March and April (with just the opposite applying in the southern hemisphere). Some factor (e.g., maternal or early infancy diet or environmental exposure to sunshine and hence vitamin D synthesis) *that varies seasonally* can apparently have a lifelong effect on the child.

How might we test the hypothesis that seasonal price and availability of foodstuffs during pregnancy affects the health and life expectancy of the child? Assuming the hypothesis is sound, how might globalization affect the relationship between seasons and maternal and infant health?

Fetal alcohol spectrum disorder (FASD), once thought to be a direct toxic effect of a mother's drinking on the fetus's brain, is now understood to have a significant epigenetic component. As Portales-Casamar and colleagues (2016) note, "some of the genes that are differently methylated between the FASD kids and the control group appear to be involved in neurodevelopment and brain development as such." Because of widespread epigenetic effects, maternal consumption of alcohol, even in small amounts, is associated with not only brain developmental issues but also offspring with small eyes; thin upper lips; small heads; abnormal growth; and vulnerability to arthritis, celiac disease, and early onset dementia (Himmelreich, Lutke, & Travis, 2017). In Canada, an estimated 10 to 15 children and youth out of every 1000 have FASD (Lange, Probst, & Gemel, 2017). Fifty per cent of FASD adults have a history of incarceration, residential drug treatment, or psychiatric hospital care as a result of the neurological and genetic damage done to them as fetuses, no doubt in combination with **cumulative effects** associated with their upbringing and unfortunate life-course pathways.

A mother's nutrition during pregnancy, and while breastfeeding, affects the length of her child's telomeres. Telomeres are found at the end of each chromosome, binding it together, protecting it, and preventing it from fusing with other chromosomes. Longer telomeres are associated with longer lives, not only for cells but also for the entire person. Shorter telomeres are associated with chronic diseases such as cancer and more rapid aging. Maternal and infant nutrition, as well as early childhood living conditions such as sense of security, stress level, and quality of family interactions, affect telomere length *and* the rate at which telomeres shorten during cellular reproduction. In sum, maternal and infant nutrition *programs* chronic disease and life expectancy.

An area of emerging research is the composition of microbial colonies in the colon. This has become a subject of great interest because of the discovery that the number, types, and diversity of gut microbes affect the immune system, the uptake of nutrients, the endocrine system, and the production of neurotransmitters, which in turn affect mood and cognition. Diet is the major determinant of which bacteria colonize the gut; however, studies of asthma uncovered a link to "seeding" of the infant's gut with maternal bacteria during vaginal birth. Bacteria from fecal matter are transferred to the newborn as it leaves the vagina, and those bacteria then become the first colonists in the newborn's previously sterile gastro-intestinal (GI) tract. A healthy colonic bacterial colony from the mother is transferred to her offspring (assuming, of course, the mother had beneficial gut microbes).

It is hypothesized that the otherwise sterile infant GI tract is susceptible to colonization by microbes inimical to its health in the absence of microbial seeding from the mother. A variety of health conditions are associated with less ideal mixes of bacteria in the infant's colon, some occurring in infancy such as diarrheal diseases and ear infections. Others are manifested not in infancy but later in life, including asthma, diabetes, obesity, depression, and inflammatory auto-immune diseases. With the rising proportion of infants born by C-section, a larger and larger portion of the population is vulnerable to a less than ideal mix of bacteria, and hence *the latent risk of disease later in life.*

In response to the popularization of these findings, some mothers have taken social media advice to "vaginally seed" their infants by swabbing their faces and mouths with vaginal fluid. Obstetricians in the United Kingdom have spoken out against the practice, suggesting, instead, that frequent handling of an infant and breastfeeding are sufficient to ensure a healthy microbial biome (Gallagher, 2017). Whether or not artificial vaginal seeding of C-section babies is an effective practice, it remains true that the early bacterial colonization of an infant's colon has lifelong implications for that infant's health. (It is also true that repeated courses of antibiotics in infancy and childhood might permanently disrupt the microbial balance in the gut, with potentially serious consequences for health.)

Critical Developmental Junctures

The concept of **critical developmental junctures** was derived from pioneering work by Huber and Weisel (1982), who reported that a kitten will become a permanently monocular cat if one of its eyes is temporarily sewn shut during the fourth to sixth week of the animal's development. The unseeing eye is perfectly normal, but the cat's brain fails to recognize its input. The reason is that the neural pathways in the visual cortex of a cat's brain are laid down around four weeks after birth. If the brain receives no environmental stimuli during the critical developmental period, no connections are formed, and none ever will be.

Animals, including humans, are born with brains that are a more or less disorganized mass of neurons. Those neurons form axons and dendrites through which complex connections are then made. Connections that are used frequently become pathways and myelinate (become protected by a myelin sheath). Connections that fail to myelinate simply disappear. Moreover, as the brain consolidates itself, neurons, as well as non-myelinated pathways that are not serving a defined function are eliminated in a process neurologists call "neural pruning." The remarkable thing is that the brain, between fetal development and age seven, literally shapes itself, determining which pathways to reinforce and which neurons to sustain and which to destroy. The process is called "neural sculpting" and is an example of **brain plasticity**, a very real physical process that can be seen in brain scans and dissection. Sculpting mostly occurs in response to the stimuli the brain is receiving from the child's interaction with his or her environment.

It would be wrong to conclude that brain plasticity is time limited and that at some point all pathways are complete and the physical brain is entirely consolidated. Even the elderly show some capacity to develop new neural pathways, for example, following a stroke. Moreover, while it was thought that no new brain cells are formed after birth, it is now known that neurogenesis, the formation of new neurons, occurs throughout life, albeit much more slowly than during fetal development.

Recent studies have shown that intense adult learning can literally reshape the human brain. London cabbies are required to memorize route details to and from every point in metro London. Learning the tens of thousands of road and lane names and their spatial relationships to one another causes measurable changes in the hippocampus, a brain region associated with memory (Maguire et al., 2000). Likewise, recent studies show that the amygdala, a part of the brain associated with emotion, is more active among adults with larger, more complex social networks (Bickart, Wright, Dautoff, Dickerson, & Barrett, 2010), presumably a neural response to social stimulation. But both the extent of changes in the brain and the ease with which they are achieved diminish sharply after the first few years of life.

Pause and Reflect   Do Physical Features in the Brain Arise from Experience?

Findings of anatomical differences in brains of taxi drivers or more intensely social people fail to tell us whether it is gaining "the knowledge" or heavy social interaction that causes those changes. What would we need to know to establish causality? How would we go about finding it out?

Some important functions in the brain are very time and context specific. For example, human face recognition and the development of normal emotional responses to human interaction require physically close interaction with a nurturing person in the first few months of life (Hertzman & Power, 2003). Children who have been deprived of nurturing human contact in early life, such as the children abandoned to orphanages in Romania, show clear signs of abnormal brain growth, in terms of both the shape and size of their brains (Mustard, 2007). When severe, no amount of subsequent stimulation can remediate the brain damage. The child's ability to relate to others, to learn, and to have a normal emotional response is permanently altered.

Early life emotional stress dramatically affects the developing brain. Severe "stress permanently blunts the ability of the brain to rein-in glutocortical secretion" (Sapolsky, 2017, p. 195). In other worlds, the brain's ability to modulate hormonal secretions is impaired. Additionally, emotional stress affects the HPA axis (our stress-response mechanism, the key link between our neurological and endocrine systems, discussed beginning on page 103), raising an infant's or young child's basal cortisol levels and disrupting normal feedback loops. The ensuing chronic high levels of cortisol are toxic to the brain, causing brain damage and permanently undermining the child's capacity for emotional regulation. The lifelong effects are lowered intelligence, heightened reactivity, chronic anxiety and aggression.

A child with adverse childhood experiences (ACE) will have

- higher basal cortisol and a more reactive stress response;
- a thinner frontal cortex, the part of the brain responsible for executive functions of planning, decision making, and regulation of emotion;
- impaired cognitive function and diminished IQ;
- diminished working memory and attention span;
- poor impulse control;
- increased propensity to anti-social behaviour; and
- increased risk of depression and anxiety disorders (Sapolsky, 2017).

The changes are permanent and lifelong, though their impact may be modified by appropriate social supports.

ACE includes a number of negative experiences, including being ignored or put down, psychological abuse, physical abuse, sexual abuse, and parenting by a drug- or alcohol-using adult. If any one of the ACE factors applies, there is an elevated risk of learning problems, difficulties with social interactions, emotional instability, substance abuse, and mental illness. The factors are cumulative; risk rises exponentially with multiple factors.

Latent Effects

Latent effects of early life experiences and contexts affect adult health independently of what happens later. For example, intellectually and emotionally impoverished early years may impair learning and social functioning over the individual's entire life regardless of the quality of schooling she or he receives from kindergarten to grade 12. Contrariwise, a nurturing and intellectually stimulating early life, either through parents or via a well-designed **Head Start**–style early childhood development program might confer life-long benefits (Hertzman & Power, 2006).

The differences in terms of intellectual stimulation between advantaged and dis-advantaged children are stunning. In the United States, a child between birth and age four in an affluent family has 30 million more words spoken to them than a child in a poor family. Exposure to language facilitates brain development as well as learning, driving up the cognitive scores of affluent children in comparison with poorer ones. In consequence of the differences in stimulation, poorer children enter school with massive cognitive defi-cits and can never catch up with children from more privileged backgrounds. Beginning in the US in the 1970s, researchers have tried to close the gap by designing and imple-menting programs that increase the exposure of poorer children to language, music, and other forms of intellectual stimulation.

American research showed that disadvantaged, inner-city residents who participated in infant and early childhood stimulation programs not only did better in school than children from similar backgrounds who did not participate but also, as adults, ended up in better jobs, were less likely to be involved in crime, and enjoyed better physical and mental health (Palfrey et al., 2005). A more recent study (Reynolds, Temple, Ou, Arteaga, & White, 2011) confirms that at age 28 people were still benefiting in terms of health, employment, and income from participating in early childhood development programs. Irrespective of what transpired after the early childhood intervention, whether the child went to a good school or a bad school, he or she did much better as an adult than children who did not participate in a Head Start program. (More on Head Start and similar pro-grams later.)

Cumulative Effects

Cumulative effects are easy to demonstrate. The longer one is exposed to negative en-vironmental, social, or dietary factors, or alternatively, the more intense the exposure to those negative factors, the worse the health effects. As noted earlier, the deeper the poverty and the longer it lasts, the worse the result.

Cumulative effects can be seen through trends. If we compare the health-related per-formance over time of children whose families become more affluent with children whose families' incomes do not rise, both height and IQ will rise at a faster rate for the children whose families' fortunes are improving (Marmot, 2010). Low-birth-weight children are at increased risk of developmental problems and poor health in adulthood, but *the risk of negative outcomes is much higher for low-birth-weight children raised in poorer families than it is for children raised in more affluent ones.* By age seven, the cognitive develop-ment, for example, of low-birth-weight children raised in affluent families will nearly equal that of normal-birth-weight children, whereas the cognitive development scores for low-birth-weight children raised in poorer families will continue to decline in comparison with those of normal birth weight (Marmot, 2010).

Edith Chen and colleagues (Chen, Martin, & Matthews, 2007) found that cumulative household income had significant effects on childhood health. Lower income over time is associated with higher odds of having, by age 10, a health condition that limits normal childhood activities.

It is important to distinguish childhood social and economic conditions from adult ones because the cumulative effects vary (Pensola & Matikainen, 2003). Behavioural risk factors such as smoking are most strongly associated with current socio-economic position, whereas physiological risk factors such as blood pressure are most strongly associated with socio-economic position at birth and in early childhood. There are, though, notable interaction effects between early childhood and adult contextual factors (Blane et al., 1996; Peck, 1994).

We saw earlier in the chapter that ACE factors are cumulative. The risk of reporting poor health in adolescence is 4.6 times greater among youth who experienced five or more incidents of violence or bullying as a child (Boynton-Jarrett, Ryan, Berkman, & Wright, 2008). Repeated episodes of childhood abuse may even stunt the growth of important regions of the brain. Brain scans show abnormal development of the hippocampus in adults who were subjected to repeated childhood abuse (Teicher et al., 2003; Teicher, Anderson, & Polcari, 2012). The amygdala, an important brain region for emotion, grows disproportionately large and is more reactive in people who encountered adversity in childhood. The enlarged and reactive amygdala contributes to reactivity, heightened vigilance, wariness and suspicion of others, anxiety, and emotions-driven decision making (Sapolsky, 2017).

We also saw earlier that violence, abuse, and other forms of early developmental adversity may also have programming implications. Researchers are finding more and more epigenetic vestiges of emotional trauma in early childhood. For example, the extent of DNA methylation (laying down of markers that influence the expression of genes) in adolescents varies with the stress levels in their homes when they were infants and young children (Essex et al., 2011). Similarly, epigenetic programming effects have been found in adults who were raised in disadvantaged families, clear evidence of cumulative effects (Borghol et al., 2011). It now appears that epigenetic patterns associated with the status of one's family at time of birth and in early childhood directly affect adult morbidity patterns and life expectancy.

Pathway Effects

Pathway effects are also easy to demonstrate. Early life experiences set the stage for future experiences, which in turn give shape to subsequent ones. For example, a rich and positive yet challenging early life experience may increase coping skills and sense of self-worth that in turn incline the child to respond favourably to future opportunities. Contrariwise, early life experience that fosters fear and timidity may set the child up for anxiety, avoidance, and acting up instead of constructively rising to challenges. Some of the factors associated with socio-economic status affecting child developmental pathways are shown in Figure 5.2.

Children show tremendous diversity in their readiness for and their capacity to benefit from school. Hertzman and his colleagues (Human Early Learning Partnership, 2005) have shown in Vancouver, Canada, that school readiness is strongly associated with family income and neighbourhood characteristics. Moreover, research consistently shows that a poor start in school is rarely overcome by subsequent events. A pathway is formed toward poor outcomes such as inattentiveness, behavioural problems in school, poor social skills, eroded self-confidence, increasingly poor academic results, and leaving school early.

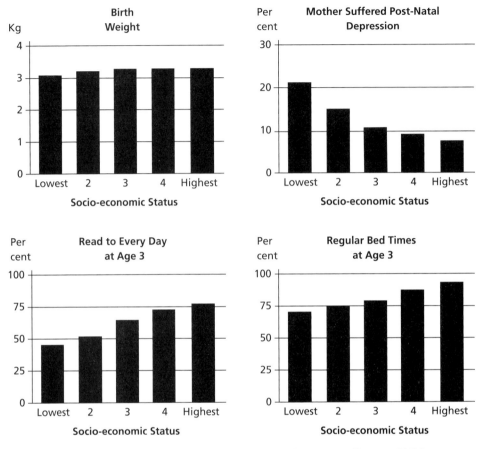

Figure 5.2 Links Between Socio-economic Status and Factors Affecting Child Development, 2003–4

Source: Jessica Allen presentation. Used with permission.

Results of the Early Childhood Longitudinal Study-Kindergarten Cohort (ECLS-K), a national [US] sample of children entering kindergarten, showed that family income is associated with children having the academic and social skills necessary for kindergarten. Compared to children in the highest-income families, children in the lowest-income families were least likely to have the needed skills, but children in middle-class families also performed less well, both socially and academically, than those at the top. (Robert Wood Johnson Foundation, 2011)

Social class of origin is a determinant of cognitive development because reading to children and passive television watching are associated with social class, as illustrated in Figure 5.3.

In sum, emotional and intellectual deprivation in childhood—not overt child abuse, but limited social interaction, being parked in front of the TV, absence of rich conversation,

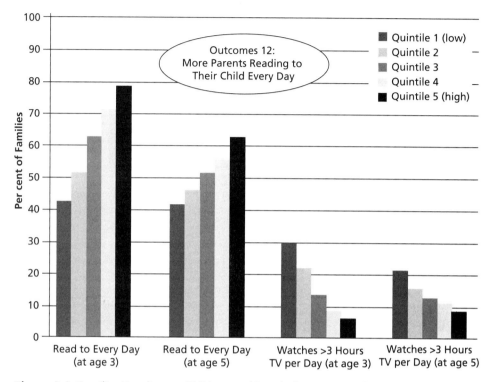

Figure 5.3 Families Reading to Children and Level of TV Viewing by Social Class (England)

Source: Angela Donkin presentation. Used with permission.

and not being read to—are strongly linked to poor educational attainment and emotional and behavioural problems over the entire life course. Poor readiness for school leads to poor performance in school, bad job and income outcomes, risky behaviours such as alcohol and drug abuse, and generally poor mental and physical health (Hertzman & Power, 2006). If childhood deprivation is combined with emotional stress and physical abuse, the outcome is even worse: **psychogenic dwarfism**. Psychogenic dwarfism is a partially reversible condition characterized by severe learning disorders, lack of normal emotional control, and acute anxiety.

While low levels of infant and early childhood stimulation and nurture are linked to low intelligence, poor learning, and emotional problems, the pathways should not be regarded as causal. They constitute risks—that is, probabilities—and obviously some children from very deprived backgrounds do develop normally. But when we look at populations of people, those from deprived backgrounds and those from affluent ones, we will see the big differences, the advantages an affluent background confers. In broad terms, we will find life-expectancy differences in men of 6 to 10 years arising from their birth weights and their early childhood experiences. The effect is thus very large.

Box 5.2   Case Study ○ Early Childhood Development and ADHD

Attention deficit hyperactivity disorder (ADHD) came to prominence in the 1970s. Researchers claimed to find a rising incidence of a syndrome among school-aged children that included distraction, forgetfulness, inability to stick to a task, problems following simple instructions, fidgeting, and difficulty staying still. By 2000, about 5 per cent of children, mostly boys, were diagnosed with ADHD. In Canada and the US, many of these children are prescribed regular doses of amphetamines, which they may end up taking for years. Up to half of children diagnosed with ADHD are expected to become adults with varying degrees of behavioural and learning disorders.

ADHD has been controversial from the start. Some claim no such disorder exists. They contend that there is a broad range of cognitive and behavioural attributes among younger children and that poorly self-regulated children are simply part of the normal mix. Immature and badly behaved children, who have always been predominantly boys, were handled in the past by behavioural measures at home and in the school. If the right measures are applied, troubled children will mature and their behaviour and performance will thus improve. From this perspective, medical intervention and treating the children with drugs are symptoms of primary schools and parents abrogating their responsibilities to guide and discipline children.

Because ADHD is more commonly diagnosed in boys who were among the youngest in their school entry cohort (due to when their birthday fell), some think ADHD children simply haven't developed enough to cope with school. Boys would be particularly vulnerable because their brain, body, and emotional development is slower than girls'. The issue, from this perspective, is mostly one of physical and emotional maturity. But the negative experience of trying to cope with situations that the child's body and brain cannot manage entrenches attitudes and behaviours that then hobble the child's performance, possibly for life.

Others agree that the disorder is likely no disorder at all, but contend that we are seeing the confluence of less tolerance for childlike behaviour with the power of organized medicine and pharmaceutical companies. A normal range of human response has been pathologized and medicalized. In other words, we are refusing to accept as normal things we find difficult or unpleasant. It's not so much the children who are immature, but rather their teachers and parents. They cannot cope with an unruly child.

Yet others believe ADHD is real and its incidence is rising. However, rather than some disease, researchers with this view contend that social changes such as disordered households, limited time spent by parents with their children, low expectations of children at home, instant gratification of children's wants, too much TV and video-game face time, small families, and limited interaction across generations all play a part.

Yet others, while agreeing that the social circumstances are important, point to possible neurological developmental issues related to the conditions under which the child was born and raised. Fundamental structures associated with emotional regulation and cognition may be underdeveloped or dysfunctional due to early childhood context and experience.

Another view is that maternal gestational diabetes is a major driver for ADHD. The latent effects of fetal development combine with early childhood poverty and deprivation to raise lifetime risk of ADHD fourteen-fold (Nigg, 2006).

And there are those who are fiercely reductionist and claim very specific causes. From this perspective, too much sugar in the diet, food additives, pesticides, or some kind of reaction to a specific trigger causes ADHD.

So far, no clear neurological basis has been found for ADHD, and even the existence of the disorder remains controversial.

How might we best make sense out of this controversy? What sorts of evidence would help us decide which of the competing hypotheses come closest to the truth? What features of this dispute make it so intractable?

Animal Studies

Primatologists have shown that emotional characteristics of a mother can affect the emotional disposition of the offspring (Suomi, 2005). About 15 per cent of the infant Rhesus macaque population is "highly reactive." They are fearful, easily provoked, unwilling to investigate new things, and consequently interact poorly with other macaques and learn less readily. They also show separation anxiety when apart from their mother or their natal troop.

Reactivity in macaques is genetic. This has been shown by deliberately breeding highly reactive monkeys. The biological mechanism is a hyperactive HPA axis causing abnormal levels of cortisol in these animals.

If highly reactive infant macaques are raised by reactive mothers, they grow up to be fearful, socially unskilled adults with behavioural and health problems. But if reactive infant monkeys are raised by calm, competent mothers (macaque females can be induced to adopt infants), even highly reactive infants will grow up to resemble normal monkeys. This provides a powerful example of the effect we saw earlier, in Chapter 1 (human genes for tallness and genes protective against alcoholism). It is not the genes that matter so much as how they are expressed, which is largely a function of context. Context and life experiences can decisively override genetic disposition.

The animal studies suggest that whatever the dispositions and biological setbacks human infants may have, competent nurturing by their mothers or other caregivers may substantially change the direction of development. That is in fact precisely what we have seen in the example of early childhood development programs and in the recognition that children with setbacks such as low birth weight do much better in more affluent and educated families than in poorer ones (Marmot, 2010).

Contributions from Psychology

Psychologists have noted for the better part of a century that children develop critical attachments to other people, usually their mother, around six months of age. But poor mothering, challenging family conditions, and abuse or neglect may prevent core attachments from developing. It is hypothesized that failure to form stable attachments in infancy makes it difficult for the individual to form meaningful relationships with others throughout his or her life.

One well-known theory based on the infant attachment hypothesis is Bowlby's **attachment theory** (1988). Attachment theory contends that the attached figure (usually the mother) provides a secure base from which the infant and toddler can "venture forth," exploring the spaces and things that make up his or her environment. Venturing forth is critical to learning. It is also critical to developing a sense of self as an independent entity along with a sense of being an effective agent in the world.

Attachment failure (or infant bonding failure) is hypothesized to cause low self-esteem, which in turn contributes to the adult being anxious, needy, ineffectual, and troubled. In extreme form, attachment failure may yield a socially dysfunctional individual, one unable to form stable bonds with others, a person experiencing an abnormal stress response and exhibiting a predisposition to depression, anxiety, and hostility.

Attachment failure is much more probable in situations where the mother is clinically depressed. Postpartum depression has been shown to be more common in lower-income than higher-income women (Marmot, 2010). Thus, the risk of attachment failure is heightened in lower-income families, especially female-sole-support families. Consequently, childhood disorders like ADHD, learning disabilities, and anti-social behaviour are consistently associated with low family income.

Bowlby thought a foster parent, a grandparent, or a neighbour might provide a surrogate for the mother and prevent attachment failure, much as a competent macaque foster mother can prevent severe anxiety in a highly reactive infant monkey. He may be right about that, but in our society, largely because of the way it is socially stratified, all too often neither children nor adults get the support they need.

Psychologists also argue, and have produced good evidence to support the contention that, mechanisms of self-control develop in early childhood. Poor environmental and social conditions may inhibit development of self-control, self-respect, and normal moral responses such as shame and empathy. The results are manifested in acting out, poor attentiveness in school (and later at work), social problems such as teenage pregnancy, efforts at instant self-gratification through substance abuse and unsafe sex, and poor interpersonal skills. Phillips and colleagues (Phillips, Hammen, Brennan, Najman, & Bor, 2005) showed that early adversity at home is predictive of depression and anxiety in adolescents. Their findings are backed by recent discoveries in neuroscience. Neurologists have shown that brain development, and areas of the brain associated with emotional regulation, are harmed by high levels of stress in early childhood (Mustard, 2007).

Early Childhood Policy

Children who have lower-cognitive scores at 22 months of age but who grow up in families of high socio-economic position improve their relative scores as they approach the age of 10. The relative position of children with high scores at 22 months, but who grew up in families of low socio-economic position, worsens as they approach age 10. (Marmot, 2010)

From our earlier discussion of early childhood, it is obvious that some of the most important measures we can take to improve the health of our populations relate to getting the best possible start in life. That includes ensuring that the outcomes from pregnancy are positive; the infant is provided with the care, sustenance, and stimulation needed for healthy development; and the child in the early part of his or her life is appropriately supported and raised in conditions conducive to his or her long-term well-being.

With such obvious importance attached to these needs, it is odd that the liberal regimes—Canada, the United States, the United Kingdom, and Australia—do so little to support infants, young children, and their mothers. Compared to social democratic Northern Europe, the liberal countries invest heavily in public schools and universities but put few public resources into infancy and early childhood. Denmark, for example, commits 1.4 per cent of its gross domestic product to child care and early childhood education. That compares with 0.59 per cent for the United Kingdom, 0.35 per cent for the United States, and 0.16 per cent for Canada (OECD, 2010).

Table 5.1 ranks selected countries in terms of their policy commitment to aspects of child development and safety. The table displays a sub-set from the total of 30 rich countries studied. Canada places roughly in the middle, scoring well on education from age six onward but relatively poorly on measures to ensure material well-being and the safety of children.

Public financial support for child care and early childhood education is reflected in use patterns. Approximately 70 per cent of Danish children under the age of three participate in formal playgroups at early childhood development centres. Less than one-third of American and Australian infants and toddlers are in comparable programs. Canada, of all developed countries, places dead last, at less than 23 per cent (OECD, 2010). Mikkonen and Raphael (2010) estimate that only 17 per cent of Canadian families have access to registered child care. Moreover, where licensed centres exist, standards in Canada and Australia (where there are approximately seven children to every staff member) are substantially lower than those in the United Kingdom and the United States (five children to every staff member). Standards in the United States, in turn, are inferior to those in European countries, Japan, and Korea (OECD, 2010).

As we saw earlier, child care programs combining high-quality early childhood education with visits to parents aimed at improving the home-learning environment have very dramatic effects on deprived children. The highly successful Carolina Abecedarian Project coupled intensive education from infancy to age five with support to the children's mothers. The children in the program later scored higher on IQ tests and did better in school. A larger proportion qualified for college admission. Similarly, the High/Scope Perry Preschool Project, launched in 1962 in Michigan, demonstrated not only higher academic achievement but major effects into adulthood, including better jobs, higher earnings, more stable family lives, and fewer arrests (Anderson et al., 2003).

Table 5.1 Comparative Policy-Focused Child Well-Being in OECD Countries (Country Rank out of 30)

Country	Material Well-Being	Housing	Education	Health and Safety	Risk Behaviour
Australia	15	2	6	15	17
Canada	14	–	3	22	10
United Kingdom	12	15	22	20	28
United States	23	12	25	24	15
Denmark	2	6	7	4	21

Large-scale public programs such as Head Start in the United States and, more recently, Sure Start in the United Kingdom, have not received the same kind of rigorous evaluation as projects like the Abecedarian Project. However, the 2008 evaluation of Sure Start, an integrated child care service that provides visits to help support parents, community health care, good-quality play, and learning centres for children at risk or with specialized needs, demonstrated significant improvement in the independence and social behaviour of participating children (Geddes, Haw, & Frank, 2010). In their evaluation, the authors comment,

> High-quality early childhood education targeted at high-risk groups from a very early age (one year or earlier) can result in significant positive cognitive and academic achievement outcomes as well as greater adult self-sufficiency. . . . The most successful programs combine intensive high-quality preschool with some home visits to improve the home-learning environment. (Geddes, Haw, & Frank, 2010)

Box 5.3   Case Study ○ Head Start and Sure Start

Using early projects like the High/Scope Perry Preschool Project as models, the US Department of Health and Human Services launched **Head Start** in 1965. Head Start was part of President Johnson's "Great Society" initiative, a grand scheme to eliminate the twin evils of poverty and racial injustice. Head Start provided federal funds to local projects that incorporated early childhood education, school readiness training, primary health care, nutrition, and support to parents. The target was high-risk children, mostly inner-city African Americans. The goal was for children from deprived backgrounds to catch up with more privileged children and thus be able to compete more effectively in school, ultimately improving equality of opportunity between the races. The Head Start program continues to this day; it costs approximately $8 billion annually.

Almost immediately, Head Start was met with a backlash from conservative Americans. The Great Society initiative in general, and Head Start in particular, were accused of undermining the African-American family, subsidizing unwed pregnancy, and fostering a generation of "welfare queens" relying on taxpayer-funded programs. In consequence, programs have failed to gain legitimacy and are of highly variable quality. That may be the reason why evaluations of Head Start typically yield mixed results. Some evaluations find large positive, persistent impacts on child development, whereas other studies claim that Head Start programs provide little or no sustained benefit.

Smaller-scale early childhood initiatives have been undertaken in Canada and Australia (the Canadian federal Indigenous Head Start program is an example). In the United Kingdom, in 1998, the Labour government launched Sure Start, an area-based intervention in neighbourhoods considered to be deprived. Sure Start includes early childhood education, school readiness, primary health care, and family support. Currently, the Conservative government in the UK is rolling back Sure Start and abandoning most program-related issues to cash-strapped local authorities.

Why do you think Head Start–type programs have proved to be so controversial? When generalized from well-funded and carefully managed projects to large-scale programs, their benefits become less clear. Why might that be so?

Good-quality, all-day kindergartens/preschools for older children (over age four) have also been shown to help reduce inequalities between children from deprived backgrounds and their more fortunate peers. The massive Early Childhood Longitudinal Study in the United States proved that preschool can compensate for learning disadvantage, but only to a much more limited degree than earlier (i.e., infant and toddler) interventions (Loeb, Bridges, Bassok, Fuller, & Rumberger, 2007). The poorest, most disadvantaged children showed the largest gain in language, pre-reading, and numeracy skills.

D'Onise and colleagues (D'Onise, Lynch, Sawyer, & McDermott, 2010) studied the question "Can preschool improve children's health?" They showed that there is good evidence that attendance from age four in preschool reduces the risk of obesity later in life, enhances social competence, improves overall mental health, and reduces the likelihood of anti-social behaviour.

Some Canadian provinces and US states are moving to all-day preschool for every child over age five, incorporating kindergarten more formally into public schooling. However, the evidence suggests that earlier interventions, beginning in infancy, have much greater impact. In 2017, the Canadian federal government began talks with provinces with a view to broadening and deepening early childhood support, at least for high-risk families. At the time of writing, it remains to be seen whether an agreement can be reached. Quebec, Alberta, and BC have made some progress independently from the federal government, with Quebec introducing subsidies for child care in 1997, making child care more accessible (but critics make claims of uneven quality). Alberta's and BC's newly elected NDP governments both rolled out early childhood care initiatives in 2018.

Should Early Childhood Programs Be Universal or Target High-Risk Families?

Interventions seeking to reduce the disparities between advantaged and disadvantaged children in brain development, social adjustment, cognitive skills development, and emotional maturation have been mostly of a targeted type like Head Start and Sure Start. Children from families where the parent(s) are low-income and have limited education and few domestic resources are targeted because those children are most at risk of poor outcomes such as low IQ, limited capacity to learn, poor social skills, and emotional difficulties. However, taking this approach raises the question Geoffrey Rose brought to prominence: might it not be better to attempt raising the average IQ (the mean level of cognitive ability, etc.) in the entire population of children rather than focusing on only the worst-off children?

Pause and Reflect   **Should Early Childhood Development Programs Be Offered Only to Children from Deprived Backgrounds?**

Should publicly sponsored early childhood development programs target at-risk children (i.e., be implemented to serve children from deprived backgrounds) or be offered to children of all family backgrounds? What are the pros and cons of high-risk versus universal approaches?

One intriguing feature of the intellectual and cognitive performance of people from different socio-economic backgrounds is that the gradients are steeper in more unequal countries. That is, in Sweden, as in the United States, people from affluent and highly educated families will score higher on literacy and numeracy tests than people from families with lower incomes and education. Scores form a gradient, just like health status, with people doing progressively better the richer and more educated their parents are. But the gradient in Sweden is much less steep than the gradient in Canada, which in turn is less steep than the gradient in the United States. Overall "countries with high-literacy scores, such as Sweden, tend to have shallower gradients" (Sloat & Willms, 2000). Again, this demonstrates Rose's point: a higher average performance in Sweden, reflecting superior programs provided to young children as well as more extensive income support for families, is the most effective way of ensuring the fewest people are at risk of poor outcomes.

In sum, having a less-affluent or a less-educated parent is not only worse for your health in the United States than in Sweden, but worse for your intellectual and cognitive ability, affecting how you do in school and consequently your ability to obtain well-paid work. This is a key reason why upward mobility and general equality of opportunity are lower in the United States than in Europe, contrary to myths about the "Land of Opportunity." Moreover, if we implement early childhood development programs targeting only the worst-off children, we will not change the overall results, as Figure 5.4 shows.

In spite of the success of the hypothetical targeted program, American children are left worse off than Swedes (indeed, even worse than Canadians). Additionally, many more-affluent Americans, receiving no benefit and having only limited compassion for the poorest and least educated of their fellow citizens, would likely resist paying higher taxes for such a scheme.

But, if instead of targeting only deprived, at-risk children, quality child care and early childhood development programming were made available universally—in other words, for all parents—every child and parent would benefit.

Raising average performance would not eliminate the need for specialized and targeted interventions for children in extreme circumstances or with special needs; but overall, as Rose suggested, a universal approach to a problem like early childhood development makes more sense than high-risk, Head Start–type approaches. In general, then, the best strategy would be one of **progressive universalism**—support for every family, with additional support going to those with greater needs (Lynch, Law, Brinkmen, Chittleborough, & Sawyer, 2010; Marmot, 2010).

Figure 5.5 provides a graphic illustrating the difference between a targeted well-funded Head Start–style program and a universal program aimed at all children.

Costs and Benefits

Economic studies on four of the early childhood intervention programmes (Perry Preschool Project, Chicago CPCs, Nurse–Family Partnership, and Abecedarian Project) showed that between $6000 and $30,000 was spent per child or family. Every dollar invested however, resulted in returns of between $3.72 and $6.89. Returns were from reductions in government spending as result of reduced use of special education services, reduced involvement in juvenile delinquency, reduced

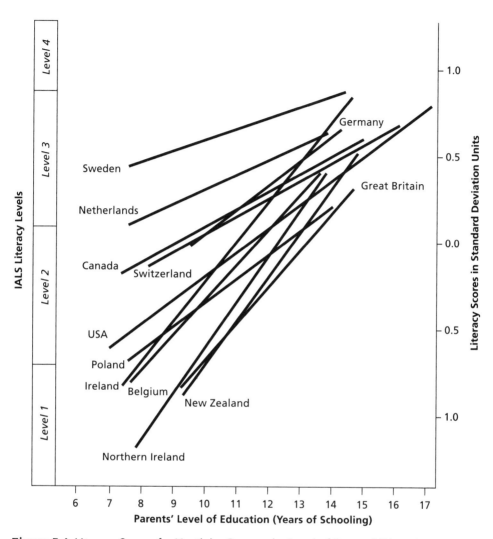

Figure 5.4 Literacy Scores for Youth by Country by Level of Parents' Education
Source: Sloat & Willms, 2000 p. 222. Reprinted with permission from the *Canadian Journal of Education*.

welfare and dependency costs, reduced criminal justice costs, and increases in tax contributions. (Geddes, Haw, & Frank, 2010)

It appears that effective, universal early childhood education would more than pay for itself, not only in terms of health and cognitive benefits for the participants, but also in overall economic terms. We must be mindful, though, of the challenges of effective implementation of large-scale programs. As Lynch et al. (2010) point out, when governments attempt to launch broad-based programs and services, they inevitably do so with less-trained personnel and in more challenging conditions than the smaller-scale demonstration projects upon which the programs were based.

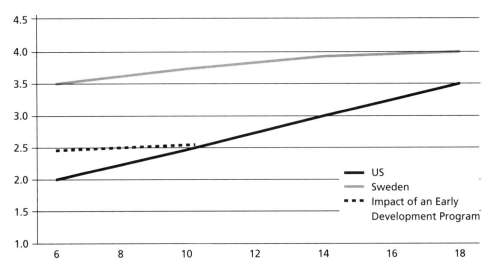

Figure 5.5 Literacy Scores for Youth by Country by Level of Parents' Education Illustrating a Hypothetical Well-Funded, Effective Early Childhood Development Program That Reaches All Deprived Children vs Hypothetical Universal Early Childhood Development Program

A Note on the Public School System

Pause and Reflect   Role of the Public School System

What role does the public school system play in a country like Canada in levelling the playing field for children born into less privileged families? How might the school system support or undermine social solidarity and community integration? What health consequences are attached to the performance of the public school system?

Readiness to learn in school follows the usual socio-economic gradient. Vocabulary, reading readiness, the ability to concentrate and stick to a task, emotional maturity, and much else correlate strongly with family income (Washbrook & Waldfogel, 2008). The public school system cannot be expected, and in reality does not, address the vast differences in school readiness and IQ of the five- and six-year-olds it admits. In fact, in spite of special education classes and other supports, the differences between children from highly educated affluent families and children from less educated poorer families grow throughout the school years (Marmot, 2010). This has partly to do with the size of the initial gap, partly with how critical the very early years are for proper brain, cognitive, and emotional development, and partly with cumulative disadvantage. Poorer children continue to live in deprived conditions whereas richer ones continue to benefit from their circumstances, increasing the size of gaps in experiences, broadening differences in exposure to healthy versus unhealthy conditions, and amplifying effects of the amount of support for learning the child receives at home. Public schools can, however, mitigate some of the injustice associated with the large socio-economic gaps in capacity to learn and flourish. Focusing on early literacy can make a large difference in the quality of a deprived child's subsequent life (Beswick & Sloat, 2006).

The social unrest that swept England in the summer of 2011 suggests that a breakdown in universal public education, affecting 5- to 18-year-olds, contributes to social exclusion and undermines community solidarity. The trend for affluent parents to place their children in private schools rather than state-run schools creates "sinks"—neighbourhood schools that serve only poor and minority children—compounding disadvantages and amplifying social cleavages. While very early childhood education is fundamental to health, we must not ignore the important role played by universal public education in enhancing equality of opportunity and bolstering social solidarity at the community level. Cutbacks in public education funding in the liberal regime countries, coupled with current policies that encourage the formation of private schools, may well have severe, unintended consequences in terms of social order and overall population health and well-being.

It is important to recognize, though, the inherent limitations of the school system. Literacy scores are much more strongly correlated with income distribution than they are with public spending on schools. "Among the wealthy nations of the OECD, additional economic prosperity and educational spending is trumped by distribution of income for its effect on adolescent reading literacy" (Siddiqi, Kawachi, Berkman, Hertzman, & Subramanian, 2012). Income distribution thus both directly and indirectly affects health by being a primary determinant of educational attainment—itself a major determinant of health and life expectancy.

Older Children and Teens

Most children are relatively stable emotionally and intellectually from the time they leave early childhood (between 5 and 7 years old, girls typically a year or more earlier than boys) and 12. Most, unless they have pre-existing conditions from birth or early childhood, also have stable health.

Puberty and entry into the teenaged years, however, are extremely disruptive physiologically and behaviourally. The body undergoes extraordinary growth and transformation as secondary sex characteristics appear under the influence of a barrage of hormones that affect virtually every body system. Most important, however, for teen health are brain development and health-relevant behaviour, and it is with those topics we will begin this section.

The Teen Brain and Behaviour

Because the brain goes through an important process of physical consolidation in the teenage years, the possibility of matters going seriously awry is increased between the ages of about 15 to 25. This is when serious mental illnesses like schizophrenia are likely to occur for reasons that likely have something to do with the interactions of predispositions, life experiences, and neural sculpting. This is also the period when there can be disconnects between important brain systems—for example, feeling emotions and the systems that regulate our responses to those feelings. Adolescent moodiness, reactivity, impulsiveness, and heightened sensitivity to criticism and social exclusion all reflect the incompleteness of brain development (Sebastian et al., 2011). If the conditions under which the adolescent is living fail to facilitate the appropriate neural consolidation, **emotional lability** and poor regulation of reactions may become life-long—i.e., the person may be permanently dysfunctional.

Novelty seeking, poor assessment of probabilities and dangers, emotional instability, difficulty keeping emotions in check, and strong bonding with peers all arise from the underdevelopment of the frontal cortex and its incomplete regulation of other brain regions which mature and "come online" sooner (Sapolsky, 2017). Incomplete frontal cortex development combined with the typical social context of teens account for the strong desire to please friends and an even stronger fear of being rejected drive "peer pressure," which in turn drives health-destructive behaviours such as taking foolish risks, excessive drinking, drug taking, smoking, fad diets, and eating disorders. Lifelong habits of smoking, neuroticism about food and dieting, and substance abuse almost always get their start in the teen years (but then, so too do almost all of our adult values, tastes, and habits, good and bad).

A number of health-related issues arise in the teen years and have implications for the length and quality of life the person will ultimately lead. The following subsections will look at four of these: accidental injury, educational attainment, health behaviour, and obesity.

Injury

Given the impulsiveness and poor judgment typical of the teen years, it comes as little surprise that injury is the leading cause of death for teenagers and the major cause of non-congenital disability. In Canada, young people aged 12 to 19 have the highest probability (27 per cent) of injury in the previous year of any population group (Billette & Janz, 2012). Although young men are much more likely to be injured than young women, the probability of an adolescent girl being injured in a given year rose from 18 per cent to 23 per cent over the past decade, presumably due to girls' and boys' behaviours and pursuits converging (more on this in the next chapter).

Using self-reported data, the World Health Organization (WHO) finds that half of Canadian boys and girls aged 15 report having had a serious accident requiring medical assistance within the past 12 months. That contrasts with about one-third of Swedish boys and girls (WHO, 2012). That shows while biological factors like brain development play a role, social ones are at least equally important. As we have repeatedly seen, health-relevant matters are rarely biological or social, but arise through interaction.

The majority of injuries are accidents associated with team sports, cycling, and skiing and nearly two-thirds of those involve falls (Billette & Janz, 2012). Young people are also more likely than older Canadians to be involved in a motor vehicle accident and sustain injury, become disabled, or die. Lack of driving experience, poor judgment, recklessness, and distractions are the primary factors.

Brain injury in sports is becoming a major matter for concern. Soccer and hockey, in particular, are implicated in multiple assaults to the brain, from falls, being struck by pucks, sticks, or balls, and "heading" the ball in soccer. While those injuries may

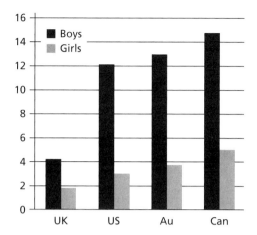

Figure 5.6 Rates of Suicide per 100,000, Boys and Girls Ages 15–19, 2008
Source: Based on OECD, 2009, p. 52.

create few immediate lasting symptoms, they are cumulative and may have powerful latent effects, contributing to stroke, dementia, and other forms of cognitive decline in later years.

The best approaches to adolescent injury are prophylactic: improved driver training; graduated driving licences; better coaching in sports; improved safety measures from enforcement of cycling and skiing helmet use; and rule changes in sports that reduce the probability of serious injury.

Suicide, another outcome from the interaction between the state of adolescent brain development and social factors, is a major cause of death for teenagers in Canada, especially boys. Comparative rates are provided in Figure 5.6. Male teen suicide rates in Canada are four times higher than in the United Kingdom. The underlying causes are complex, but the availability of guns and lax gun controls play a part. Because suicide rates among young Indigenous Canadians are extraordinarily high, we will look more closely at the range of factors driving adolescent suicide in Chapter 8, on Indigenous health.

A recent study (Swanson & Colman, 2013) shows a clear association between teens knowing about the suicide of another youth and future suicidal ideation (thinking about killing oneself) and suicide attempts. The phenomenon is called "suicide contagion" and involves a spike in numbers of attempted and successful suicides following the death of a schoolmate. The contagion effect is strongest among young teens (12- and 13-year-olds) but remains significant until age 17.

Education

Educational achievement by 15-year-olds is highly variable, both between and within countries. Figure 5.7 below shows the tremendous range of literacy scores. On this measure, Canada ranks near the top and the US at the bottom of wealthy countries. But within Canada, literacy varies from province to province, school district to school

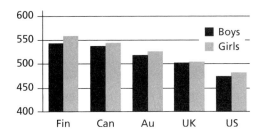

Figure 5.7 Average Literacy Score, 15-Year-Olds, Finland, Canada, Australia, United Kingdom, and United States (2006)

Source: Data from OECD, 2009, p. 52.

district, and especially between poorer Canadians and richer ones and between Indigenous and non-Indigenous people. This variability matters because a person's lifelong prospects in terms of employment and general satisfaction with life depend on literacy level. And, as we have seen, individuals' lifelong health depends mostly on their lifelong wealth, which, for most people, is a function of their education.

Health Behaviour

Many health-relevant attitudes and behaviours are formed in late childhood and the teenage years, not through influences from family of origin, but rather from peer reference groups and the social network in which the person is embedded. Level of interest in sports, skill development in physical activities, dietary preferences, and patterns of use of alcohol, tobacco, and illicit drugs are all shaped during this portion of the human life course. The variability from peer group to peer group, neighbourhood to neighbourhood, region to region, and country to country is huge.

One determinant of health-relevant behaviour is the effectiveness of communications between parents and their adolescent children. Rates of alcohol consumption, drug use, unsafe driving, and unsafe sex can all be modified through effective intergenerational communications. A recent study (WHO, 2012) shows that ease of child–parent communications varies among affluent countries. Ninety per cent of both boys and girls report easy, open communication with their mothers in the Netherlands, but the proportions drop to 73 per cent for boys in Canada and 64 per cent for boys in the US. The percentages in the latter two countries for girls reporting easy communication with their mothers are slightly better, at 74 per cent and 70 per cent respectively. Communications between fathers and sons, as one might expect,

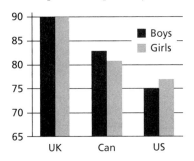

Figure 5.8 Per Cent of 15-Year-Olds with Three or More Close Friends

Source: Adapted from WHO, 2012.

are worse than communications between mothers and their children. Only 71 per cent of Dutch male teens report easy communications with their fathers, compared with fewer than half of Canadian teenage boys.

Another, probably more significant, determinant of adolescent health is the size and density of the teenager's social network. First, it is substantially more probable that teens from affluent families have large friendship circles (WHO, 2012, p. 29). Second, the number of friends a teenager has depends on place of residence. Some international data is provided in Figure 5.8.

As we will see in Chapter 7, social support (measured through number of friends) is an important determinant of human health and well-being.

Older children and teens experience substantial stress associated with school and from their interactions with their peers. Fifteen-year-olds in Canada and England report significant school-related stress (between 55 and 65 per cent of girls and between 45 and 50 per cent of boys). Oddly, adolescents in what are usually regarded as the stricter and more demanding European schools report less stress (less than one-third of girls and less than 20 per cent of boys in the Netherlands, for example). Part of this variance may have to do with the support teens receive from their peers.

Not surprisingly, figures for life satisfaction follow the same trend. Ninety-six per cent of Dutch male teens report high life satisfaction, compared with 87 per cent in Canada and 85 per cent in the United States (WHO, 2012).

Dietary behaviour is a major determinant of health and well-being. Recent data (WHO, 2012) show that 75 per cent of Dutch 15-year-old girls eat breakfast every day, compared with less than one-half of Canadian teenage girls and only one-third of US female teens. Regular consumption of breakfast is a key element in preventing eating disorders and obesity, as well as a general determinant of overall health and vitality.

A major health threat to US teens is the consumption of sugar-sweetened soft drinks. One-third of American teens consume soft drinks daily, compared with approximately 15 per cent in Canada and 5 per cent in Scandinavian countries (WHO, 2012). Soft drink consumption correlates strongly with dental disease, obesity, and diabetes.

Smoking rates among teens have fallen sharply in Canada and the US and now stand at about 8 per cent (defined as having smoked at least once in the past week). Smoking rates remain relatively high in parts of the UK, roughly 15 per cent in Scotland for example

Pause and Reflect   Social Media and Teenage Health

Teens and young adults heavily use mobile phones and computers for staying in contact with other people. Researchers contest the health effects of electronic media contact. Some argue that teens feel increased social pressure and experience elevated stress because they are made so vividly aware of what others are doing through social media sites. Others point to harassment and other negative aspects associated with social media. Still others think use of electronic media encourages superficiality, narcissism, and expectations of instant gratification. But many researchers think there may be positive mental and physical health effects from "being connected," analogous to the positive effects of face-to-face contact with other people.

Recently, the potential destructive side of the Internet made worldwide headlines. The case involves the alleged cyberbullying of Amanda Todd, a 15-year-old Port Coquitlam, BC, teenager. Todd committed suicide in October 2012 after posting a video on the Internet chronicling her experience with online intimidation, insults, and harassment.

What are the positive and negative impacts on adolescent health of cellphone and social media technologies? What measures related to electronic media might enhance the health and well-being of adolescents?

(WHO, 2012). Fortunately, most teenage smokers quit by age 25, minimizing damage to their health.

Alcohol consumption, however, has remained fairly stable. About 15 per cent of Canadian 15-year-olds report drinking at least once a week, substantially more than Americans, but substantially less than the English. Nearly one-third of English male teens report drinking at least once a week (WHO, 2012). The problem with adolescent drinking in the UK became acute over the 1990s and the first decade of this century. Accidents, violence, and even deaths from liver failure have skyrocketed among children aged 12 to 20 in England, Scotland, and Wales, an increase mostly attributable to the fashion of binge drinking.

Obesity

The subject of obesity will be covered in more detail in Chapter 11, on food and nutrition. At this point, it will suffice to emphasize some of the precursors for adult obesity. We already mentioned low and high birth weights as predisposing conditions (latent factors) and intrauterine and early life conditions as programming infants epigenetically for weight gain, diabetes, and heart disease. Infant feeding is also important. Breastfeeding is associated with normal body weights for both the infant and the person when he or she reaches adulthood, whereas bottle (formula) feeding is associated with infant, childhood, and adult obesity. In Canada, breastfeeding follows a distinct socio-economic gradient, common among affluent and rare among disadvantaged mothers. Countries also vary in terms of rates of breastfeeding.

We also noted earlier how few Canadian and American teenagers regularly eat breakfast, an omission that predisposes toward disordered eating and obesity. It comes as no surprise that the United States and Canada have, alongside Greece, the world's worst obesity record for 15-year-olds. Twenty-seven per cent of girls and 34 per cent of

Box 5.4   Case Study ○ Uncomfortable in Our Own Skin

Girls and young women feel tremendous social pressures to have perfect—which means *very thin*—bodies. While the evidence is mixed, it appears that depression and anxiety levels are rising among tweens and teens, mostly arising from concern about their body shapes and weight. There are increasing media reports of normal girls and women feeling so uncomfortable about their appearance that they refuse to go to the gym, beach, or swimming pools. Canadian and British girls report smoking in order to control their weight. Eating disorders, while perhaps not more prevalent than a few years ago, are commonplace. Mostly, many young people suffer from self-loathing and a lack of confidence, in other words, a serious decline in their sense of well-being. Commercial interests play into this, flogging bad ideas and harmful products to the vulnerable.

How serious do you believe the body-image problem to be in Canada? How is it affecting the health and well-being of Canadian girls and young women? What steps might public authorities take to reduce the pressure on girls and women?

boys aged 15 in the US report they are overweight or obese, compared with 17 per cent of girls and 24 per cent of boys in Canada. In the Netherlands, the comparable figures are 5 per cent and 11 per cent. American and Canadian teens, ironically, are among the most physically active, with between one-quarter and one-third reporting a minimum of one hour of moderate to vigorous activity a day, compared with approximately 15 per cent of Dutch teenagers. Similarly, the Dutch teens spend more time watching TV, playing video games, and using their mobile phones than Americans or Canadians, yet remain substantially thinner (WHO, 2012). Obviously predisposing factors such as infant nutrition and current caloric intake are more important than exercise in terms of obesity incidence.

Theoretical Considerations

Hypotheses involving the concepts of latency, programming, cumulative effects, and pathways require a "life-course approach." That means individuals must be tracked over time to see if the hypothesized effects occur in individuals who have been putatively affected. To establish validity (truth) and causality (versus simple association between variables) prospective cohort studies are required. The cleanest, most bias-free way, to conduct such a study is through **birth cohorts**—enrolling all infants at birth born in a particular year and tracking events occurring in and around them as well as health-relevant outcomes for the entire life of each person. The United Kingdom has been a pioneer in conducting these studies, the oldest (still ongoing) being the 1946 cohort study. Much of the richest data has come from the 1958 birth cohort study (also ongoing) and more recently from the 1970 and Millenium (2000) birth cohort studies. Having four spaced studies allows for estimations of temporal change and intergenerational effects. Important theoretical components such as the Barker hypothesis can be tested only through these expensive, complicated, and time-consuming studies.

The point was made in this chapter that we must interpret program evaluation studies cautiously. It *appears* that early childhood development programs have large effects, both immediately and latently. However, most programs that have been evaluated were carefully controlled pilot projects, well resourced and staffed by highly trained personnel. That means rolling out such programs in the real world may not have the same magnitude of effect because their implementation will inevitably be more messy. In the real world, politics, funding levels, availability of committed well-trained staff, and a host of other practical matters bedevil social program implementation.

Summary

An individual's start in life has major and lasting implications for how well she or he will do over her or his life. Being born fully mature for gestational age, an outcome significantly influenced by the age, nutrition, health, and fitness of the mother, confers a distinct advantage. Contrariwise, being born small for gestational age is associated with health problems such as diabetes and heart disease in later life, as well as with measures such as unemployment and low income, suggesting lifelong brain and emotional developmental issues relating to low birth weight.

Most of the disadvantages of low birth weight can be compensated for by early life experiences. Children in affluent and nurturing households can overcome infant deficits. However, children in poorer and less nurturing households will experience cumulative disadvantages.

Child readiness for school is a function of their home environment and neighbourhood. That is principally due to the critical development through which the human brain must go in the years between birth and age three to five. Not only basic cognitive skills, but also capacity for facial recognition, ability to understand the emotions and states of mind of other people, emotional development, achieving self-control and a sense of self-mastery, capacity to concentrate and stay on task, and many other critical life skills are learned and incorporated, not only as habits, but organizing principles within the brain itself.

Apart from nurturing and intellectual stimulation, infants and young children are also very sensitive to nutrition. Food insecurity hampers intellectual and emotional development of young children. Children born large for gestational age (usually to overweight or diabetic mothers), are prone to excessive weight gain, especially if bottle fed (which is most likely in lower-income families). Such infants, once they reach adulthood, are susceptible to obesity, diabetes, renal disease, and heart attack.

Stress and neglect of infants and young children can cause permanent changes in key biological mechanisms, including the HPA axis and the immune system. Severe cases of abuse or neglect may be manifested in highly abnormal brain development and profound lifelong intellectual and emotional effects.

Maternal health and nutrition, maternal obesity, and challenges in infancy and early childhood may induce epigenetic changes (DNA methylation). Those epigenetic changes are associated with adolescent and adult disease, obesity, and premature mortality.

In order to improve the lives of children, more effective measures must be taken to mitigate material inequality in society, especially income inequality. This requires co-ordinated taxation, income support, and employment policy—such as, progressive taxation and progressive public policies.

Low income, unaffordable housing, and food insecurity among young women of child-bearing age could be subject to targeted interventions through measures such as improved tax credits and affordable housing strategies to ensure that women are healthy going into and coming out of pregnancy. In general, if we are serious about improving health, priority should be given to accessible, high-quality primary care for young women in their child-bearing years, before, during, and after pregnancy.

Parents cannot adequately support their children, especially in the first few years of life, if they both have to work. Paid parental-leave provisions in Canada are weak by international standards, although are planned to be extended for fathers in 2018.

Financial support to women with young children should be enhanced through improved child tax credits or similar mechanisms (e.g., a return of family or child allowances).

Governments should ensure the provision of high-quality affordable child care for all women. In North America, only Quebec has made progress in this regard. The promised Canadian federal–provincial initiative collapsed with the election of a Conservative federal government in 2004 (though, as of the summer of 2017, it may be revived).

In 2013, 70 per cent of Canadian women with children under the age of three were in the workforce, but only 22 per cent could find a space in a regulated child care centre. Less than one-third of Canadian children under six from families in the lowest income quintile participate in out-of-home child care. Only three provinces regulate child care fees (Manitoba, PEI, and Quebec). Full-time monthly fees for a two-year-old in BC average $850, whereas the federal tax credit totals $100 per month ("Child Care by the Numbers," 2013).

The principle of progressive universalism should be applied to early childhood development programs. Those programs should span infancy to age four and include home support as well as child development centres. Governments should also expand access to quality preschools and kindergartens for four- and five-year-olds.

Governments should continue to support and invest in public schools, paying special attention to early reading and literacy programs. However, it must be recognized that socio-economic conditions in general, and social inequality in particular, undermine the effectiveness of schools in liberal regime countries.

Community resources that support child literacy, such as public libraries, should receive adequate funding and support.

Governments at all levels should be more mindful of the needs of teenagers and young adults. Especially important in this regard are possibilities for positive socializing with peers and affordable access to recreation and sport.

Critical Thinking Questions

1. Why, in light of the mounting research evidence, do countries such as Canada invest so little (apart from public schools) in supporting women, children, and families?

2. Would universal child development programs broaden or narrow the range in health and cognitive outcomes in the population? How might programs be organized to reduce the gap?

3. Adolescence is the critical bridge between childhood and an independent adult life. What measures might a country like Canada take to assist teens in safely transitioning to a healthy adulthood?

Annotated Suggested Readings

The most comprehensive review of research, programs, policies, and services relating to early childhood development may be found in the World Health Organization's report *Early Childhood Development, A Powerful Equalizer*, available at www.who.int/social_determinants/resources/ecd_kn_report_07_2007.pdf.

A recent American policy paper, *Early Childhood Experience and Health*, provides an accessible overview of research in the field, as well as describing and evaluating US efforts to deliver developmental programs for high-risk children. This Robert Wood Johnson Foundation report is available at www.rwjf.org/files/research/1%20Early%20Childhood%20Issue%20Brief.pdf.

Canada Research Chair in Population Health and Human Development Clyde Hertzman has published widely in the area of early childhood development. The book chapter he co-authored with C. Power provides a good overview of the life-course perspective, emphasizing the importance of the early years. Hertzman C. and C. Power (2005), "A Life Course Approach to Health and Human Development." *Healthier Societies: From Analysis to Action.* Eds. Heymann J., Hertzman C., Barer M.L., and Evans R.G. New York: Oxford University Press, pp. 83–106.

The World Health Organization report *Early Childhood Development: From Measurement to Action* includes detailed reviews of longitudinal studies examining the effects of early childhood development programs, including programs and projects in Canada. The report is available at www-wds.worldbank.org/external/default/WDSContentServer/WDSP/IB/2007/09/20/000020 439_20070920154913/Rendered/PDF/409250PAPER0Ea101OFFICIAL0USE0ONLY1.pdf.

Annotated Web Resources

Medical Matters
www.bbc.co.uk/programmes/b0137z06
The excellent BBC *Medical Matters* three-part program "First 1000 Days: A Legacy for Life," along with the links to other relevant research resources found on this site, illustrate the strengths of a life-course approach in explaining the variable susceptibility of adults to chronic disease, obesity, and premature death arising from fetal development and early childhood. The programs provide interviews with the world's leading researchers in the field of fetal and early childhood determinants of adolescent and adult health.

Human Early Learning Partnership
http://earlylearning.ubc.ca
Housed at the University of British Columbia, this rich site provides links to information on epigenetics, determinants of child readiness for school, and latent, cumulative, and pathway effects on the health of older children and adults.

"Romanian Orphanage Babies: 21 Years On"
www.bbc.co.uk/iplayer/episode/b015p62y/
    All_in_the_Mind_Romanian_Orphanage_
    Babies_21_Years_On
For those interested in the fate of the Romanian orphans and the extent to which early developmental delays and subsequent brain damage may be reversed, the BBC *All in the Mind* program offers this follow-up.

**"How Childhood Trauma Affects Health
    Across a Lifetime"**
https://www.youtube.com/watch?v=95ovlJ3dsNk
This TED Talk by Nadine Burke Harris discusses how childhood trauma affects lifelong health.

"The Healthy Child: Assembly Required"
https://www.youtube.com/
    watch?v=fXf3CCyhLGU
This TEDxUNC Talk by Kathleen Gallagher discusses early childhood education.

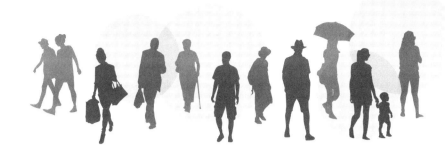

6   Gender and Health

Objectives

By the end of your study of this chapter, you should be able to
- distinguish between sex- and gender-relevant implications for health;
- understand that reproductive roles are important but are not decisive determinants of health;
- appreciate how relations between genders affect the health of men and women;
- recognize that binary conceptions of sex and gender inadequately capture human diversity.

Synopsis

Chapter 6 opens with a discussion of the differences and similarities in the health of women and men. A summary of the "morbidity paradox" follows, reviewing findings and hypotheses related to the apparent worse health (but longer lives) of women. We then turn to a discussion of the effects of long-term relationships on the health of men and women, before discussing the health implications of increased gender equity. A short section on gender, sexual orientation, and intersexuality follows. The chapter ends with a discussion of body image and anorexia nervosa.

The Health of Women and Men

We noted in Chapter 1 that it is wrong to focus on either sex or gender as fundamental to resilience or susceptibility because sex and gender are inextricably bound together. Health outcomes are neither biological nor sociological but rather arise in the interplay between biology and social environment. For simplicity, though, this chapter will use mostly the language of "gender" (men and women) rather than the more awkward, albeit more accurate, expression "interaction of gender and sex."

Pause and Reflect   Health-Relevant Differences

Apart from obvious physiological differences, in what ways do men and women in North America differ? Which of those differences are important for health? Why?

Men and women can differ in several health-relevant ways. Women may differ from men in terms of typical exposures, usual risks, and specific vulnerabilities. The nature, severity, or frequency of health problems may vary systematically between men and women. Women and men may differ in how they understand health problems and in the extent to which they seek help from others. If they access treatment, men and women may differ in terms of their compliance with prescribed treatment. Which of these things apply and in what way will depend on context.

Women have more robust and reactive immune systems than men. This has an upside in terms of lower rates of infection and generally less severe infection than in men. But it has a downside. Women are more susceptible to auto-immune conditions such as lupus and rheumatoid arthritis.

Women's brains are smaller and wired differently than men's, but the differences have been wildly exaggerated. There is no typical male or female brain, men's brains aren't connected front to back and women's side to side, and women aren't dominated by their right-brain hemispheres and men by their left. More importantly, there are no discernable differences in intelligence, creativity, or even math and linguistic abilities. Girls in Iceland, a relatively gender-neutral country, actually outperform boys on math. Gender gaps in math and reading are displayed in Figure 6.1. It is clear from the data that the gaps are more socially than biologically driven.

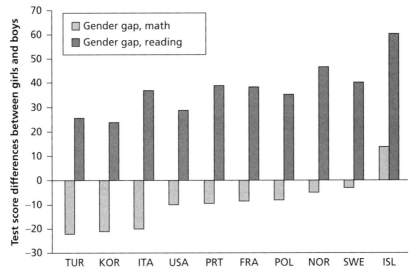

Figure 6.1 Gender Gaps in Math and Reading

Source: Reproduced in Sapolsky, 2017, p. 267.

Hormones are also not destiny in terms of personality and behaviour. Testosterone, for example, is more closely associated with optimism and sociability than "masculinity" or aggression. How hormones, estrogen, testosterone, oxytocin, serotonin, and dopamine influence personality and behaviour is contextually dependent (Sapolsky, 2017).

Babies with predominantly male sex traits outnumber babies with predominantly female sex traits. The ratio differs from place to place and time to time. It currently runs in the 52 per cent range of live births in North America and over 53 per cent worldwide (World Bank, 2018). But infant and childhood deaths are higher among boys than girls, leading to near equality by gender in adolescence and early adulthood. The reasons for this are unknown but may lie in the greater genetic complexity and lack of genetic backup in males combined with the apparent preferential nutrition provided to female fetuses by the placenta, meaning that fewer male infants are viable than females, a situation that is compensated for in human biology through a larger number of male births. This is about as far as biological determinism runs.

Risk taking by boys and young men, combined with higher activity levels and social expectations of participation in more dangerous endeavours, mean injuries and deaths are higher among teenage boys and young men than among girls and women. Violence by men against men in warfare and crime causes more death, disability, and injury to men than do violent acts against women. Men also run higher risks than women from behavioural/social factors. Men are more exposed to smoking, alcohol and illicit drug use, dangerous driving, and dangerous employment settings. Women, however, are more likely than men to be sedentary and engage in little vigorous physical exercise. Women are also vulnerable to assault by men. Nearly one-quarter of women in affluent countries, including Canada, have suffered violence from a partner ("Violence against Women," 2013).

Women, *qua* females, run higher sexual and reproductive risks, ranging from greater susceptibility to bad health outcomes associated with sexually transmitted infections to potential threats to health arising from complications of pregnancy and childbirth. Both of these—sexually transmitted disease and childbirth complications—remain major threats to women in poorer parts of the world, notably sub-Saharan Africa, where HIV/AIDS and complications of childbirth are major causes of mortality among women. They are, however, relatively minor health threats in Canada, the United States, the United Kingdom, and Australia (but see Box 6.1 below). Thus, the focus on gender and health in this chapter will be on health issues apart from sexual/reproductive health. It is worth noting, though, that even in sub-Saharan Africa, reproductive health issues are not entirely sexual as opposed to gender: high rates of female HIV infection and maternal mortality persist because of gender inequality, women's inability to control their own fertility or give/withhold consent for sexual activity, and a general lack of resources on the part of women, notably education and health care services. To regard the problem as biological, or reproductively determined, is absurd. Women's health problems do not exist in the same way and to the same extent in North America and Europe, not because men and women are different from those in Africa, but because our societies are differently organized and our gender roles are different. Women, however, are especially vulnerable to violence within the family. The vast majority of people injured in the 95,000 cases of family violence reported in Canada each year are women. Half of murder-suicides involve men killing their spouse (see Figure 6.2).

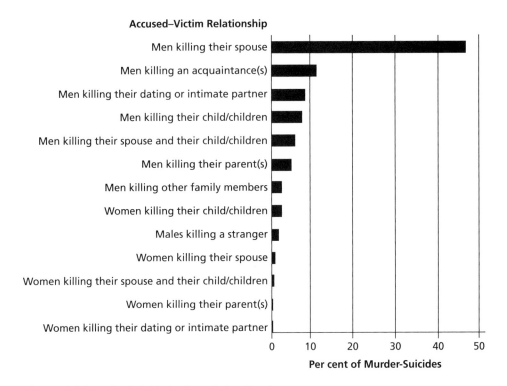

Accused–Victim Relationship

Figure 6.2 Murder-Suicide in Canada by Gender
Source: Statistics Canada, 2013. http://www.statcan.gc.ca/daily-quotidien/130625/dq130625b-eng.pdf

Box 6.1	Case Study ○ Maternal Health in the United States: Preventable Death and Mortality Amenable to Health Care

While Republicans and Democrats are engaged in apparently abstract debt reduction talks, it's worth noting that a cascade of federal, state, and local spending cuts has already taken its toll on the health of pregnant women, mothers, and babies. Between 2003 and 2007, the average maternal mortality rate—defined by deaths that occur within 42 days of childbirth—has risen to 13 deaths per 100,000 live births, approximately double the low of 6.6 deaths per 100,000 live births recorded in 1987. Today, the United States ranks 41st in the world for maternal mortality, one of the worst records among developed countries. "Near misses," complications so severe that a woman nearly dies, have increased between 1998 and 2005 to become common—at one woman every 15 minutes.

These disturbing trends are even worse for African-American women and poorer women. Nationally, African-American women are three to four times more likely to die of pregnancy-related death than white women. States in which poverty rates exceeded 18 per cent had a 77 per cent higher rate of maternal mortality than states with lower rates of poverty. (Daguerre, 2011. Copyright Guardian News & Media Ltd 2011.)

How can public policies and government-funded programs affect (positively and negatively) maternal and infant health in advanced countries like Canada, the United States, the United Kingdom, and Australia?

In rich Western countries and Japan, over the past century, increases in life expectancy of women outstripped those of men, mostly because women's social position dramatically improved (see Table 6.1). In the United States, for example, the life expectancy for a woman is currently 4.8 years longer than for a man. However, there is some preliminary evidence that the gap between life expectancies of men and women has shrunk slightly in recent years, at least in Canada. It is too soon to know if it is a trend and, if so, to offer an explanation, but it is sensible to assume that as the conditions under which men and women live and work equalize, so will (eventually) life expectancies.

It is important to note that the income inequality gap in remaining life for women reported in Table 6.2 is smaller than it is for men (4.8 years compared to 7.1 years—Quintile 5 minus Quintile 1). Notice also that the life expectancy/income gradient is less pronounced and less consistent for women than for men. This finding is consistent across studies and between places. The reason may be that women and men have different levels and kinds of social support, which can modify the health impact of other variables (more on this in Chapter 7). Women appear less susceptible to socioeconomic impacts on health than do men, because of the **buffering** effects of their gender roles within families and communities. Women, in most societies, are far more connected with their immediate family, their family of origin, and their neighbours than are men. They also have larger circles of friends. In consequence, women, in contrast to men, have more instrumental and emotional support to draw upon.

Note that the income-related health gap reported in Table 6.3 is less for women than men. The difference between the HUI for the highest quintile and the lowest is 0.078 for women versus 0.087 for men. But more significant is the fact that women *report poorer*

Table 6.1 Life Expectancies at Birth: Women and Men

Country	Women	Men
Australia	84.4	80.3
Canada	83.8	79.6
Japan	86.8	80.5
United Kingdom	83.2	79.5
United States	81.3	76.5

Source: OECD data, 2017.

Table 6.2   Remaining Life Expectancy at Age 25 by Gender and Income, Canada

Income Quintile	Years Remaining, Men	Years Remaining, Women
1 (lowest)	48.2	55.0
2	51.4	57.4
3	52.9	58.5
4	53.9	59.2
5	55.3	59.9

Source: Statistics Canada, 2015. http://www.statcan.gc.ca/pub/82-003-x/2011004/article/11560/tbl/tbl1-eng.htm

Table 6.3   Health Utility Index (Perfect Health = 1) Men and Women Aged 25–34, Canada

Income Decile	Men	Women
Decile 1 (lowest)	0.864	0.865
2	0.893	0.885
3	0.907	0.892
4	0.922	0.905
5	0.922	0.913
6	0.933	0.915
7	0.927	0.930
8	0.938	0.925
9	0.936	0.935
10 (highest)	0.951	0.943

Source: Adapted from MacIntosh, Fines, Wilkins, & Wolfson, 2009.

health than men at every income level except the lowest. This rather perverse finding, women reporting poorer health but living longer lives than men, is referred to as the **"morbidity paradox."**

The Morbidity Paradox: Why Do Women Appear Less Healthy than Men but Live Longer?

Pause and Reflect   Women Report Poorer Health but Live Longer

Why might women in advanced countries such as Canada report worse health than men yet live longer lives? How might this apparent paradox be resolved?

We have known for a long time that there is an apparent "disconnect" between women's self-reported health and their life expectancy (Verbrugge, 1985). This has been referred to as the morbidity paradox—a paradox because sicker people presumably ought to die sooner. One way of resolving the paradox is to appeal to the fact that women experience higher rates of distress, emotional disorder, and depression (Bird & Rieker, 1999). Another is to appeal to the higher probability of older men suffering from life-threatening diseases compared to the non-fatal degenerative conditions more common among women (Verbrugge, 1985). Older men, for example, are more likely to have a sudden, fatal heart attack; older women are more likely to have a non-fatal but disabling stroke.

Self-reported disability tends to be higher among older women than men. Sixty-six per cent of women aged 85 or older report one or more functional limitation compared to only 50 per cent of men the same age (Gorman & Read, 2006). Gorman and Read (2006) speculate that higher levels of depression and anxiety among women might skew self-reported health and disability in a negative direction. Strangely, though, the "health gap" between men and women actually narrows over the life course. Young men report much better health than young women, but the differences in self-reported health among elderly men and women in the United States are more alike (Gorman & Read, 2006). Ross and Bird (1994) reported no significant differences in self-reported health between elderly men and women in the United Kingdom or the United States. Recent evidence of this sort suggests that the problem—the apparent paradox—might lie in the measure of health, *self-reported health*, rather than in the objective state of health of men and women. That is, women may *for social reasons,* such as greater sensitivity to health issues and more frequent consultation with health care providers, tend to report worse health. Different, more objective measures of health, such as clinical assessment of pain and disability instead of reliance on self-reports, would likely show a convergence of health status between men and women.

Younger women report issues associated with menstruation varying from mild discomfort to significant pain (Grandi et al., 2012). A proportion of middle-aged women have moderate to severe symptoms associated with menopause (Dennerstein, Dudley, Hopper, Guthrie, & Burger, 2000). Pelvic floor weakness and/or torn pelvic floor muscles caused by pregnancy and delivery can cause bladder leakage and prolapse, distressing but not life-threatening conditions (MacLennan, Taylor, Wilson, & Wilson, 2005). These sex-linked genito-urinary conditions may account for some of the morbidity reported by younger women. But they are likely partly or wholly offset by urinary urgency and frequency, nocturia, and urinary incontinence in older men.

Is the Health of Men and Women So Very Different?

Thus, it is fair to say that health differences between men and women in Canada, the United Kingdom, the United States, and Australia are not very large and appear, in the last few decades, to have shrunk. Obviously some specific diseases do vary on gender lines, with, for example, some auto-immune diseases such as lupus and other forms of arthritis occurring more frequently in women. Parkinson's disease and a host of conditions related to behaviour, including brain trauma, spinal cord injury, lung cancer, and chronic obstructive pulmonary disease (COPD) and cirrhosis of the liver, are more common in men (but lung cancer, COPD, and cirrhosis rates in women have been closing in on men's rates in recent years).

Breast cancer occurs in both men and women but is very much more common in women. In Canada, female breast cancer incidence (approximately 25,000 new cases per year) is almost exactly equal to male prostate cancer incidence and so are deaths—approximately 5000 men and women each year (Canadian Cancer Society, 2010). Overall incidence rates and deaths from cancer have been falling for both men and women, with the exception of lung cancer in women.

Estimated deaths from cancer in 2017 totalled 42,600 for men and 38,200 for women in Canada. Total incidence for cancer is identical for Canadian men and women, 103,000 cases diagnosed annually in men and women (Canadian Cancer Society, 2017). The two leading causes of death, cancer and heart disease, are the same for men and women in all affluent countries, but the third leading cause of death in Canada and the United States is accidents and violence for men and stroke for women.

Overall death rates have continued to decline for both men and women in Canada, albeit more slowly in recent years for women. In the United States, death rates for both men and women have been increasing since 1996, reflecting falling life expectancy (National Center for Health Statistics, 2017). Of rich countries, only the United States appears to have experienced a significant reduction in life expectancy, though the most recent data from the UK government suggest that life expectancy has stalled or may have even declined in the United Kingdom in recent years. It is worth noting in this context that the United States and the United Kingdom are among the most unequal countries, and poor economic performance, public program cuts, and reductions in taxes on the affluent since the mid-1990s may be differentially affecting their populations due to that inequality. Denney and colleagues (Denney, McNown, Rogers, & Doubilet, 2012) show that not only has the trend to longer life in the United States flattened out, but also that the gaps in life expectancy between the poorer and the richer are growing.

One exception to the generally similar pattern of disease in men and women in Canada is mental health, particularly anxiety and depression. This is most evident in younger Canadians, as can be seen in Figure 6.3.

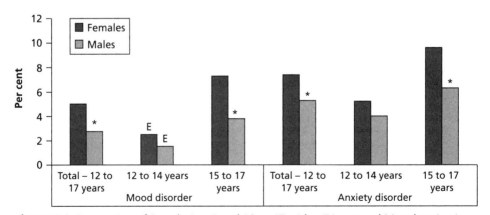

Figure 6.3 Proportion of Population Aged 12 to 17 with a Diagnosed Mood or Anxiety Disorder, by Age Group and Sex, Canada, 2013/14

Source: Statistics Canada, The Girl Child, 2017. http://www.statcan.gc.ca/pub/89-503-x/2015001/article/14680-eng.htm

There are mounting concerns in Canada and the United Kingdom that the emotional health of girls and young women is declining for unknown, but almost certainly social, reasons (Centre for Longitudinal Studies, 2018).

The Gender Convergence of Health-Related Behaviour

In rich Western countries like Canada, the differences in behaviour between men and women are shrinking. More men are becoming as sedentary as women, more women are as active in sports as men, smoking and drinking behaviour is converging, and more women are working in dangerous occupations. Further, women are "no less promiscuous and no more chaste than men" (Baranowski & Hecht, 2017). They take as many risks, albeit of a different kind than men. We would therefore expect health outcomes to become more alike.

Perhaps most concerning from the point of view of behaviour and their health, women in Canada and the United States are now drinking large amounts of alcohol more frequently, sparking concern over a new, major public health risk. The US Centers for Disease Control and Prevention (2016) reports women are more prone to brain atrophy, heart disease and liver damage than men. Women's smaller mass means that a similar amount of alcohol drives a much higher blood concentration of alcohol than is the case with men. US data show that the phenomenon of heavy, health-damaging drinking is prevalent among affluent, more-educated white women. A similar pattern of heavy drinking among affluent white British women has also been noted. This presumably reflects the aggressive marketing of wine ("mommy's time out") to women, combined with the idea that wine is a safe, possibly even healthy, beverage. Instead, wine drinking is associated with breast cancer, liver disease, colon cancer, brain damage, and heart disease, especially in women (OECD, 2015). This could be one of the reasons why breast cancer has a reverse gradient in Canada. Affluent women may have a higher incidence rate of the disease because they are drinking more alcohol (see Figure 6.4).

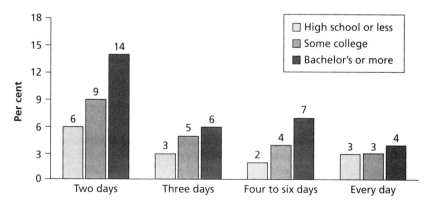

Figure 6.4 Percentage of American White Women Drinking Multiple Times per Week

Source: *Washington Post*, Dec. 23, 2016, https://www.washingtonpost.com/news/national/wp/2016/12/23/nine-charts-that-show-how-white-women-are-drinking-themselves-to-death/?utm_term=.bfa00b74808f

Box 6.2	Case Study ○ Gender Parity and Alcohol Consumption

Several period studies by the National Institute of Health in the US have found that while male consumption of alcohol has remained stable, the consumption of alcohol at all age groups for women has increased. Some examples of their findings:

> In a single decade—from 2002 to 2012—the proportion of women who drank rose from 44.9% to 48.3%, while the proportion of male drinkers fell from 57.4% to 56.1%.
>
> A survey conducted by the Centers for Disease Control and Prevention (CDC) between 2011 and 2013 indicated that 53.6% of women ages 18 to 44 were drinking, and 18.2% were binge drinking. The CDC followed up with an alert that three million US women were at risk of increasing the likelihood of sudden infant death syndrome and fetal alcohol spectrum disorders.
>
> According to the National Institute on Alcohol Abuse and Alcoholism (NIAAA), the gender gap has closed among teens, with about 20% of 17-year-olds drinking regularly and 13% binge drinking. (Merz, 2017)

Why might this closing parity gap be worrying?

The Effects of Stable Long-Term Relationships on Health

One of the most hotly contested areas in social epidemiology is the health effect of marriage (or any form of long-term partnership) on men and women. Early research dating from the 1960s suggested that men benefited from marriage but women did not. Later research in the 1970s and 1980s suggested that both men and women benefited from stable relationships but that men benefited more (and were harmed more by relationship termination through death of the partner or separation/divorce). It was hypothesized that the effects arise mainly through social support, both instrumental support in terms of making more resources available to the partners and emotional support. In conventional marriages, women benefit from access to additional income, better housing, and so on; men benefit from the domestic work provided by women, as well as from emotional support. Running through the analyses was the chronic problem of confounding—it was possible that people who form and are able to maintain stable relationships with a partner are better adjusted, have better mental health, or are more resilient in some way than people who remain single or whose relationships break down. The only clear fact was that married men and women have better health than single, divorced, or widowed men and women.

Martikainen and colleagues (Martikainen, Martelin, Nihtila, Majamaa, & Koskinen, 2005) argue that the benefit of marriage to both men and women has been increasing over time. But others, such as Liu and Umberson (2008), have suggested that the health value of marriage is actually declining, especially for men. That gave rise to the rather contentious hypothesis that marriage supports the health of women by providing them with more material resources and, at one time, supported the health of men (but no longer) through the domestic work of women. It is plausible that since the 1970s the domestic work of women has declined with the erosion of the traditional gender division of labour, making marriage less supportive instrumentally of men than it once was. Because women are now more economically independent, their benefit from marriage may also now be declining, narrowing the gap in health between married and unmarried men and women.

There now seems to be no doubt that the health benefits of marriage for men and women in terms of self-reported health and longevity are shrinking (Liu & Umberson, 2008), at least in North America. But the health of women who are separated or who experience the death of a partner has worsened relative to married women. It remains unclear as to whether the effect is mostly due to changes in resources available to widowed or separated women or to stress arising from the change in status (Liu & Umberson, 2008).

Recent Secular Trends Regarding Relationships

In Canada, the United Kingdom, and Australia (but less so in the United States), marriage and fertility rates have dropped and separation and divorce rates have risen. Both men and women—if they marry—marry at a substantially later age than their parents and grandparents did. The related results are that (1) more people are living alone and (2) household sizes are shrinking (see Figure 6.5). The trends might be expected to reduce health, first because living alone suggests lower levels of social support and second because smaller households (as we noted in the earlier chapter on income) mean higher per capita costs for food, housing, and other requisites of a healthy life. However, as we noted in the previous section, the health advantages of living as couples or in family units are disappearing, likely due to more equal participation rates between men and women in the paid workforce and the declining costs to young adults who are remaining childless or supporting no more than one child.

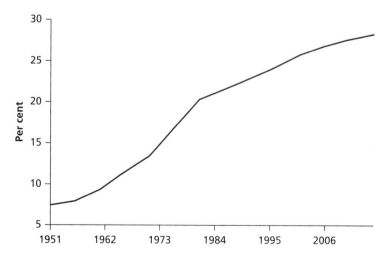

Figure 6.5 Percentage of One-Person Households in Canada, 1951 to 2016

Source: https://beta.theglobeandmail.com/news/national/census-2016-statscan/article35861448/?ref=

For women, delaying or foregoing childbirth raises the risk of breast, ovarian, and uterine cancers, but lowers the risk of negative health consequences associated with pregnancy and delivery. This relationship has been known for over a century and was first noted in a comparison of nuns to the general population. The effect arises because of lifetime exposure to hormones, particularly estrogen (just as the risk of breast cancer rises or falls depending on menarche, the age of first onset of periods, again because of lifetime exposure to hormones). Additionally, for the same reason, women taking contraceptive pills have significantly lowered overall mortality rates and reduced risk of ovarian and uterine cancers, without risking elevated rates of breast cancer due to improved formulation of the "pill" (Britt & Short, 2012). These factors taken together help to explain why today's childless singles, particularly single women, are healthier than the generation before.

Not only may remaining single in contemporary Canada, the UK, and Australia (as well as Western Europe) enhance your health, but remaining childless may also (today, unlike in the past) lead to greater happiness and health. Most, but not all, recent research suggests childless individuals and couples are happier and healthier than those with children (see, for example, Council on Contemporary Families, 2015; Deaton & Stone, 2015). Somewhat paradoxically, researchers are finding that women, in particular, are happier without children. Although research has yet to disclose why singles and the childless are happier, the effect likely arises from greater freedom, less economic stress, and the material benefits accruing to people who do not have to allocate income to child raising. It may be symptomatic of living in a materialist, consumption-oriented society.

Box 6.3   Case Study ○ Gender Differences Vary Across Dimensions of Relationships

While current involvements and recent breakups are more closely associated with women's rather than men's mental health, support and strain in an ongoing relationship are more closely associated with men's than women's emotional well-being. (Simon & Barrett, 2010)

This is quite a remarkable and controversial finding. Men appear to be more sensitive to the current dimensions of their romantic relationships than are women. This suggests that the nature of the supports intimate relationships offer differ between men and women. Why might that be so?

Distress Among Women

Among the explanations offered for women suffering more from anxiety, depression, and debilitating conditions than men is the psychosocial hypothesis relating to gender inequity. Gender differences reflect differentials in status and power, and women continue, even in affluent Western countries like Canada, the United States, the United Kingdom, and Australia, to occupy inferior positions. In addition, women may be differentially exposed to stresses arising from the multiple demands made upon them in juggling roles of mother, spouse, employee, and community member.

While intuitively plausible, the hypothesis that women experience excess stress due to gender inequity is hard to reconcile with the fact that women who are occupying multiple roles—partner, parent, employee—are actually healthier than women who have fewer roles and fewer potential role conflicts. The idea of a lack of power contributing to stress also runs up against the evidence that women who face high demands and low control in the workplace fare better than men and better than women who are not working (Denton, Prus, & Walters, 2003). Moreover, women do not report higher levels of stress in the workplace than men (Crompton, 2011). This leads some researchers to conclude that women rely heavily on social support to buffer the various stresses. But that leaves unexplained the clear differences in distress reported by women compared to men.

Having a higher income, working full time, having a spouse and family, and having social support have all been shown to be stronger predictors of women's health rather than men's (Denton, Prus, & Walters, 2003). This suggests a materialist explanation for differences in women's health—the health drivers are primarily resources not psychosocial factors such as stress. However, the questions arising from women reporting higher levels of distress and more emotional difficulties than men are far from answered. As noted earlier in this chapter, the apparent increase in mental health issues in recent years among younger women is not understood.

Gender Equity

Pause and Reflect   Gender Equity and Health

Greater gender equity could lead to convergence of the health and life expectancy of men and women due to growing similarities in living conditions. Or, growing gender equity could magnify the advantage women have over men by interacting positively with sex-related advantages such as cellular conserving features of estrogen and genetic advantages of chromosomal duplication. Which is more likely? Why?

There is no doubt that Canada, the United Kingdom, and Australia have made great strides in improving gender equity. Canada was recently ranked fourth in the world on the United Nations' gender-related development index, an aggregate measure of legal, civil, employment, and health measures (United Nations Development Program, 2010, p. 326). The US placed sixteenth and Australia placed second.

However, Canada has a very long way to go to match a country such as Sweden. Some additional data from the UNDP's Human Development Indicators (2010) include the following:

- women in parliament, Canada placed forty-fourth;
- life expectancy, women, Canada placed nineteenth;
- female education, Canada placed twelfth;
- income gaps between men and women, Canada placed fortieth;
- employment participation rates, female, Canada placed forty-first.

Presumably, improvements in gender equity in Canada will tend to increase the gender gap by differentially benefiting women through improved access to resources and greater control over their lives; but also, the convergence of lifestyles and health behaviours between men and women could harm the health of women, bringing health outcomes more in line with those of men. We have already noted that COPD and lung cancer rates are converging for men and women. The actual outcomes for health and life expectancy for men and women will depend on the balance between the two sets of factors.

Education and the Health of Women and Their Communities

One of the strongest relationships discovered through research into the health of populations is the correlation between educational level of women and a variety of measures of population health. The overall health of neighbourhoods, cities, regions, and countries varies in response to how much education girls and women receive.

Education for either men or women has individual-level health effects that show up in population-level data such as average life expectancy. We have seen that education is an important dimension of the health gradient. But in the case of women, the health effects of education extend beyond the individual woman.

The principal reason why female education has such profound health effects appears to be the additional control education gives women over their fertility. Control over fertility both reduces the number of children women bear and increases the age of first pregnancy. Fewer pregnancies and avoiding teenage pregnancy are associated with substantial gains in women's health, and, importantly, they are also associated with better health outcomes for the infant. In addition, greater female education increases the material resources available *not only to women but also to each of their children*. Fewer pregnancies beginning at a later age directly improve the lifelong health of the mother *and* the health and well-being of each child, each of whom is better nourished during fetal development and early childhood, and enjoys more resources and maternal attention.

Apart from increased reproductive control and enhanced access to material resources, education improves the personal autonomy and control over other aspects of the woman's own life, decreasing gender inequality. The women themselves, their families, and their communities also benefit from knowledge, skills, and capabilities gained through increased educational opportunities. Consequently, in the field of global health, improving the educational level of girls and women is a top priority.

Gay, Lesbian, Bisexual, and Transgender People

Gender Versus Sexual Orientation

Up to this point, the discussion has assumed adults have one of two genders grounded in their biological sex—they are men or women depending on their dominant sexual characteristics. However, gender—the sexually related roles and behaviour people adopt—is a social construct and hence inherently complex. First, a person's own sense of whether he or she is a woman or a man may not accord with his or her dominant birth sexual characteristics. A person who is anatomically male might perceive herself to be a woman; equally, a person who is anatomically a female might perceive himself to be a man. In other words, a person's "gender identity," his or her sense of whether he or she is a man or a woman, may not accord with his or her biological sex. Such people are referred to as "transgender." Second, gender has a public as well as a private dimension. People express their gender through adopting particular roles, behaving in certain ways and choosing certain forms of dress and hairstyle. "Gender expression" is the way in which people signal to others their gender identity. Transsexual people may seek to alter their bodies through surgery and hormones to improve the alignment of gender identity with gender expression. We do not know why some people are transgender. We do know that there is no simple answer. Biological and social factors both seem at work. Genetics, prenatal conditions, and experiences in childhood all appear to influence our sense of gender identity.

Quite separate from gender identity is sexual orientation. Traditionally, people have been classified as heterosexual, homosexual, bisexual, or asexual. "Heterosexual," meaning "different sex," refers to men and women who are sexually attracted to people whose gender is the opposite of their own. "Homosexual," meaning "same sex," refers to men sexually attracted to men and women sexually attracted to women. "Bisexual," meaning "two" or "both" sexes, refers to men and women who are sexually attracted to both men and women. "Asexual," meaning "no sex," refers to men and women who are indifferent to sexual activity.

Box 6.4	Case Study ○ Health Disparities

The distinction between gender identity and sexual orientation is important. A biological male who perceives herself to be a woman, for example, could be sexually attracted to men or to women or to neither. This fact raises some social issues. For example, some women are uncomfortable with transgender women using women's toilet facilities and locker rooms, at least partly because the question of sexual orientation is unresolved. Some university campuses have explicitly confirmed the right of transgender people to use the toilet facilities and locker rooms with which they are the most comfortable. Others believe that the individual's anatomical characteristics ought to determine access.

What are the issues at stake in this controversy? Is there a transgender policy on your university campus? Do you agree with your school's policy? Why or why not?

A History of Hostility

Traditionally, women sexually oriented toward other women have been classified as "lesbian" from the Greek myth of Lesbos, the isle of women. Consequently, the now virtually archaic term "homosexual" is most often applied to men. It developed a deeply negative connotation, with the expression "homo" becoming a common slur in the English-speaking world. In response, men's sexual rights groups advanced the use of the alternative term "gay." Women have preferred to retain the older expression "lesbian"; hence North American advocacy groups are sometimes referred to as gay–lesbian alliances (or, increasingly, gay–straight alliances, to signal solidarity between gay and non-gay people). Gay–lesbian groups often belong to coalitions that include bisexuals and transgender people—lesbian, gay, bisexual, transgender, queer (LGBTQ) or "rainbow" coalitions. While the term "gay" replaced "homosexual" in the vernacular, the negative connotations remained. In the 1980s and 1990s, use of the word "gay" as a disparagement or insult became commonplace among youth in North America.

Attitudes toward sexual orientation have differed over time and place. The Abrahamic (Judeo-Christian-Islamic) religious tradition has been hostile to men having sex with men, but indifferent to women's sexuality. The difference arises because Abrahamic theology and law regard anal sex to be "an abomination." Penalties for anal sex have been severe. England's *Buggery Act* (in force from 1533 to 1861) made sodomy (anal sex between men) a hanging offence. The death penalty still applies to sodomy in Iran, much of the Arab world, and parts of Africa. Penal codes specify life imprisonment for sodomy in Bangladesh, Pakistan, and Malaysia. Criminal penalties applied in the United States until 2003, when a Supreme Court ruling overturned state sodomy laws. Elsewhere, even when decriminalized, gay sexual behaviour is highly stigmatized. In Russia, for example, protests recently broke out over rock musicians purportedly "promoting homosexuality" by including lyrics in songs that advocated greater tolerance of LGBTQ people.

But not all religions and cultures have taken such a hard stance regarding men's sexual behaviour. Hinduism, Confucianism, and Taoism generally disapprove of non-vaginal intercourse, regarding it to be impure, but none of them prohibits sex between men. Ancient Greeks encouraged pederasty—sex between higher-status, older males and lower-status, younger ones—provided the higher-status male performed the penetrating role. But in general, sex between men has been taboo, highly stigmatized, and, wherever possible, punished until recent times.

Women who do not conform with prevailing gender norms have faced discrimination, abuse, and, in some cultures, severe punishment. Outward expression of gender (compliance with social conventions) has typically been more important in the case of women than private sexual behaviour.

Liberalization has occurred only in the affluent, secular, social democratic Northern European and liberal regime countries, and even there to a limited degree. In other words, gay men have been, and continue to be, persecuted in spite of recent advances in human rights in countries such as Canada. (Canada repealed laws against homosexual behaviour in 1969 and introduced same-sex marriage in 2005.) Canada is a world leader in respect of gay and lesbian rights, with most other countries lagging a considerable distance behind. But even in Canada, discrimination and violence against gay men and intolerance toward women who deviate from gender norms remain serious problems.

Attitudes toward homosexuality vary considerably depending on education, race, and gender. In North America, university-educated whites, particularly white women, are generally supportive of same-sex rights (Pew Center, 2011). Because views differ across socio-economic, racial, and gender lines, the subject is politically divisive. Conservative political parties take advantage of the fragmentation of the electorate by fanning the flames of intolerance toward same-sex and other "non-conforming" relationships.

Demographics, Health Behaviour, and Partner Support

The LGBTQ community is a minority population. In Canada, about 2 per cent of adults are gay or lesbian or bisexual. Approximately 2.1 per cent of men are gay and 1.7 per cent of women are lesbian (Statistics Canada, 2009). Gay men in North America are an unusual population because they are more highly educated and more affluent than the general population. In Canada, 76 per cent of gay men have a post-secondary education, compared to 65 per cent of heterosexual men; 30 per cent of gay men are in the highest income quintile, compared to 23 per cent of heterosexual men (Statistics Canada, 2009). Lesbian women are more similar to heterosexual women, but bisexuals tend to have lower education and lower incomes than the general population. As one would expect, based on socio-economic status, the health of gay men is better than the general population, the health of lesbian women is comparable to the general population, and the health of bisexuals is worse than the general population. As one would also expect, people who self-identify as homosexual congregate in the more tolerant urban centres, notably Paris, London, Sydney, New York, San Francisco, Vancouver, Toronto, and Montreal. (Gay men often establish affluent enclaves such as the Castro in San Francisco or English Bay in Vancouver. Some estimates place the proportion of San Francisco residents who are gay at over 6 per cent.)

Like most sub-populations, homosexual people have developed distinctive cultures and lifestyles. Some aspects of gay culture are potentially health promoting, such as greater attention to body mass index, diet, and exercise (though that may contribute to the risk for body image and eating disorders) (Kaminsky, Chapman, Haynes, & Own, 2005). Other aspects, such as smoking among gay and bisexual men, are unhealthy. An estimated 32 per cent of gay and bisexual men smoke, compared to 21 per cent of the general population (American Cancer Society, 2012). Lesbians are more likely to smoke and be overweight, and less likely to exercise, than heterosexual women. Use of illicit drugs and alcohol is more prevalent in the LGBTQ community than in the general population.

Gay male sexual behaviour also poses special health risks. Oral–anal contact (in straight and lesbian couples, as well as between gay men) elevates risk of hepatitis A, E. coli, and other forms of gastrointestinal disease. Anal sex is a much more efficient mode of transmission than vaginal sex for sexually transmitted infections, ranging from syphilis to HIV.

As noted earlier in the chapter, heterosexual marriage is generally health conferring on both partners. It is now thought this is mainly due to instrumental reasons such as division of labour, sharing of resources, and providing help and support to one another. In theory, then, persisting same-sex relationships should confer similar benefits, and early evidence suggests that may be true. However, partners—both same sex and opposite sex—also promote unhealthy behaviour and habits—and they may do so differentially depending on whether the intimate partnership is heterosexual or same sex. In general, LGBTQ relationships appear to be less likely to involve actively supporting the other person to pursue healthier habits (seeing health behaviour more as a matter of personal responsibility) and may be more likely to involve "pleasure seeking through concordant unhealthy habits," such as overeating, drug taking, or unsafe sex (Reczek, 2012). Nevertheless, stable same-sex relationships ought to confer health advantages analogous to, and generally arising from the same causes as, heterosexual unions.

Gay men in stable relationships are an affluent demographic. In most gay couples, both men work and, as men, typically earn higher salaries than women. Thus, that their household income exceeds that of heterosexual couples is not surprising. What is surprising is the *size* of the difference. Statistics Canada (2017) reported in a 2017 income study that gay couples have a median household income of $100,707 compared to a median income of $87,605 for heterosexual couples. Presumably this finding reflects differences in income stemming from education. Recall that, in general, gay men have more education than heterosexual men. These very high household incomes explain the health advantage gay men have over other Canadians.

Discrimination and Health

Members of the LGBTQ community face discrimination, harassment, and sometimes physical violence and criminal sanctions. The LGBTQ community usually refers to the hostility it faces as "homophobia"—literally "neurotic fear of the same." Others have taken issue with that characterization. The Associated Press, for example, claimed in November 2012 that "homophobia" is a misleading term because it implies that people who oppose homosexual activity have a mental disability (Strudwick, 2012). It is better, the Associated Press contends, to use less loaded language, such as "anti-gay."

Regardless of terms, it is clear that some segments of society are deeply hostile to homosexuality, especially toward men who have sex with men. The consequences for gay people are enormous. Hostility, social exclusion, bullying in schools and the workplace, and the threat of violence create stress, fear, and resentment. Adolescents just awakening to their sexual orientation feel especially besieged and vulnerable. Adolescent suicide among gay youth is a substantive risk.

Health of the LGBTQ Population

Given the discrimination faced by homosexual people, it is surprising that their self-perceived health is comparable to that of the heterosexual population. Bisexuals, however, are more likely than gay men and lesbian women to report poor health (Statistics Canada, 2009). Homosexual and bisexual people are more likely than the general population to report chronic disease or disability. All members of the LGBTQ community are more likely to report mood disorders such as anxiety and depression (Statistics Canada, 2009), and bisexuals are more than twice as likely as heterosexuals to report mental health problems. Gay men use more health care and mental health services than heterosexuals, but lesbian women use comparatively less health care. Neither gay men nor lesbian women are any more likely than the general population to report unmet health care needs (Statistics Canada, 2009). In general, lesbian, gay, and bisexual health is comparable to the general population, apart from increased incidence of mental health problems and sexually transmitted infections. However, transgender women are 20 or more times more likely to be living with HIV in Ontario (an estimate based on limited data; worldwide, the ratio is estimated to be 49 times more likely), as well as more likely to experience discrimination, stigma, and violence, and to be confronted by barriers to accessing appropriate health care (Bauer, Travers, Scanlon, & Coleman, 2012; WHO, 2017).

Intersex People

Throughout the text, we have noted that today's biologists and sociologists regard neither sex nor gender as binary. Human physiology—and social responses to physiology—are complex and varied. Sexuality is best understood as a continuum rather than two categories. Males share female characteristics just as females share male ones; men have feminine attributes just as women have masculine ones; gender identities and sexual orientations, in human populations, are quite varied. Moreover, physiology does not drive gender, though biology clearly affects emotion and behaviour, as well as how those are mediated through social relations. There remains, however, resistance to a non-binary understanding of sexuality and gender in the Judeo-Christian-Islamic world (due to its view of God and creation). Elsewhere, fluid conceptions of sexuality and gender are part of the cultural inheritance. Indigenous peoples in the Americas recognize "two-spirited" people, and societies in southern and southeast Asia accept more than two genders (for example, "kathoey").

As we have noted, physical appearance, cognition, emotional (including sexual) responses and behavioural patterns, are influenced by nutritional, hormonal, and other chemical exposures in utero. Intra-uterine conditions substantially affect primary and ultimately secondary sexual characteristics, perception and information processing, as well as lifelong emotions and behaviour. Alone these do not determine gender or sexual expression, but they do interact with social and environmental conditions following birth to give rise to mature gender and sexual orientations. Conditions in utero also influence later body shape and size, endocrinal function, and fertility.

Sexual determination and differentiation also have genetic components. Over 99 per cent of people have 46 chromosomes in 23 pairs, one pair being either XX ("female") or XY ("male"). This is referred to as 46XX (women) and 46XY (men). Usually, a Y chromosome is dominant, and its presence will drive male sexual characteristics—the growth of a penis and formation of testes, for example. But this isn't always the case; variation in the Y chromosome may result in the emergence of female (the default) physiological characteristics in a 46XY fetus. Moreover, it is now understood that there are genes in parts of the human genome other than the X and Y chromosome that affect sexual phenotype, including genitalia.

Forty-six chromosomes in 23 pairs is usual, but not everyone is 46XX or 46XY. The most common variation is 47XXY (Klinefelter syndrome). About 1 in 600 men have few secondary male sexual characteristics, produce very small amounts of testosterone, and are infertile. Men can also inherit an extra Y chromosome, 47XYY. Such men may be unaware of any difference between them and other men, although there are differences in physiology and testosterone production. Prevalence is approximately 1 in 1000.

Women may inherit an extra X chromosome, 47XXX. Such women generally have some physiological differences from 46XX women, typically being taller and slimmer. Prevalence is about 1 in 1000.

The sexual determination by chromosome may be missing entirely. Some people are born 45X (Turner syndrome), a relatively rare variant. With no Y chromosome, individuals will be phenotypically female, but they do not develop secondary sexual characteristics, are small for their age, and sterile.

In addition to chromosomal variations, other genetic variations also cause differences in sexual phenotype. Two are relatively common ones: adrenal hyperplasia and androgen insensitivity. In the case of the former, 46XX girls develop with a male appearance because of a genetically low level of cortisol production. In the case of the latter, genetic variation in 46XY males makes them insensitive to hormones that drive male sexual physical characteristics. They thus develop female genitalia and may also develop secondary female sexual characteristics despite being genetically male.

In short, there are many human variants. Unfortunately, social and religious pressures, particularly in the United States where some states continue to deny legal status to anyone except a man or a woman, led to the practice of sex and gender assignment. Surgical and drug interventions were, and in some places still are, deployed to make sexually ambiguous infants and children conform to either a male or female stereotype. The thinking was that making physical changes to genitalia combined with rearing in accordance with the sex assignment would create a "normal" boy or girl. Hormones and other drugs could be used to foster secondary sexual characteristics, erasing the sexual ambiguity completely. While some people have developed to be happy and well adjusted to their assignment, others have not. How to approach the issue of infants whose bodies do not conform with binary sex beliefs remains controversial.

Body Image and Health

Anorexia nervosa is often regarded as a modern condition arising from contemporary social pressures on girls and women to look slim. However, self-starvation by women is well documented in the ancient world and female "holy anorexics," some of whom were sainted following their deaths by starvation, were fairly commonplace in medieval Europe. Mary Queen of Scots (1542–87) is thought to have suffered from anorexia from the age of 13 (McSherry, 1985). The English doctor Richard Morton described the condition in detail in 1689 (Pearce, 2004). One of Queen Victoria's physicians coined the expression anorexia nervosa in 1873 for a condition more frequently referred to in nineteenth-century Europe as a variety of female hysteria.

Today, anorexia nervosa remains a mostly female condition, affecting somewhere around 1 per cent of the female population in Canada, the United States, the United Kingdom, and Australia. There are male cases, about 10 per cent of the total incidence, but those tend to be less severe and to have better prognoses than female cases (Stoving, Andries, Brixen, Bilenberg, & Horder, 2011). It is a very serious disease, chronic and debilitating, leading to death in an estimated 10 per cent of cases.

Anorexia nervosa is characterized by an effort to maintain a body mass far lower than is considered normal or healthy for the person's age and height. Sufferers have an intense fear of weight gain. Social norms and attitudes promoting thin female body types appear to play some role, as do personal traits of perfectionism, anxiety, and a need for control. Anorexia is often associated with compulsive exercising, self-imposed social isolation, and highly unrealistic perceptions of body image.

The cause of anorexia is unknown, though there may be links to estrogen (Young, 2010) and epigenetics (Frieling et al., 2009). Bouts of dieting may trigger altered gene expression. Social factors play a role. The incidence of anorexia was found to be most common in wealthy white families, especially where the parents have professional occupations (Linberg & Hjern, 2003); however, more recent research suggests that eating disorders (bulimia, excessive dieting, anorexia) are quite widely distributed among social classes, ethnicities, and races (Mulders-Jones, Mitchison, Giros, & Hay, 2017). Thus, the condition remains poorly understood.

Theoretical Considerations

Women in Canada, the United States, the United Kingdom, and Australia continue to have less access to many resources than men, advanced education being the most important exception. Women also typically face a more complex set of demands under conditions of less control than men do—family, friends, community, maintaining a household, as well as employment all compete for time and energy. We have seen that resources and control are key determinants of health. Thus, we would expect to find that women suffer worse health than men because of gender differentials in opportunities—i.e., gender inequities—and excessive demands coupled with inadequate control. In short, we would expect, on theoretical grounds, that women's health would more closely resemble that of disadvantaged populations. Some feminists, Verbrugge for example, have suggested this is the case and can be seen in the incidence of degenerative diseases, emotional and mental health, and reported distress among women, even though it remains true that women outlive men. More recent research has called the health differences between men and women into question. The newer suggestion is that "buffering effects," such as those that might arise from better social support among women than among men, might be protective of women's health. This is becoming an important new line of research.

We need also to recall the continuing large differences in health behaviour and health care–seeking behaviour between men and women. While not able to account for the size of observed health differences, accidental death, violence, suicide, and deaths associated with smoking, alcohol use, and substance abuse are all contributors to an excess burden of illness and premature death in men. We might expect, on theoretical grounds, to see a convergence of life expectancies and health outcomes as women's lifestyles come to more closely resemble men's, and we are beginning to see this in the recent data.

The nature of human interaction is becoming a central theme of research. For example, the size, density, and other characteristics of women's networks versus those typical of men has become a topic of enquiry. Likewise, the nature of the relationship between men and women—how they pair and bond, and how tasks and resources are shared within relationships—has now been recognized as an important set of health variables.

The study of pregnancy has led to conclusions that imply "biology is destiny"—i.e., genes, hormones, and our evolutionary history drive our values and behaviour. Examples include studies documenting the common experience of craving certain foods and suddenly abhorring others, and studies of "nesting" (the frequently observed behaviour of cleaning and organizing domestic spaces in the final months of pregnancy). Pregnant women have also been observed to become more wary of strangers and to associate more closely with those whom they trust most. But overgeneralization is surely at work here. There may be some biological factors at work; in fact it would be surprising if that were not the case. But, importantly, the behaviour of pregnant women remains highly context-dependent, and the choices made by women are highly contingent on culture, the nature of their households, education, income, and a host of other non-biological determinants.

In short, behaviour is not hormonally driven. In other words, health-relevant behaviour, like virtually everything else of importance to health, must be understood in terms of the *interaction* between biology and context.

Summary

Apart from different reproductive risks, the drivers of health, disease, and life expectancy in men and women are surprisingly alike. There may be some cellular conserving effects of estrogen in women (and cellular destructive effects of testosterone in men), but the consequences are small. There may be some genetic advantages to a double X chromosome versus a single X (due to duplication of genetic sequences and thus something of a "failsafe" in women), but very few health outcomes are straightforwardly genetic or sex-linked. Mostly the big differences between women's and men's health arise from context and context-shaped health behaviours.

Men and women do appear to have significant differences in susceptibility to socio-economic variables. Men's health is more affected by income and education than women's health. Men are more subject to health problems associated with social breakdown than women. And men are more likely to fall ill or die if a partner becomes seriously ill or dies. The leading hypothesis explaining this key difference is the different levels and nature of social support between men and women. Women are typically more integrated into their families and communities and typically have larger and denser social networks. The resulting differences in social support may buffer women from the consequences of some health risks.

While life expectancies of men and women in rich countries diverged over the twentieth century, they now appear to be converging. This appears to be for social reasons, the outcome of a range of important changes ranging from better control over fertility, falling birth rates, smaller family units, greater gender equity, and trends in the relationships between men and women (e.g., marriage).

Hormone levels and other sex-related biological features are relevant to health. Women experience the world differently than men and have different concerns. Brain and muscle development are different in men than in women, and those differences affect aptitudes, attitudes, and behaviour. Hormonal levels also affect mood and behaviour. But all of these effects are socially mediated through gender roles. The behavioural and health outcomes arise not directly from the biology, but instead from the interaction of biological variables with social ones. Thus, in more gender-equitable societies, with women's levels of education and earning power reaching parity with men's, health differences between men and women will decrease.

We have come to appreciate in recent years that sex and gender are not binary. Male and female characteristics, biological and behavioural, exist in both men and women. It remains a struggle to achieve universal recognition and tolerance, though some countries such as Sweden have made enormous progress, not only in the pursuit of gender equity, but also in the broader field of human rights associated with identity and sexual preference. The current federal government in Canada has committed itself to making similar progress.

Critical Thinking Questions

1. On 1 December 2011, the BBC reported ("Gay Marriage 'Improves Health,'" 2011) that gay marriage improves health. The report claimed that US research shows less use of health care facilities and a reduced number of health complaints among gay men who were recently married compared with those who were single or in conventional longer-term relationships. Assuming the evidence for this is sound, what might account for these findings?

2. In Sweden, arguably the most gender-equal country in the world, life expectancy for men and women is converging quite rapidly. Over the past 10 years, men have gained two years of additional life expectancy, compared with only one and one-half years for women. Why might that be happening?

3. A study by Statistics Canada (Ramage-Morin, 2008) shows that older women in Canada report worse self-reported health, greater distress, more perceived pain and lower levels of happiness than older men. What accounts for the difference?

4. "Body image is a subjective experience of appearance. It's an accumulation of a lifetime's associations, neuroses and desires, projected on to our upper arms, our thighs. At five, children begin to understand other people's judgement of them. At seven they're beginning to show body dissatisfaction. As adults 90% of British women feel body-image anxiety. . . . Many young women say they are too self-aware to exercise; many say they drink to feel comfortable with the way they look; 50% of girls smoke to suppress their appetite. . . ." (Wiseman, 2012) Uncomfortable in our skin: the body image report, *The Guardian*, Sunday 10 June 2012)
Is socially-driven anxiety harming girls and women?

Annotated Suggested Readings

A good resource on the topic of gender and health is the excellent book by Chloe Bird and Patricia Rieker, *Gender and Health: The Effects of Constrained Choices and Social Policies* (New York: Cambridge University Press, 2008). As the title suggests, the authors not only summarize research on gender and health, but also explicate the cumulative impacts of the social shaping of choices made by men and women. Unlike most comprehensive treatments of the subject, Bird and Rieker adopt an explicitly theoretical approach to their work that neatly demonstrates the complex interaction between biological and social factors. Best of all, the book is well written and accessible to the general reader.

An excellent resource book on LGBTQ health was published in 2011, *The Health of Lesbian, Gay, Bisexual, and Transgender People: Building a Foundation for Better Understanding* (Washington: National Academies Press, 2011). The book is available as an open book at http://books.nap.edu/openbook.php?record_id=13128. While based on US research and social settings, the findings are generalizable to the rest of the affluent countries of the Western world.

The Journal of Men's Health (Elsevier) covers a wide range of issues relevant to men's health and gender medicine.

Annotated Web Resources

Gender and Health Collaborative Curriculum
http://genderandhealth.ca
A superb learning tool has been created by the Gender and Health Collaborative Curriculum Project. The interactive curriculum covers a wide range of gender and health topics, including how to understand the difference between sex and gender, how gender works as a determinant of health, and a range of specific gender and health issues (cardiovascular disease, depression, lung cancer, and sexual diversity).

"Health Portfolio: Sex and Gender-Based Analysis Policy"
https://www.canada.ca/en/health-canada/corporate/transparency/corporate-management-reporting/Health -portfolio-sex-gender-based-analysis-policy.html

For general information on gender-related health and disease in Canada, the Health Canada website includes information on integrating gender-based analysis into policy and program development. It also provides four case studies (cardiovascular disease, mental health, violence, and tobacco).

CNN: Research on Childlessness and Happiness
https://www.cnn.com/2016/12/06/health/parents-happiness-child-free-studies/index.html
A fascinating discussion of the health and happiness benefits of remaining childless can be found on this CNN program site, which includes links to videos discussing research on childlessness and well-being.

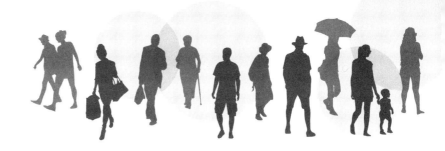

7 Social Support, Social Capital, Social Exclusion, and Racism

Objectives

By the end of your study of this chapter, you should be able to
- understand how social support and community cohesion provide a protective effect, mitigating the potential harm of risk factors;
- comprehend the potential health effects of social networks;
- describe and analyze the various forms of social support;
- appreciate the potential ill health effects of social exclusion.

Synopsis

Chapter 7 explores how our relationships with others may enhance or harm our health. It reviews the health significance of norms and group engagement, the health-protective effects of social support, the significance of social networks, the concept of social capital, and the deleterious health effects of social exclusion and racism.

Social Norms, Predictability, and Human Health

"Suicide varies inversely with the degree of integration of the social groups of which the individual forms a part."

—Émile Durkheim (1897)

It has been widely accepted since Durkheim wrote *Suicide* that the extent of social integration has effects on the well-being of the individual. Durkheim himself saw social integration as a function of attachment and regulation. By **attachment,** he meant the extent to which an individual maintains ties with others. By **regulation,** he meant the extent to which an individual is governed by the prevailing social beliefs, values, and norms. We already encountered a modern application of Durkheim's ideas in Bowlby's theory of attachment. Bowlby contends that an individual's capacity to attach to others in society, and be governed by societal norms, critically depends on an infant's primary attachment or bonding with a caregiver, a process that is necessary for emotional stability over the individual's life course.

Male residents of an Italian immigrant community in the eastern United States were found to have an unusually low incidence (compared to other Americans) of coronary heart disease. What factors could account for such a finding?

Research into the health of people in Roseto, Pennsylvania, increased interest in ideas associated with social integration, social support, and health. We noted earlier that in the 1970s a great deal of attention was paid to the epidemic of heart attacks among middle-aged American men. The community of Roseto stood out as an exception to that trend. The incidence of coronary heart disease among men in Roseto was, for some unknown reason, much lower than in surrounding communities—a fact that had been noted quite accidentally by a physician who treated patients from the locality.

Residents of Roseto were recent immigrants from a small region in southern Italy. Given knowledge of risk factors at the time, researchers initially focused on diet as a probable cause of the difference in heart-attack rates between the Italian immigrants and the broader population of Pennsylvania. The story of Roseto is partly a story of the emergence of the idea that a Mediterranean diet rich in olive oil, fish, and red wine protects men from heart attack. However, it was soon evident that the diet of men in Roseto was not healthy, but like most Americans' diets was based on high-fat and high-carbohydrate foods. Moreover, with respect to other risk factors, obesity and smoking for example, residents of Roseto should have had more rather than fewer heart attacks than people in surrounding communities.

Researchers eventually looked to the characteristics of the community of Roseto for an explanation. It was clear that Roseto had some unusual norms. Among those were a sense of collective responsibility for raising children, an aversion to embarrassing neighbours by conspicuous consumption, an ethic of sharing, and a strong sense of social solidarity. Ultimately, by elimination of risk factor explanations, researchers concluded that it was features of social support and social cohesion that accounted for the remarkable difference in health status between Roseto's men and those of nearby communities.

Social and economic disruption soon provided a test for the social-support hypothesis. An economic downturn and layoffs at the quarry where most of the men from Roseto worked changed the complexion of the town. As the norms of mutuality and cohesion broke down, heart-attack rates in Roseto rose, soon up to and then (as one might expect given the risk factors) to levels that were higher than surrounding communities. The reversal of trends has been interpreted to mean there is a **protective effect** associated with social support. Community-level characteristics, it was now believed, could offset risk factors for disease. Those protective effects, stemming from social support and social cohesion, are often referred to as the **"Roseto effect"** (Egolf, Lasker, Wolf, & Potvin, 1992).

Recently a natural experiment has been interpreted to confirm the Roseto effect. The collapse of communism in Russia and Eastern European states in the late 1980s brought with it unprecedented social and economic change. The rapid transition away from a structured economy with guaranteed housing and employment to a competitive market economy uprooted much of the labour force and drove many people out of their homes and neighbourhoods. Just as Durkheim predicted, disruption of existing attachment and regulatory mechanisms ushered in widespread stress and anxiety, crime, suicide, and alcohol abuse. Heart-attack rates soared. The life expectancy of Russian men fell by approximately six years and continued to fall even after economic growth resumed. Life expectancy in Russia, Ukraine, and other post-communist states remains substantially lower today than it was in the 1970s (Shkolnikov, 1997; Plavinski, Plavinskaya, & Klimov, 2003).

Roseto and Russia tell us that supportive, predictable, social norms can be protective of human health and well-being. They also tell us that widespread social and economic disruption, and the associated collapse of norms, can have extremely deleterious health effects.

Box 7.1   Case Study ○ Integrated Societies

Denmark, Sweden and Norway have healthy life expectancies of approximately 73 years. Japan, the world leader, has a healthy life expectancy of just over 74. The United States is near the bottom of developed counties, with a healthy life expectancy of around 70. Denmark, Sweden, Norway, and Japan share a characteristic in addition to being more equal societies than the United States. Japanese and Scandinavian societies are well integrated, with high levels of social co-operation. Solidarity, the sense that an individual's success or failure is linked to the success or failure of others, is a strong value in all four countries, but a very weak one in America. Danes, along with their Scandinavian neighbours, have an ethos of "hygge," which roughly translates as finding contentment in the moment, particularly in the context of time spent with friends and family. Norwegians and Swedes subscribe to the principle of "lagom," which emphasizes moderation and balance, core values in Japan. Both the Scandinavian countries and Japan emphasize sharing, teamwork, and collaboration. Social harmony is highly prized (but has a downside in fostering conformity). These cultural features interact with income equality to create a supportive social context that supports human health.

It had been thought that the values of both Scandinavia and Japan, and their high degree of social solidarity, were functions of homogeneous populations. Today, the values and solidarity persist, yet Denmark and Sweden are very diverse societies, with many different ethnic and racial groups comprising the population.

As in Roseto, culture and values supporting social integration are key variables explaining healthy life expectancy, albeit less significant ones than income distribution and public programs.

Social Networks

Social Network Theory

In contemporary society, we are encouraged "to network" in order to get ahead. This advice is sound because size, density, and other characteristics of a person's **social network** influence the information, resources, and access to opportunities available to him or her. Knowing and regularly interacting with a large number of people, and having access to influential people, substantially improve personal knowledge and influence. Moreover, a person's social network affects behaviour. The characteristics of our interactions with others set constraints on some behaviour and licence others. For example, in France, drinking alcohol is expected and normal, but drinking to excess is regarded as a sign of poor self-control. As a result, most people in France drink alcoholic beverages, but public drunkenness is uncommon. Effects like these can be significant from a health point of view. Another example: if social norms are to eat regular meals with friends and family and overeating in those social contexts is frowned upon, then obesity is likely to be uncommon compared with societies where people often eat alone and large portion sizes and second helpings are regarded as normal.

Observations such as those noted above lead to two linked hypotheses:

1. the richer (larger and denser) your personal network, the better your physical and mental health because of (a) improved access to resources and (b) enhanced control over your life prospects; and
2. networks discipline members into adhering to norms, beliefs, and values, many of which are potentially health-enhancing (e.g., social networks typically discourage "abnormal," high-risk behaviour).

Both hypotheses are supported by considerable evidence. But, of course, some types of social relations can be extremely harmful. Belonging to a cult or to a community of IV drug users is anything but health enhancing. Moreover, health-destructive norms such as smoking or overeating can be communicated through social networks, as we shall see later. In general though, rich, regular, social relations improve an individual's life prospects and overall health.

Box 7.2	Case Study ○ Networking

Mary is the centre of attention. She has many friends, a crowded and active Facebook page, and ongoing connections with a large number of diverse groups in her community. Sally, in contrast, is relatively isolated. While in a similar occupation and having similar earnings to Mary, Sally has only one close friend (an associate at work), little contact with her family, and little community engagement. How might Mary's and Sally's health and well-being be affected by their differing levels of social engagement? Why?

Social Support and Social Networks

It is useful to distinguish between social support and social networks.

Social support is about the qualitative nature of the interaction. Are others lending emotional support such as empathizing with us over some setback? Most of us think having someone show that they care and having someone listen to us talk about our emotional upsets are helpful to us. There is some evidence that such emotional support facilitates recovery from trauma (Gabert-Quillen et al., 2012). Most of us can readily see how others can help us by giving us information or advice. When making a difficult decision or dealing with something we feel we know very little about, we often rely on the advice and experience of others. Having to decide something on our own, without help and guidance from others, can be extremely stressful, and the consequences of error can be serious. Even more obvious is that other people might be doing something tangible, providing us with material assistance of some kind. Examples would include lending us money or use of a car, or physically helping us to eat or dress if we are disabled. Such instrumental support has been shown to be important in recovery from heart attack and in overcoming trauma arising from assault (Barth, Sneider, & von Kanel, 2010; Gabert-Quillen et al., 2012).

In sum, social support has been shown to have several probable health-relevant effects. Those include

- lowering stress level;
- raising self-esteem;
- facilitating cognitive development;
- encouraging and supporting better health behaviour;
- decreasing anxiety. (Karademas, 2005)

Social networks, on the other hand, are about the amount of interaction—the number of contacts and the frequency of those contacts matter. In addition, the characteristics of the network itself are significant. If the network is characterized by frequent, regular interaction among large numbers of its members, it is dense. The importance of this lies in the fact that contact with one member can help put the individual in contact with, or in a position to be influenced by, a great many other members.

It is important to understand that being embedded in a social network is not only about receiving information and support from others; equally, and perhaps more, important is providing emotional, informational, and instrumental support to others. Social relations are transactional; they involve reciprocity. A substantial part of our sense of self-efficacy and control stems from being able to support others. Moreover, we not only find ourselves influenced in our tastes and behaviours by those with whom we interact; we also exert influence over the others with whom we are in contact.

The characteristics of social support and social networks are laid out in Table 7.1.

Table 7.1   Characteristics of Social Support and a Social Network

Social Support	Social Network
Emotional support	Number of contacts
Informational support	Frequency of contacts
Instrumental support	Density of the network

Social Network Theory and Human Health

Christakis and Fowler (2009) showed that characteristics of social networks affect the health-relevant behaviour of, and outcomes for, their members. Associating with an obese person—or even associating with a non-obese person who associates with an obese one—affects the probability of someone becoming obese. Similar effects have been found for smoking and the cessation of smoking. Behaviours and outcomes travel through networks of people in much the same way as viral diseases with clusters of "cases" forming. Presumably those effects arise from changes in norms—exposed individuals change their beliefs and values with respect to some state (being overweight or underweight) or some behaviour (smoking or exercise) due to social influences communicated to and through them by their social contacts. From the point of view of health promotion, social network findings are vital. If we are most influenced by the people with whom we are in contact, as opposed to being influenced by what we read or see on television, then informational and advertising strategies—health education messages—are unlikely to have much impact. Obviously this is well understood by commercial advertisers who increasingly rely on social marketing and "viral campaigns" to promote consumer products. Companies know it is more effective to have a well-connected person wear their athletic shoe than it is to pay a celebrity to claim allegiance to that brand.

Pause and Reflect   Behavioural Epidemics?

Social network theorists examine networks through measuring the number of members and the extent and frequency of their interaction. Mapping networks to illustrate who is in contact with whom is a helpful tool. Social network theory has been deployed in examining health-relevant norms such as smoking and eating habits. Dr Nicholas Christakis, a Harvard-based physician and sociologist, has posted several social network animations on the website http://christakis.med.harvard.edu. These animations show how things as diverse as taste in music, loneliness, smoking behaviour, and obesity are shaped by the pattern of our interaction with others.

Dr Christakis contends that beliefs and norms are transmitted through social networks. Health-relevant behaviour is "communicable" in similar ways following similar patterns to epidemics. Controversially, he is associated with the idea that it is your friends and associates who "make you fat." If your friends, or even the friends of your friends, become obese, your risk of obesity rises by over 50 per cent. How could this possibly be true? Can you think of any examples of beliefs, norms, or behaviours that have spread from person to person through contact?

Evidence That Our Fundamental Attitudes Are Shaped by Our Social Interactions

An important recent application of network theory is found in the research program of Miles Hewstone and the Oxford Centre for the Study of Intergroup Conflict. To appreciate the importance of their work, we need to review the thinking on ethnic diversity and **social capital**.

It has long been recognized that individuals who routinely interact with the same people develop common ideas, values, and ways of doing things. That is partly because people are more comfortable associating with people similar to themselves and partly because many of our ideas and values are heavily influenced by social interaction. This phenomenon is especially easy to see in the case of "cliques" in high school—groups that define themselves differently, listen to different music, adopt a style, and differentiate themselves from other non-clique members. Sociologists talk about the formation of intra-group solidarity—thinking and acting alike, with members of the group supporting one another—and extra-group hostility—each group having little to do with other groups and acting to exclude their members.

Social capital theory as developed by Robert Putnam and others contends that the divide between groups can be bridged through the development of norms of trust and reciprocity, and that these are most likely to arise in more equal societies. (Social capital theory is discussed in more detail in the following sections). Contrariwise, in unequal, hierarchical societies, extra-group hostility is likely to intensify, possibly to the level of violence or blood feuds. As we have seen, higher levels of social capital, associated with greater equality and social engagement, are theorized by Putnam, Kawachi, and Wilkinson to be a key determinant of population health. Putnam saw social diversity, equality, and social engagement to be hallmarks of healthy societies.

However, in 2007 Putnam radically changed direction when he contended in an influential paper that growing ethnic and religious diversity in countries such as Canada and the US undermines social capital, increases conflict, and degrades quality of life. Putnam's contentions depend on evidence supporting the ideas that similar people will form groups that act to exclude others, usually understood as intra-group solidarity and extra-group hostility (referred to by sociologists as "**conflict theory**"). Putnam claimed his recent US data confirm the anticipated extra-group hostility but in addition show that, under threat from diverse groups, intra-group solidarity also breaks down. In other words, instead of groups rallying and becoming more integrated in the face of perceived threats from other groups, they are falling apart. For example, instead of Hispanics banding together to confront racism and efforts to deport them from the US, solidarity among Hispanics has been replaced by infighting, and the fracturing of the larger group into established long-term residents, new arrivals, conservative elements versus liberal ones, and so on. Individuals risk being set adrift; they can no longer seek security and confirmation in their group, but they deeply distrust people unlike themselves. The result is a bleak universal intra- and extra-group hostility, something Putnam calls "hunkering down." Essentially, Putnam sees a society of atomized individuals, nursing hostility and resentment, conditions that are not only deeply unhealthy but also politically dangerous—indeed, fatal to democracy.

Against this bleak assessment, "**contact theory**" contends that as individuals and groups gain experience with those different from themselves, norms of tolerance and co-operation develop. Putnam explicitly denies this. Instead, in a "hunkered-down society," people become increasingly materialistic, withdrawn, and suspicious—a nation of anti-social, television watching, non-participating, obese, and emotionally disturbed people.

Hewstone and colleagues take on Putnam in a series of articles. Schmid, Hewstone, Kupper, Zick, & Wagner (2012) show that not only does contact between individuals from different groups positively influence their attitudes about one another, but also, stunningly, simply seeing people from a group with which they identify interacting positively with a member of some different group can markedly shift attitudes and subsequent behaviour. An example of these "**secondary transfer effects**" would be a Canadian of Scottish ancestry walking by a market stall where he observes another person (who looks much like him) buying produce from a traditionally dressed Sikh. In such cases, Hewstone's research finds *positive* shifts in attitude and *stronger* senses of solidarity. That, of course, is very good news for our increasingly diverse communities.

The key points to extract from this discussion are that humans are influenced by the people they interact with, and are influenced, possibly even more heavily, by interactions they simply observe or otherwise find out about. "Secondary transfer effects" explain Christakis's rather puzzling finding that if your spouse interacts with obese people it is more likely to lead to you becoming obese rather than your spouse. Recall that Christakis's research team discovered that if friends, siblings, friends of friends, or friends of your spouse become obese, your probability of becoming obese rises by 57 per cent, but if your spouse becomes obese your risk rises by only 37 per cent (Christakis & Fowler, 2009, p. 357).

Social Support and Health

An important question arising from social-support research is "Does having and maintaining positive relationships with others really improve health?" Studies, such as those showing that people in stable relationships with a spouse or partner live longer than people who do not maintain stable relationships, suggest the answer is "yes." But it is surprisingly difficult to be certain. It is possible that some attribute of the person, such as being well adjusted, contributes to them building positive relations with others and those in turn help support healthy living ("**mediated relationship**," see Figure 7.1). Or it is possible that being well adjusted independently gives rise to better physical and mental health as well as making it easier to develop positive relationships ("**confounded relationship**," see Figure 7.1). Or it is that being well adjusted leads to both better health and more positive relationships and good health and positive relationships reinforce each other ("**independent relationship**," see Figure 7.1).

Recent brain research (Bickart, Wright, Dautoff, Dickerson, & Barrett, 2010) has in some ways further muddied rather than clarified the relationship among the variables. Our brains show marked differences depending on the amount of social contact we have had. Those differences can be shown both in spatial configuration of the brain and in scans of brain activity. But those results raise the question of whether people with certain brain characteristics are more inclined and better able to make friends or, alternatively, whether having lots of friends changes the structure and function of our brains. It would appear that making and keeping friends induces changes in brain structure and function, but the exact nature of the relationship remains poorly understood, and will remain so until prospective studies can be conducted to determine the direction of causality.

Nevertheless, there are plausible reasons regarding why social support can affect health. Other people may affect our behaviour in positive ways. Our friends and associates may help us to drive more cautiously, wear our seatbelt, eat less, moderate our alcohol intake, exercise more, and so on. Family members may help one another to take their

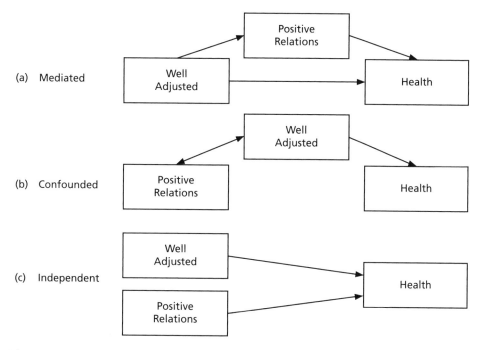

Figure 7.1 Mediated, Confounded, or Independent Relationship

medication as prescribed, and elderly spouses remind each other of how much each has eaten and drunk and when another meal is in order. Moreover, interacting with others may increase our sense of efficacy and self-worth.

Indirect effects of social interaction may also matter to health. As noted earlier, emotional support or receiving information and advice may lead to a constructive re-evaluation of our situation, reduce stress, or help in dealing with the consequences of stress.

Pause and Reflect   Recovery and Social Support

How probable is it that seriously ill people will recover faster and more completely if provided with more rather than less emotional, informational, and instrumental support? Might support be more important for some conditions and under some circumstances than in others? Think about cancer and depression as examples of serious illness where support might help, but in different ways.

But in spite of the remarkable stories of Roseto and Russia, the evidence that social support directly enhances health remains elusive. One very dated Swedish study (Orth-Gomer & Johnson, 1987) linked social integration to longevity, but few have since. A number of studies link the lack of friends and low levels of social engagement to poor mental health. Social isolation does seem detrimental to health, not only for people but also for all primates. Moreover, people in stable, long-term relationships tend, on average, to be healthier and to live longer than people who live alone. But studies have failed to exclude the possibility that underlying personality factors might be responsible for some or all of the differences in health outcomes. It remains possible that people who have few friends, engage little with their communities, and remain single are hostile, anxious, or have low self-esteem, and it is those personality features and/or their correlates that are the main determinants of their poor health.

Where social-support effects have been found, they tend to be associated with mental health and coronary heart disease but not cancer or other chronic diseases. Men seem to be more sensitive to social-support effects, possibly because men in Anglo-American societies generally have smaller social networks and fewer close friends than women. Hence, the loss of a friend or spouse is more significant in emotional and health terms for men than it is for women.

Efforts to test for positive social-support effects in experiments have yielded mixed results. Improving social support for male patients after a heart attack helps prognosis, but this does not appear true for women or for other illnesses (Barth, Sneider, & von Kanel, 2010). Death rates for people with no social supports are higher than for people with substantial social support, but that is likely due to instrumental reasons. Crisis-support intervention and social support for cancer survivors, while popular and commonplace in our society, have not been shown to yield consistent results. Moreover, poorly designed or poorly executed interventions, such as grief counselling, can actually do substantial harm (Jordon & Neimeyer, 2003). In reality, many people do not benefit from talking about painful episodes, and doing so may deepen their trauma (and could be the cause rather than a prevention of chronic problems such as post-traumatic stress disorder).

An important study by Kroenke and colleagues (Kroenke, Kubzansky, Schernhammer, Holmes, & Kawachi, 2006) showed that women who were recently diagnosed with breast cancer and were socially isolated were at elevated risk of death. However, the study showed there is no relationship between social support, community engagement, religiosity or church attendance, or having close confidantes and breast cancer mortality. Extreme isolation is harmful, but social integration and social and emotional supports do not appear helpful, at least in terms of prognosis.

Social Isolation Among Older Adults

Many older Canadians are socially isolated. They no longer belong to a sizable social network. If previously married, their spouse has pre-deceased them; children may live in distant communities or otherwise no longer be in regular contact. For men in particular, most of their social network when younger may have been work related, and connections quickly weaken upon retirement. Consequently, older adults often have little instrumental social support for transportation, information, monitoring for diet and adequate hydration, ensuring medications are taken properly, and helping keep their residence clean, safe, and properly maintained. Meanwhile, their independence, sense of confidence in their abilities, physical strength, and cognitive function all decline. Lack of informational support and advice creates vulnerability to fraud. The isolated frail elderly thus become a highly vulnerable population—vulnerable to poor diet and dehydration, medication error, scams, falls, and house fires.

Older adults are also vulnerable to loneliness. Many have very little social contact beyond visiting caregivers and staff in grocery stores and pharmacies where they shop. Hearing problems inhibit the ability to interact with others. Limited social interaction speeds cognitive decline and depresses mood. Inability to get exercise and be outdoors increases risk of serious depression.

Social isolation of older adults is strongly associated with early mortality (Holt-Lunsted, Smith, & Layton, 2010). Interventions such as friendly visitation, regular telephone calls from volunteers, and invitations (and arranged transportation) to seniors' centres and adult day care programs all have demonstrated effectiveness in reducing risk of disease and premature death. Pets, especially dogs, have been shown to be effective surrogates for human emotional support, and have the added benefits of forcing their owner to take walks, which not only provides needed exercise but also increases opportunities for social interaction with other people.

Holt-Lunsted and Smith (2016), based on a large meta-analysis of research papers, claim that loneliness and social isolation are more dangerous to health than smoking, heavy drinking, or obesity.

Box 7.3   Case Study ○ Social Support

In our society, it is widely believed that greater social support yields better health outcomes, yet the evidence for that belief is quite weak. In particular, we expect to see a **dose response** between a causal independent variable and the dependent variable, and it is precisely the dose response that appears to be missing. People who are socially isolated suffer, but it does not follow that a person with normal supports will become more functional, experience elevated well-being, or enjoy better health outcomes if additional support is forthcoming. The natural history of diseases, such as cancer, does not appear to be changed by social support. The odds of recovery, length of survival, and other *hard outcome measures* fail to respond to increased social support, though the recipient may report feeling better in light of increasing aid and compassion. Should the non-linear, non-causal nature of social support affect our responses to others? Does the lack of a dose response suggest changes in the design and expectations of our health and social service interventions? Is there still an important purpose to be served in striving for higher rather than lower levels of social support for members of our society?

In sum, we know social stability and predictability are important for cardiovascular and mental health, presumably because of the stress caused by uncertainty. We know that social networks influence people's health-relevant behaviour through transmission of norms. The effects can be positive—for example, cessation of smoking—or negative—the spread of obesity. We know social isolation harms mental health and probably negatively impacts physical well-being, though physical health effects, as opposed to emotional ones, may arise from purely instrumental means, such as lack of assistance with daily living or being out of an important communication loop. We know that outcomes for men and women differ when they lose a close friend or spouse. Loss of friends and death of a partner affect men more than women, presumably because of the smaller size of a typical male friendship circle.

What remains uncertain is whether community-level variables, such as high levels of social cohesion or large amounts of social capital, matter to human health. Roseto and Russia suggest they do, and some theorists including Kawachi (1999; Kawachi & Berkman, 2000; Kawachi, Kennedy, Lochner, & Prothrow-Stith, 1997) and Wilkinson (1996; Wilkinson & Pickett, 2009) think that social integration in affluent societies is the factor that matters most. Social cohesion and social capital play large roles in their work.

Social Cohesion

Social cohesion is the broader of the two concepts (social cohesion and social capital) and is usually operationalized through measures of participation in community affairs, the number of community-based organizations, the level of interpersonal trust, and crime statistics. Dating back to the Roseto study, researchers have found correlations between disease incidence and life expectancy and the various measures of social cohesion. For example, communities where lost items are likely to be returned to their owners (rather than being appropriated by the finders) rank more highly on health indices.

The idea that social cohesion is health conferring is attractive, but, as a contextual variable, social cohesion has come under considerable attack. The main problem is confounding. In other words, is it social cohesion that improves health status or is it some other variable that gives rise to both social cohesion at the community level and better health at the individual level? Income and education have both been suggested.

Populations of higher income and/or more highly educated people generate many more organizations and higher levels of social networking than populations of lower income and/or less highly educated people. They have more resources individually and more resources to share among themselves. Additionally, psychologists have shown that richer, more educated people are more trusting of other people and more optimistic about their futures. Better-educated people are more inclined to report high levels of support from others than less well-educated people. In short, the supposed collective effects of social solidarity may simply be reflections of individual-level resources such as income and education.

Notice this is a variant of the dispute about whether equality itself matters or whether income distribution matters only because of the resources available to individuals. Social solidarity theorists point to the fact that more equal societies are healthier societies and attribute this to the relationship between equality and solidarity. More equal societies do tend to demonstrate more solidarity, as we noted earlier. Or to put the point the other way around, people in very unequal societies tend not to support one another—they do not perceive a common interest and it is difficult to generate public goods like parks and publicly funded health care. But these effects, real as they are, can be largely explained by the income held by individuals. It is the composition of the society, the numbers with and without various resources that matter, not the income distribution per se (but see Kondo, 2009, whose meta-analysis found modest income inequality effects when the GINI index exceeds 0.30).

As we noted earlier, in Chapter 4, the dispute has ramifications. If the only meaningful story to be told, as we saw Lynch argue against Wilkinson, is about resources available to individuals, then real resources—money, educational opportunities, health care access, decent housing, and capabilities such as powers of decision making in the workplace—must be redistributed. The only ways of transforming a population's health and well-being are (a) income transfers from the rich to less rich via progressive taxation together with provision of public programs and services and (b) power transfers from supervisors to subordinates in the workplace. Notice the close association of these policy goals with liberal and social democratic politicians.

But if social solidarity is important in its own right, then cultural programs, state support for strengthening families, and voluntary organizations and policing to reduce anti-social behaviour are meaningful strategies for improving population health and well-being. Notice the close association of these policy goals with conservative politicians such as past president George W. Bush in the United States.

The dispute is not easily resolved by appealing to the evidence. For example, Wilkinson objects to including education in the category of "individual resource" because it is such a socially laden concept (Wilkinson & Pickett, 2009). From Wilkinson's perspective, talking about education makes little sense except in a relative way by comparing one person's or group's educational level with another's. Thus different stances and values are at work, making the academic dispute at least partly ideological and not purely scientific.

There is some, albeit limited, direct evidence supporting the social solidarity thesis. For example, aggressive policing of anti-social youth in the United Kingdom, at least in some neighbourhoods, improved levels of social engagement and co-operation. Researchers have made the link from improvements in neighbourhood functionality to reduced stress on the part of individuals (Wilkinson & Pickett, 2009). Thus, it is at least plausible that social solidarity at the community level is health conferring but of less significance than access by individuals and households to resources for healthy living.

Table 7.2 identifies some values associated with the two principal political ideologies of the liberal regime countries: conservatism and liberalism. Health-related hypotheses that emphasize social stability, hierarchy, status, security, and non-interference with families and individuals appeal to people with a conservative orientation, whereas health-related hypotheses that drive conclusions that we need social change and should embrace diversity, create fresh opportunities for individuals and groups, and take steps to improve the circumstances of less well-off people appeal to those with a liberal orientation. Psychosocial theories thus align with conservative values, whereas materialist ones align with liberal values.

Table 7.2 Psychosocial Account of "Cohesive Healthy Society" Appeals to Conservatives; Materialist Account Appeals to Liberals

Conservative	Liberal
Preserving "heritage"	Embracing social change
Promoting social integration	Promoting diversity, tolerance
Supporting traditional family, religious groups, charities	Championing rights of minorities, women, gays
Law, order, and security	Education, support, and rehabilitation
Enhancing predictability of social life	Enhancing opportunities for development
Leaving people to decide what they want to do with their money and property (i.e., "volunteerism"; small government)	Taxing the more affluent to provide programs and services for the less affluent (i.e., regulation; larger role for government)

Social Capital

Social capital theory is a sub-set of the social solidarity literature. "Social capital is defined as those features of social structures—such as levels of interpersonal trust and norms of reciprocity and mutual aid—which act as resources for individuals and facilitate collective action" (Kawachi & Berkman, 2000).

As was noted earlier, the concept has roots in American social science. In the 1960s, much was made of "civic culture," the idea that democratic norms were grounded in stable family life, community-level voluntary organizations, church membership, engagement in the local economic marketplace, and children participating in organizations like amateur sporting clubs. This rather US-centric set of ideas later found its way into economics, where social capital was identified, literally, as a form of capital—something a community could build up, bank, or lose depending on the nature of engagement among its members. Meanwhile, American criminologists developed a similar hypothesis about crime rates: communities with weak integration, low levels of trust, and lack of community engagement in daily life were hypothesized to have high crime rates. Interest in this line of thinking, and the specific concept "social capital," was revitalized in the 1990s following the publication of American political scientist Robert Putnam's *Making Democracy Work* (1993).

Putnam and most later academics operationalized social capital by measuring (a) participation rates through things like voter turnout in elections, (b) levels of trust through surveys, and (c) community engagement though counts of community clubs and organizations. Kawachi and colleagues (1997) applied the concept of social capital in this classic form to US states and found that all-cause mortality is inversely correlated with measures of social capital, as in the example provided by Table 7.3. They included among their measures membership in churches and hobby groups, trust in neighbours, and voter turnouts.

Although the concept is still seen in the literature, interest in social capital has waned since the late 1990s. The first problem is the familiar one of confounding discussed above under "Social Cohesion." The principal difference between areas of low social capital and high social capital appears to be income, suggesting that income may be the main determinant of both social capital and health measures. Also, the social capital literature is almost entirely American. This is a problem because US population-health data is badly confounded not only by income but also by race. In the United States, neighbourhood characteristics are also strongly associated with racial composition, making segregation,

Table 7.3   "Most people would try to take advantage of you if they got the chance": A Measure of Social Capital

US State	Proportion of Adult Population Agreeing with the Statement	Age-Adjusted Mortality Rate
Washington State	12% agree	800/100,000
Louisiana	43% agree	1000/100,000

Source: Adapted from Kawachi et al., 1997.

social exclusion, and resource availability at the neighbourhood level additional confounders. Second, some theorists claim social capital theory is inherently ideological—simply a cover for the economic and social injustices rooted in unequal access to resources (Navarro, 2002). Third, the concept has been challenged as lacking theoretical coherence. There is a hint of this even in Kawachi's definition. Recall that he started with social capital comprising "features of social structures," but he ended the definition with "resources for individuals." This suggests a key ambiguity—are we really talking about social facts, features of collectivities, or, alternatively, are we talking about things individuals can make use of such as money, education, parks, and health care? If the latter—resources—the position collapses into materialism. From a theoretical standpoint, without clear evidence that the level of social trust directly affects something biological (such as stress hormones), we have a set of statistical associations derived from aggregated population data but no obvious causal pathway.

Navarro is not mistaken in sensing a whiff of right-wing ideology in social capital theorizing. President George W. Bush in the United States, for example, extolled the many virtues of civic organizations, service clubs, and churches, claiming them to be the backbone of healthy communities. Bush insisted that shrinking government would increase space for non-government actors such as small businesses and charities, thereby building up communities through more robust markets and volunteerism. Also on the political right, the American conservative columnist David Brooks (2011), who was seen as a major influence on the British Conservative government ("Please Explain," 2011), emphasized community, civic order, and smaller government. Like Bush, Brooks thinks dismantling public programs (except for schools, which he thinks we need but should reform to become stricter) will remove motivational barriers that currently inhibit co-operative action. He goes so far as to claim that joining a bowling club will improve the average person's happiness more than receiving additional money, a belief that supports his hostility toward fairer tax rates for America's wealthy.

This affluence-friendly woolly thinking took concrete shape in the United Kingdom. Prime Minister Cameron's Conservative government cut programs and transfer payments that support the UK's least well-off while claiming it was laying the foundations for a "Big Society" that values volunteerism, civic duty, and traditional families. Indeed, according to Cameron, the route to stronger families and more functional neighbourhoods is through smaller government, a surprising English echo of George W. Bush. Meanwhile, many of the voluntary organizations upon which a Big Society would depend went bust because of the loss of government core funding. And, as one would expect, life for the average person did not get better; rather, the quality of life both at the individual and community level degraded rapidly.

The now retired archbishop of the Church of England felt compelled to comment on social capital–inspired politics in England:

> In the run-up to the last election as a major political idea for the coming generation, [increasing social capital] has suffered from a lack of definition about the means by which ideals can be realized. Big society rhetoric is all too often heard by many as aspirational waffle designed to conceal a deeply damaging withdrawal of the state from its responsibilities to the most vulnerable. (Helm & Coman, 2012)

Network Social Capital

There is a second, and more academically robust, strand of social capital theorizing that has recently come to the forefront. The first approach, Putnam's and Kawachi's, focuses on social cohesion and is interested in the "capital" comprising the amount of trust and reciprocity available to social groups. It is implicitly or explicitly psychosocial in that societal trust and reciprocity are linked to reduced stress at the individual level. Living in a relatively equal community with lots of volunteer organizations and high levels of trust in one another (e.g., San Jose, California) engenders a positive endocrine response (low stress) and hence better health than living in divided and hostile community (e.g., Louisville, Kentucky). We already noted that the existence of this causal pathway is in question.

The second approach focuses on "**network capital,**" composed of informational and instrumental supports embedded in an individual's social network (Legh-Jones & Moore, 2012). A well-organized support group, for example, could function to provide information, companionship, emotional support, and instrumental assistance, such as transportation, for its members. Each member is a beneficiary of the "capital" created by the network. This is clearly a variant of neo-materialist theory, linking health outcomes to resources available to the person, in this case from the characteristics of the networks in which he or she participates. Researchers are currently exploiting network social capital theory to understand issues like maintaining healthy body mass indices and supporting healthy physical-activity levels in groups.

Sense of Community-Belonging

A fellow traveller of social capital theory is researchers' interest in the relationship between the "strength of sense of belonging" and health outcomes:

> Community-belonging—the degree to which an individual is, or perceives to be, connected to their community—has been a central element in a number of theoretical conceptualizations regarding how community contextual factors might be linked to health-related behaviours. Community belonging may influence the likelihood of undertaking behavioural changes through: (1) the exposure to health-related behaviour norms and attitudes in the community; (2) pychosocial mechanisms such as self-esteem, social status, control and social stress; and (3) access to material and other types of community resources. (Hystad & Carpiano, 2012, p. 277)

Community-belonging is strongly related to community-level capacity for healthy behavioural change. Thus it is regarded as "an important component of population health" (Hystad & Carpiano, 2012).

Social Exclusion

Some of the biggest health gaps exist between dominant populations and racialized groups captured within them. African-American men live eight years less than American white men (Centers for Disease Control and Prevention, 2010). Australian Indigenous men live 12 years less than Australian non-Indigenous men (Australian Institute of Health and Welfare, 2011). In the United Kingdom, Pakistani men live seven years less than non-Pakistani men (Wohland, Rees, Nazoo & Jagger, 2015). Twenty-six per cent of British Pakistani men report an activity-limiting illness compared to 15 per cent of white British men (Wohland, Rees, Nazoo & Jagger, 2015). And, of course, Canada's most prominent excluded population, Indigenous people, suffer the worst health in the country.

"Social exclusion" refers not only to the economic hardship of relative economic position, but also incorporates the notion of *the process of marginalization*—how individuals come, though their lives, to be excluded and marginalized from various aspects of social and community life (Shaw, Dorling, & Davey Smith, 2006). It is about power and the nature of social relations, hence social exclusion is a *process* arising from social structures rather than a stable artifact. It is thus a health-relevant feature that can only be understood appropriately and completely from a life-course/population-health perspective.

In Europe, in particular, social exclusion arrived in the early 2000s, at the top of many countries' policy agendas. Several social-policy concerns converged. One was the increasing presence of racialized and linguistic minorities in Western European countries as peoples from the Middle East, Asia, and Africa migrated into more affluent countries. Another was the growing significance of the religious divide between Muslim and non-Muslim Europeans combined with the potential for radicalization of the former into enemies of the latter. A third was the mounting evidence that health and social inequalities were particularly large and intractable between groups who were not fully integrated into broader society and the host population. Thus, in countries as diverse as Denmark, Germany, France, and England, remedies for social exclusion were sought ranging from increasing educational and employment opportunities to combatting racism to enforcing greater conformity by minorities to the practices of the majority.

Dealing with social exclusion, then, was seen as important but approaches have differed sharply. In France, the objective was to make everyone a secular French citizen adhering to core French values, whereas Scandinavian countries have tried to bridge ethnic and racial gaps by implementing policies aimed at improving the income of and access to public services by people of differing backgrounds, values, and interests. Both integrative (France) and multicultural policies (Scandinavia) seek to make it easier for different groups to co-operate and to share in the opportunities the country has to offer. And both, depending on how they are applied, can be reduced to efforts to assimilate. As such, policies may trivialize differences that are of fundamental importance to people, and consequently damage rather than enhance some of the factors important to human health.

Canadian research on the exclusion of racial and ethnic minority populations is underdeveloped. The earnings of immigrant cohorts are tracked over time by Statistics Canada, but how well minority populations are faring in terms of their mental and physical health is not. Officially, Canada has an inclusionary policy that formally values multiculturalism and diversity, but there is little evidence that minorities are well supported in Canada nor that much effort is made by any level of government to ensure groups are not excluded. Canada has arguably the strongest human rights and anti-hate laws in the world, but remains weak on ensuring access to good housing, employment opportunities, and safe, culturally appropriate health, education, and policing services.

While solutions are plainly not easy, and certainly not without controversy, the problem is obvious and growing. Migrants virtually everywhere have worse life prospects and worse health than members of the host society. Whereas in the 1950s and 1960s, migrants tended to achieve standards of living comparable to those of their host neighbours within a generation, sluggish economic growth has made this no longer true. Thus, while migrants may initially have better health than the host population ("**healthy immigrant effect**"), in today's world, the longer migrants stay in Canada, the US, the United Kingdom, and Australia, the worse their health becomes.

Box 7.4	Case Study ○ A Young Man from India

Nirav recently arrived in Canada from India via England. He is 19 years old and his family has just moved into a basement suite in Surrey, British Columbia. Nirav was an excellent student in his home community and something of a hero as a star midfielder on his high-school soccer team.

What health challenges—emotional, mental, and physical—might Nirav face over the next 10 years of his life in Canada?

Health prospects for minorities trapped within the host population are generally poor. But minorities who are able to group together in sizable numbers, creating their own communities and shared resources, such as the Chinese in British Columbia's lower mainland or Hispanics in New York, do better than migrants living in small enclaves (Stafford, Newbold, Bruce, & Ross, 2011).

In Canada, when compared to whites, South Asians and black Canadians have twice the risk of diabetes (Chiu, Austin, Manuel, & Tu, 2010). In the United States, infant mortality rates, a fairly reliable marker of the health of populations, vary substantially by ethnicity and place of residence.

Visible minorities generally face greater exclusion, greater difficulty in accessing services, getting jobs, and decent housing than cultural minorities. Since the economic downturns of the 1990s and 2000s, "new arrival," "visible minority," and "economically deprived" have become almost synonymous in Canada, the United States, the United Kingdom, and Australia. Today's immigrants to these nations are mostly from Africa and Asia, and a growing proportion are Muslim. The rising immigrant and refugee numbers, their ethnic, racial, and religious composition, and the poor performance of world economies since 2007 mean many affluent countries are facing something of a crisis. The alignment of race, ethnic difference, religion, and poverty with ongoing lack of opportunity and the hostile attitudes of the host populations is a toxic and explosive mix. Consequently, the United States is (again) contemplating stronger immigration restrictions and stepped-up deportations; Canada has imposed new limits on immigration and deportation appeals; and the United Kingdom has started advertising, telling potential immigrants that they are not wanted and job opportunities do not exist for them.

When sub-cultures of marginalization develop, especially among minority youth, the chasm between the excluded minority group and the dominant society grows. For example, in August 2011, black Caribbean neighbourhoods in London, England, erupted in riots and looting. Paris has seen similar ethnic and racial unrest. Along with rising social unrest, the health gap between the marginalized populations and the general population continues to grow. The size of that gap, and its variability, can be seen in the Table 7.4 data comparing white, African-American, and Hispanic infant mortality rates in different locations in the United States.

Table 7.4 Infant Mortality Rates per 1000 live births, United States, Selected States

State	White	African American	Hispanic
Alabama	6.8	13.6	7.7
California	4.6	11.4	5.0
Dist. of Columbia	3.4	17.2	7.2
Indiana	7.1	15.1	6.8
Massachusetts	4.0	10.0	6.5
Minnesota	4.3	8.9	4.2
New York	4.6	11.8	5.5
Washington	5.0	9.0	4.9

Source: Adapted from Henry J. Kaiser Family Foundation, 2009, p. 1.

Racism

Racism has biological roots. First, humans immediately recognize, in milliseconds, people who are of a different race— and react emotionally *before* they are even conscious of having noticed them. Second, functional MRI brain scans show that people react less strongly to people of a different race from themselves suffering pain than they do to people with whom they share racial characteristics (Sapolsky, 2017). However, innate reactivity is of little or no social consequence because higher brain functions, executive brain activity in the frontal cortex, can correct, modify, and override these innate reactions. The real trouble begins when beliefs, values, and social structures *reinforce the innate reactions,* producing "racism"—*social discrimination based on racial characteristics.*

The foundational belief grounding racism is "Those people are different from us, not only in skin colour and some other physical characteristics, but also in terms of their capacity for reason, regulation of their emotions, and moral behaviour." In short, "those people" are not fully human, they lack some critical capabilities, and that lack justifies "us" subjecting "them" to our control and regulation. Such beliefs get traction when there is significant advantage arising from subjugating and exploiting "them" in order to commandeer their labour (enslaving Africans) or to expropriate their lands (restricting indigenous peoples to reservations). Beliefs and values fuse to justify the exercise of power over other people, to exploit them to our advantage.

An institution like slavery (or the reserve system) entrenches the beliefs, values, and privileges of the dominant race. Now subordinated, immiserated, living and working under inhuman conditions, and denied educational and health care resources, the enslaved indeed look more and more like inferiors, while their exploiters prosper, growing the gap between "them and us." Attitudes, roles, and relationships persist even after the abolition of the institution that fostered them. Systems of privilege reproduce over generations via the intergenerational transfer of differences in wealth, education, income, and employment opportunities. Ideas such as a particular race's alleged propensity to criminality and violence persist because of the persistence of poverty, lack of opportunity, poor housing, and differential law enforcement.

Racism is not an adverse distinction between one person with a set of characteristics versus another; that is simply discrimination. The real significance of racism, and its huge impact on health, arises in its structural aspect. "Structural racism" refers to "the totality of ways in which societies foster racial discrimination through materially reinforcing systems of housing, education, employment, earnings, benefits, credit, media, health care, and criminal justice" (Bailey et al., 2017). These "ways" generate, perpetuate, and reinforce negative beliefs, while simultaneously determining the (unfair) distribution of resources.

In America, neighbourhood segregation affects housing quality, as well as neighbourhood characteristics such as availability of affordable, high-quality goods, parks, good quality of schools, health care, and much else. Differential access to high-quality education translates into differential access to high-quality, good-paying jobs. Employer prejudice already means, in America, that identically qualified black applicants will be called for an interview half as frequently as white ones (Pager & Shepherd, 2008). When employer prejudice is combined with real and perceived differences in education and training, the racial effect on employment is considerably amplified. Growing up in a segregated, deprived neighbourhood is predictive of a bad job, living in adulthood in poor housing in a bad neighbourhood, and harassment by police.

Racist police practices such as "carding" (demanding identification from people who have committed no offence) and provisions in statutes that differentially affect one race such as heavy penalties for crack cocaine (used mostly by blacks in inner cities) and light ones for powdered cocaine (used mostly by whites) and virtually no penalties for abusing prescription drugs (again mostly a white practice) skew criminal enforcement and contribute to disproportionate numbers of racial minorities being imprisoned. In America, sentences for crimes vary by race; the darker a defendant's skin, the longer his/her sentence (Sapolsky, 2017). Infamously, the probability of being beaten up or shot by police in America is a function of race.

Health effects of racism are well documented. Total loss of life expectancy ranges from 5 to 12 years; loss of healthy life expectancy is much greater. Racial minorities have elevated rates of coronary heart disease, anxiety, depression, obesity, and diabetes. Some of the effect is psychosocial and arises from the stress associated with continual vigilance, perceptions of lack of control and worth, and abuse by others. But much of it is resource or material based, in denial of access to high-quality education and job training, employment opportunities, fair credit at fair interest rates, decent housing, health care, and the opportunities that better-quality neighbourhoods accord their residents.

Policies of desegregation and improving opportunities through preferential admission to schools and employment can, and have, made some difference, but it is very difficult to shift informal practices through laws and policies. For example, the increasing segregation of cities like Detroit and Chicago has occurred in spite of desegregationist policy and civil rights laws— privileged people are using their privilege to establish their own, privileged, enclaves. Community development initiatives, infrastructure spending targeting less well-off neighbourhoods, efforts to improve schools in deprived areas, re-housing programs that move less privileged people to better neighbourhoods, and criminal justice reform that ends discriminatory arrest and sentencing all show promise. Unfortunately, progress is going to take time and considerable, persistent effort.

> **Pause and Reflect   Are You Racist?**
>
> Marlon James, the acclaimed Jamaican writer, posted the following video in 2015: https://www.theguardian.com/commentisfree/video/2016/jan/13/marlon-james-are-you-racist-video. In it, he challenges viewers to see that "not being a racist" is inadequate; we have a deeper obligation "to be anti-racist."
>
> Most people do not believe they discriminate or that they harbour racist beliefs and attitudes. Harvard University has devised a test for *implicit racism*—a test for values, beliefs, and motivations of which we may not be aware. You can access the test at the following URL: https://implicit.harvard.edu/implicit/Study?tid=-1

Theoretical Considerations

We can see at least five theoretical strands at work in the discussion of social support. The first may be typed "individual-level psychological," and depends on the provision by a person or persons of emotional, informational, or instrumental support. Essentially, the recipient of support is hypothesized to benefit from an enhanced ability to cope due to the aid he or she receives. And that enhanced ability, it is further hypothesized, should improve health, either through modifying the recipient's behaviour (e.g., taking their medication as prescribed) or by reducing their stress.

The second possibility is theorized as "collective-level psychosocial." Societal features such as norms of trust and reciprocity or functional community organization are hypothesized to produce protective effects, presumably through reducing the stress experienced by community members. Social capital theory fits this description.

A third possibility draws from social constructionist theory and focuses on the features of social networks rather than community organization. Here it is hypothesized that networks exert interactional effects on their members, influencing beliefs, values, and behaviours. Networks shape individuals' identity, practices, and conceptions of normalcy, and through those processes, impact on health and well-being.

"Collective-level materialism," a form of neo-materialism, is another theoretical possibility. Networks remain the unit of analysis, but the focus is now on the distributional effects of networks—how resources like information and instrumental support are apportioned among members. Health effects stem from the opportunities that arise for individuals from their engagement in social networks.

Finally, this chapter discussed a collective-level psychosocial hypothesis based on the concept of "sense of belonging." Here, it is hypothesized that a strong sense of community-belonging, which can be constructed both as a community feature and as an emotive state of individuals, enhances community empowerment and individual self-efficacy. Community empowerment and individual self-efficacy facilitate (and possibly are necessary conditions for) collective and individual change (e.g., adopting higher activity levels).

It is important to note that the psychosocial and materialist theoretical perspectives are not mutually exclusive. It is possible both sets of causal pathways operate in a given context. Moreover, it is difficult theoretically and operationally to pry them apart. Good-quality studies have found evidence in support of each of the five theoretical perspectives outlined above. In general, material and instrumental effects appear to be the most significant, and may arise at the individual level (direct support from other individuals) or collectively through networks and societal institutions.

Summary

Severe disruption of social structures, norms, and expectations for the future can have devastating effects on human well-being. For example, the ex-communist bloc continues to struggle with elevated coronary heart disease, mental health problems, and addictions.

It is less clear whether stable, supportive social relations improve health prospects, although there is some evidence to suggest that social solidarity and social cohesion have protective effects—in other words, may mitigate the harms of other health risks.

Social network theory has emerged as an important area of inquiry. Norms of health-relevant behaviour appear to be transmitted through our societies much like communicable diseases. Findings such as these are important in understanding how best to address problems like obesity and sedentary lifestyles.

Networks are also important social vehicles for the transmission of information and other health-relevant resources. Individuals embedded in rich, dense networks derive substantial health advantages, partly through direct resource benefits (e.g., enhanced income, enhanced self-efficacy) and partly through indirect means (e.g., better health information, effects on health behaviour).

In general, people benefit from social support and are harmed by social isolation. Mostly this appears to arise from material effects—receiving assistance, guidance, and information from others. Emotional support may play some role in heart and mental health, but does not appear to play a role in cancer incidence or prognosis.

Social exclusion is becoming a major social problem, one with serious health effects, particularly for racialized minorities. Canada, the United States, Australia, and Europe are all struggling with the potentially divisive and health-damaging effects of recent migration patterns. In this regard, it is worth recalling the dispute between Putnam and Hewstone over "hunkering down." Against Putnam, Hewstone argues that well-ordered neighbourhoods and constructive public policy can ensure that ethnic and racial diversity lead to more vibrant, more tolerant, more supportive, and hence, healthier communities.

Critical Thinking Questions

1. We now know that our membership in social networks has a major impact on our health-related beliefs, values, and behaviour. How might this discovery be used to address some of the big issues currently confronting health promotion, notably obesity and low levels of physical activity?

2. The evidence for effectiveness of disease-support groups (e.g., cancer survivors, diabetics) is mixed. Why might this be? Based on the research presented in the chapter,

how might support groups best be organized to achieve the goal of improving the mental and physical health of their members?

3. Canada and Australia have aimed at creating multicultural societies, whereas the US and France have pursued policies of assimilation. How might the different policy approaches to ethnic and racial diversity affect the health of the relevant populations?

Annotated Suggested Readings

The bestseller *Connected* provides an excellent overview of social network theory and various hypotheses regarding how our contacts with other people affect our ideas, our values, and our behaviour. N. Christakis and Fowler, J. *Connected: The Surprising Power of Social Networks and How They Shape Our Lives*, New York: Little Brown, 2009.

For Putnam's views on the destructive forces in contemporary advanced countries, the best resource is his highly readable 2006 Johan Skytte Prize Lecture, reprinted as the paper "*E Pluribus Unum*: Diversity and Community in the Twenty-First Century," *Scandinavian Political Studies*, 30(2):137–74. This paper is also available at www.utoronto.ca/ethnicstudies/Putnam.pdf.

Social Support and Physical Health: Understanding the Health Consequences of Relationships (B. Uchino, New Haven: Yale University Press, 2004) includes a comprehensive overview of the biopsychosocial model of human health and explores the complexity of the concept of social support. The book is especially strong on the problems of operationalizing social support as a variable and the validity and reliability of various approaches to measurement.

Annotated Web Resources

Connected: Slides
www.connectedthebook.com/pages/slides.html
Christakis and Fowler, the authors of *Connected: The Surprising Power of Social Networks and How They Shape Our Lives*, have posted a remarkable set of slides.

Center for Advanced Studies in Behavioral Sciences, Stanford University lecture, "Impact of Diversity on Intergroup Relations,"
https://www.youtube.com/watch?v=zrP6XPhvGTw
The lectures presented in this video include a discussion of Robert Putnam's and Miles Hewstone's divergent findings on conflict and diversity.

"Obesity and Social Networks: Health Matters"
www.youtube.com/watch?v=OTyZ7Kagh5I
The University of California produced an interesting video outlining the evidence for network effects on obesity incidence in the United States. Professor Fowler, co-author of *Connected*, discusses the research.

"The Secret to Living Longer May Be Your Social Life"
https://www.youtube.com/watch?v=ptlecdCZ3dg
Susan Pinker describes the secret to longer living as our social life in this TED Talk.

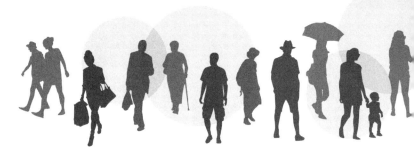

8 Health of Indigenous Peoples

Objectives

By the end of your study of this chapter, you should be able to
- appreciate the diversity of Indigenous people in Canada and the factors impacting on their health;
- understand the process of social exclusion and the means through which it adversely affects the health of excluded populations;
- apply the concepts of macro, intermediate, and individual-level health determinants.

Synopsis

Chapter 8 provides a profile of Indigenous people in Canada and the adverse impact of colonization by European settlers. The chapter outlines the negative health implications of discriminatory practices and racism, and then turns to the development of a conceptual framework for understanding the determinants of Indigenous health. The chapter concludes with a discussion of recent progress in addressing health inequities between Indigenous and non-Indigenous populations in Canada.

Pause and Reflect	Causes of the Health Gap between Indigenous and Non-Indigenous Populations

What factors contribute to the poor health and reduced-life expectancies of Canadian Indigenous people living on reserves? What steps could be taken to reduce the disparity between Indigenous and non-Indigenous health?

Who Are the Indigenous Peoples?

The Indigenous peoples of Canada were and remain very diverse. The peoples of the Arctic, the Pacific Northwest, the Prairies, Central Canada, and the Eastern seaboard have distinct histories, languages, and cultures—indeed unique civilizations. "There were as many as fifty or sixty different languages in Canada at the time of European contact in the fifteenth century" (Waldram, Herring, & Young, 2006, p. 6). Even peoples less separated by geography, such as the Dene tribes of the northern Canadian boreal forest, have little contact with, and remarkably little similarity to, the physically contiguous tribal groups such as the Cree further south. But tribal groups do not, and historically did not, exist in splendid isolation. Tribes migrated within the Americas and complex trading patterns developed, as did less peaceful struggles for territory, goods, and influence.

Exactly when the various groups arrived, and from whence they came, are still disputed matters. It appears the first humans settled in the Americas and then began to move south down the west coast around 20,000 years ago. They were followed by other groups of people migrating from what is today Siberia across the land bridge that existed at that time.

There is nothing unusual about these human migrations. Groups of people fanned out all over Africa, Europe, Asia, and the South Pacific 40,000 years ago, mingling with or out-competing earlier human arrivals, and settling down or moving on. Indeed, large-scale migrations of people continue to this day.

The Legacy of Racism and Colonization

Social exclusion associated with socio-economic status, ethnicity, religion, or race has deleterious effects on human health due to the familiar impact on (1) social status and self-esteem (psychosocial factors) and (2) constraints on resources for healthy living (material factors). Indigenous peoples in Canada, the United States, Australia, and many other parts of the world have been—and still are—socially excluded populations. Through historic conquest and colonization, they have experienced a process of marginalization, being pushed into small parcels of often remote and unproductive land. They continue to face racism and denigration.

Colonization of Indigenous lands by Europeans uprooted the peoples living there, undermined their means of subsistence, called into question the legitimacy of traditional beliefs and cultural practices, imposed religions and alien modes of thought and enquiry, established economic and social priorities without consultation, and supplanted the languages spoken by the indigenous tribes. All these changes came suddenly and relentlessly. They were experienced as a full-on assault to the culture and identity of the subjected peoples.

The pattern of subjection and exploitation, followed by efforts to Europeanize, began with the Spanish and Portuguese invasions of the Americas, extended northward to the French and English invasions of North America, and reached Australia and New Zealand in the eighteenth century. Colonization followed invasion. The support and assistance of Indigenous people were initially sought, but as the numbers of colonists grew, oppression and even efforts at extermination supplanted coexistence.

Indigenous people's capacity to resist the forces of colonization was severely curtailed by the diseases brought by the settlers. Measles and smallpox killed children and sickened adults. Famines associated with the loss of lands and environmental degradation lowered immunity and increased the death toll. In the United States, when Indigenous people resisted the loss of land to foreign settlers, the colonists began hunting or enslaving them. Later, with US independence, organized militias and armies attempted to exterminate them. In Canada, seeking to use the Indigenous people as a force against the anti-English expansionary-minded Americans, the British Crown offered promises and treaties, but in one-sided deals with tribes under extreme duress. The terms were misrepresented, and the Crown unilaterally abrogated many agreements.

In more recent times, with the settlers entrenched, virtually all land and resources controlled by the new arrivals and their companies, and European-style institutions from law to education to health care to governments firmly in command, consideration turned to dealing with the residual "Indian problem." It had become apparent that the containment of Indigenous peoples on small parcels of land set aside for their use and the maintenance of their cultures was not a sustainable solution. The reserves were simply not large enough and did not contain enough resources to maintain their peoples, and changes to the natural environment wrought by European agriculture, hunting, fishing, and forestry made traditional life impossible in all but a few locations, such as the Far North and the Arctic lands of the Inuit. Health and general living conditions were plainly deteriorating, and socio-economically sensitive diseases like tuberculosis (TB) were becoming epidemic.

In the US, Canada, and Australia, policy-makers came to similar conclusions in the immediate post–Second World War period. Basic health, education, food security, and housing services needed to be provided to Indigenous people. Doing so, however, presented a logistical challenge given that the Indigenous people did not typically live in easily serviced, large, year-round settlements. The obvious answer (at least, obvious to governments in the social engineering heyday of the 1950s) was to relocate people to purpose-built settlements composed of inexpensive, Western-style houses. The project of relocation, however, proved problematic because many people did not want to move, did not see any benefit in the prefabricated towns, and (correctly) saw the relocations as a further nail in the cultural coffin. Undeterred, governments forced the moves, uprooting Indigenous peoples yet again.

With the new government-provided health centres and hospital ships, it became easy to diagnose TB, but not so easy to treat it. In the 1950s and 1960s, the only approach to managing the disease was residential care in a sanatorium. Sanatoria in small Indigenous communities were impractical, so large ones were built in urban centres that were hundreds, or even thousands, of kilometres distant. Indigenous people were understandably unsettled by government chest X-ray campaigns that could, and did, lead to mothers being sent away from their children for six or more months, and to children being separated from siblings and parents. Between 1953 and 1961, over 5,000 Inuit were sent to southern TB hospitals; at the time, the entire Eastern Arctic had a population under 12,000. And, of course, while in the sanatoria, the patients were exposed to TV, priests, educators, and health care providers, few of whom exhibited cultural sensitivity or made any effort to preserve and protect Indigenous culture and language.

Also beginning in the 1950s, foodstuffs were trucked, flown, or shipped in by boat to the newly created Indigenous communities. Those foodstuffs were cheap staples such as flour, sugar, and canned goods, products that upended traditional diets and provided far too much energy and far too little nutrition. Obesity, large-for-gestational-age babies, and diabetes quickly ensued.

Residential Schools

The worst assault on Indigenous people, however, began much earlier—in the 1870s—when Canada and Australia (following the US example) decided that education in general, and vocational training in particular, would be the most effective route to ending poverty and social problems in Indigenous communities, while simultaneously smoothing the way for the complete integration of the remaining Indigenous populations into Western society. Because schools and technical institutes were impractical in very small Indigenous settlements, the answer lay in building regional facilities, in this case residential schools. The initiative required removing children from their families. That was not an accidental, but rather an essential, part of the policy. Separating the children from their communities and families would divorce them from their language, culture, way of life, and ties to land, preparing them for assimilation into the English-speaking, Christian, market economy.

The Canadian federal government wanted to spare the taxpayer the enormous expense of such a social engineering project and turned to churches to undertake the work. Essentially contracting out Indigenous education to ecclesiastical organizations, governments took a hands-off approach, failing utterly to ensure proper standards, the respectful and safe care of the children, and ignoring completely the psychological trauma to families and their children embedded in the residential school model.

Unfortunately, pedophiles and child abusers are drawn to all work involving children, especially in residential contexts, and particularly when standards are lax and oversight absent. Residential schools proved no exception. The churches also took full advantage of their situation to proselytize, justifying the approach as "saving souls," but destroying Indigenous culture and spirituality in the process. In many schools, using Indigenous languages or following an Indigenous practice was met with punishment. Thus, while it is true some residential school teachers were caring and ethical, the model itself was vile and fundamentally flawed; hence, enormous damage was done to thousands of children and their families.

The effects were cumulative. The historic uprooting and undermining of Indigenous people; the assault on their subsistence and culture; the decimation of populations by disease, famine, and genocide; the forced relocations; the sanatoria; the food-aid programs; and the residential schools worked synergistically to harm the mental and physical health of Indigenous populations. By the time the relocation of Indigenous communities and residential school projects were finally abandoned in the 1990s, enormous damage had been done.

The Indigenous Peoples of Canada

In Canada, governments refer to "status Indians," "non-status Indians," "treaty Indians," "Métis," and "Inuit" as comprising Indigenous peoples. A status Indian or a *registered status Indian* refers to someone who has the legal status of an Indian under Canada's *Indian*

Act (1876). Not all registered status Indians are culturally, genetically, or self-identified as Indigenous: until 1985, status could be acquired by women through marriage. "Non-status Indians" refers to people of Indigenous ancestry who either never qualified for registration or lost their legal status under the *Indian Act*. Treaty Indians are registered status Indians who have rights under a settled treaty. Treaties involve relinquishing rights to the land in return for land set aside for exclusive use and a variety of governmental undertakings. All treaty Indians are registered (status Indians) but not all status Indians are covered by treaty. In fact, in parts of Canada, notably British Columbia, very few are covered, and negotiations between government and representatives of registered status Indians regarding land and government obligations ("land-claims negotiations") are ongoing. Indian bands and tribal councils operating under negotiated treaties are referred to as "First Nations," and the expression "First Nations people" is more or less synonymous with "treaty Indian." Métis are culturally linked to Indigenous peoples and they self-identify as "Indigenous." Mostly, they are mixed-race descendants of Scottish and French traders. Inuit live in the high Arctic and are a distinct population.

The Health of Indigenous Peoples

From a health perspective, the picture is a bleak one. Millions of Indigenous people died from infectious diseases communicated by the new arrivals. North American Indigenous peoples had no immunity to the commonplace European viruses smallpox and measles. Millions more died from food insecurity as the result of environmental change wrought by European settlement. The introduction of firearms and the European appetite for meat and hides decimated the prairie herds of bison. European overfishing destroyed salmon and other fish stocks, virtually eliminating the historic food sources of many North American peoples. Forestry and agriculture changed the landscape, reducing substantially the production of wild foods. A much-reduced Indigenous population found itself dependent on European foodstuffs, especially cheap staples like lard, flour, and sugar.

Conditions stemming from poor nutrition, poor housing, and overcrowding on the lands set aside for First Nations people, and social problems such as alcoholism and family violence arising from poverty, marginalization, and the residential school experience combine to create the poor health profile of First Nations people today. Diabetes, tuberculosis, respiratory diseases, heart disease, cirrhosis of the liver, and death by suicide and violence are all much more common among today's First Nations people living on reserve than among non-Indigenous people.

Premature deaths among Indigenous people in Canada are reflected in the projected life expectancies at birth in Figure 8.1.

Table 8.1   Indigenous Health, Off Reserve, Over 20 Years Old, Canada, 2007

Self-Report	Non-Indigenous	First Nations*	Métis**	Inuit
Excellent or very good health	58.7%	51.3%	56.7%	49.2%

* Self-identified as being associated with a tribe.
** Self-identified as of Scottish/French/First Nations heritage.
Source: Adapted from Garner, Carriere, & Sanmartin (2010), p. 3. Available at http://publications.gc.ca/collections/collection_2010/statcan/82-622-X/82-622-x2010004-eng.pdf

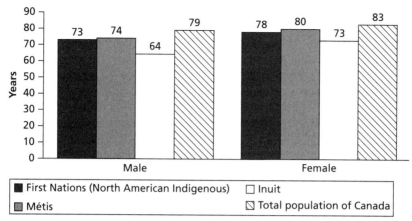

1. Estimated data

Note(s): 'Life expectancy' is an estimate of the number of years a person is expected to live, for a given year. Most often reported as life expectancy at birth, but it can be reported at any age, for different population groups.

Figure 8.1 Projected Life Expectancy at Birth by Sex, Indigenous Identity, 2017[1]

Source: http://www.statcan.gc.ca/pub/89-645-x/2010001/c-g/c-g013-eng.htm

The life expectancy of Indigenous peoples has been increasing more rapidly than that of non-Indigenous residents of Canada. Thus, since 2000, there has been some convergence. However, in parts of Canada, and on rural reserves in particular, there has not been a trend toward improvement. In Alberta, the health situation of First Nations people has actually deteriorated (see Figure 8.2).

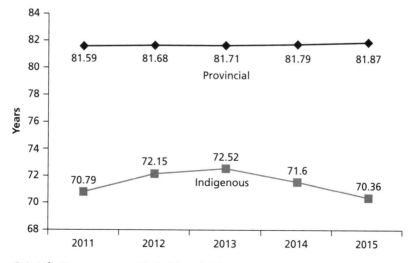

Figure 8.2 Life Expectancy at Birth (Years), Alberta

Source: http://www.afnigc.ca/main/includes/media/pdf/fnhta/HTAFN-2016-05-31-LifeExp2.pdf

Discrimination and Health of Indigenous Peoples

The word "discrimination" comes from the Latin *discriminare,* "to divide, separate, distinguish." In current usage it refers to "the unjust or prejudiced treatment of different categories of people" (OED, 2011). At issue are (a) practices of dominant groups to maintain privileges they accrue through subordinating the groups they oppress and (b) the ideologies they use to justify those practices. Practices may include differential access to resources like education, health care, and job opportunities. Ideologies include beliefs such as that Indigenous people are "primitive" or that they have a different "child-like" orientation to the world that justifies subordination to whites.

Discrimination between groups of people is more pervasive than is apparent on first consideration. People under-report their negative social attitudes because they realize that admitting to such attitudes would cast them in a poor light. Moreover, dominant groups typically deny that discrimination exists. Rather, they regard themselves as dominant because of their alleged superior education or intelligence or work ethic. The hallmarks of contemporary discrimination, then, are not expressions of hostility, but rather are paternalism combined with an expression of friendly feelings alongside a denial of responsibility for the plight of oppressed peoples. What matters from a health point of view is not what the dominant population believes but rather the experience of the oppressed minority. Currently, nearly 40 per cent of First Nation adults living on reserves in Canada report they have experienced one or more instances of racism in the past 12 months (Reading & Wien, 2009).

Pathways embodying discrimination include the following:

- economic and social deprivation such as unemployment and substandard housing;
- segregation, such as the reserve system in Canada, the United States, and Australia;
- exposure to toxic substances such as the tar sands pollution of the Athabasca River in northern Alberta (the people affected downstream are tribes of Indigenous people);
- socially inflicted trauma such as residential schools and related assimilation policies;
- targeted marketing of unhealthy items, such as the historic targeting of Indigenous people by whisky traders;
- inadequate health care, education, and social services.

Economic and Social Deprivation

The median income of Indigenous people in Canada is 30 per cent lower than that of non-Indigenous Canadians (Wilson & Macdonald, 2010). The 2010 unemployment rate for Indigenous adults (15 to 65 years old) was 13.9 per cent, compared with 8.1 per cent for non-Indigenous Canadians (Statistics Canada, 2010). Housing conditions on most Canadian reserves and throughout Nunavut are poor. Housing, in general, is in bad condition and is typically overcrowded. Low income combines with poor housing; the cumulative risk to Indigenous health is substantially greater than either low income or poor housing alone.

Segregation

Reserves serve to isolate their residents from mainstream Canadian society and, most importantly, from the resources available to non-Indigenous communities. Critical public services, such as quality education, health care, fire protection, transportation, potable water systems, sewers, and organized refuse collections, are either missing or underdeveloped on reserves. Many reserves and Inuit Arctic communities are very isolated, meaning that goods and services are scarce and expensive.

Relations between reserves and adjacent non-Indigenous communities are frequently strained, with non-Indigenous communities often withholding fire, ambulance, and police services because residents of Indigenous reserves do not contribute to local government taxes. Indigenous people leaving the reserve may face significant prejudice from non-Indigenous people, who often embrace negative stereotypes of Indigenous people, regarding them as unemployed welfare recipients. The lack of support from, and not infrequent hostility of, the non-Indigenous population has dual, synergistic effects on health—first by denying resources readily available to non-Indigenous populations, and second through the stress and dehumanization experienced as a consequence of racism.

The reserve system, continuing discrimination, and the lack of educational, social, cultural, and employment opportunities reinforce the exclusion of Indigenous peoples from mainstream Canadian life.

Exposure to Toxic Substances

Because Indigenous communities in the past enjoyed very little status and power, their interests have frequently been compromised by industrial developments, such as mining, petroleum extraction, forestry, and pulp and paper manufacturing. Affluent and politically connected communities can successfully block prejudicial development, but marginalized communities cannot. Thus, we see many examples in Canada where industrial developments have been planned to protect non-Indigenous communities but harm Indigenous ones. A case in point is the pulp and paper mill in Powell River, British Columbia. The mill was situated so that the toxic and very unpleasant plume of stack effluent would be directed away from the (non-Indigenous) town but directly into the adjacent Indigenous community. It is doubtful that anyone intended to harm the Indigenous people. Instead, these people did not count in the planning because they had no effective voice. Oil sands development in northern Alberta, and mining operations in British Columbia and northern Ontario, have been justly accused of similar indifference. This is not a uniquely Indigenous issue. Marginalized communities find toxic landfills or nasty industrial activities popping up in their neighbourhoods, whereas their richer and better-connected neighbours do not.

Box 8.1   Case Study ○ Mercury Crisis in Ontario

Reed Paper dumped mercury into the English Wabigoon River in the 1960s, contaminating the water, and hence the fish, downstream. The people of Grassy Narrows and Wabaseemoong First Nations relied on the fish for food and the river water for drinking. Before the contamination was discovered, there was widespread mercury poisoning of local Indigenous peoples. Today, 90% of those people show signs of mercury poisoning and the river water is still contaminated, despite repeated promises and remedial measures by the federal and the Ontario governments. The Ontario government contends that disturbing the river sediments in an effort to undertake a thorough clean-up will make the contamination worse. Environmentalists and the First Nations disagree. ("Ontario Knew about Mercury," 2017)

Socially Inflicted Trauma

A great deal has been written about socially inflicted trauma associated with Canadian assimilation policies, particularly residential schools. Although assimilationist policies were reversed in the 1980s and 1990s, a generation of Indigenous people has been born to parents whose family lives and connections with Indigenous traditions were forcibly severed. The sequelae in Canada include elevated levels of family abuse, substance misuse, and mental health problems.

Over the course of the life of residential schools in Canada (1879–1996), more than 20 per cent of Indigenous children, roughly 150,000, were taken from their families and communities (Schwartz, 2015). In 2006, the Indian Schools Settlement Agreement was concluded, and the prime minister, Stephen Harper, apologized on behalf of Canadians to First Nations people. A $2 billion compensation package with an average lump-sum payment of $28,000 was put in place for all former residential school students. The agreement also allocated $60 million for a Truth and Reconciliation Commission charged with documenting the experiences of past students.

Targeted Marketing of Unhealthy Products

In the nineteenth and early twentieth centuries, Indigenous people in Canada and the United States were subjected to heavy commercial pressure from whisky traders and tobacco merchants. Government efforts to protect Indigenous communities from those activities were sporadic and generally ineffectual, establishing legacies of excessive alcohol and tobacco use. More recently, US food-aid policies led to the dumping of unhealthy foods made up of refined carbohydrates, lard, and sugar on Indian reservations. Currently, Canadian provincial and territorial governments ensure uniform pricing of alcohol but not of foodstuffs. Thus, a bottle of whisky costs the same in remote northern Yukon as it does in Vancouver, but a litre of milk may cost two or three times as much.

Inadequate Health and Social Services

The Canadian federal government is responsible for health care, education, and social services on reserves. In general, it has not discharged this function well. The health care provided is basic, primary care, provided mostly by outpost nurses. Professional staff turnover is high and morale is often low. Nursing stations, cottage hospitals, and federal regional Indian hospitals have a poor track record, and are underfunded and understaffed. The severely ill or injured must be evacuated to larger centres, often incurring delays that compromise well-being. Social services are often next to non-existent beyond welfare and housing services of varying quality administered by Indigenous governments.

Drinking Water

Because of poor drinking-water infrastructure (using surface sources combined with inadequate treatment and distribution systems), 70 First Nations communities in Canada have been under long-term, more or less permanent, boil-water advisories. The drinking water, simply put, is unsafe. The current federal Liberal government, elected in 2015, promised to end boil-water advisories on reserves, and did manage, by August 2017, to lift 18 of them. But 12 new ones have been added. Nearly $2 billion was included in the 2016 federal budget to upgrade systems and train local people to maintain them; that has been added to the $3 billion over eight years committed by the previous government (Tunney, 2017).

The Health of the Indigenous Population in Canada

As you would expect from their economic position, Indigenous people in many parts of the world are marooned on the demographic and epidemiological transitions. Birth rates remain high, but death rates, especially infant mortality, have come down. Hence, Indigenous populations are very young and are growing rapidly, from roughly 4 per cent to about 5 per cent of the Canadian population over the past few decades. Nearly one-half of the Indigenous population in Canada is under age 25 (Garner, Carriere, & Sanmartin, 2010).

Infectious and parasitic diseases such as TB, scabies, sexually transmitted infections, and head lice remain serious problems, but chronic diseases are also commonplace. Indigenous populations thus face, in many on-reserve situations, the effects of high rates of heart disease and diabetes combined with high rates of respiratory and other infectious diseases such as HIV/AIDS. On-reserve age-standardized diabetes rates currently stand at 19 per cent, compared to 5.2 per cent for the Canadian population as a whole (Health Canada, 2011).

Some years ago, the health transition for Indigenous peoples in Canada was described as shared with other populations undergoing rapid socio-cultural change. This description of key features experienced by the Inuit remains true for Indigenous people today:

> The health transition experienced by the Inuit is shared by many other populations undergoing rapid socio-cultural change. Its key features are
>
> (1) the precipitous decline in infectious diseases (such as tuberculosis), which have stabilized at a level that remains higher than in the general, national population;
> (2) a corresponding increase in the chronic diseases such as heart disease;
> (3) the most important group of health problems, however, is the so-called social pathologies: violence, accidents, suicide, and alcohol and substance abuse. (Bjerregaard, Young, Dewailly, & Ebbesson, 2004)

Death rates in Inuit Nunangat (the Inuit homelands of Nunavut, northern Quebec, and northern Labrador) are disturbingly high. The age-standardized mortality rate at ages 1 to 19 stands at 188 deaths per 100,000, compared with 35 deaths per 100,000 in the rest of Canada. Death rates for unintentional (accidental) injury stand at 40 per 100,000 in Nunangat, versus less than 8 per 100,000 for the rest of Canada. Death rates for intentional injury (suicide) stand at 75 per 100,000 in Nunangat, versus 3 per 100,000 for Canada as a whole (Statistics Canada, 2012).

Conditions under which many Indigenous people live on reserves in Canada are more comparable to living conditions in impoverished parts of the world than to those of non-Indigenous people in their own country. Reserves frequently have only the most basic health care and education services and next to no potable water, sewage, road, electrical, or communications infrastructure. Many are isolated, rural, and remote. In Canada, more than one in six reservations is currently under a boil-water advisory (Health Canada, 2011), meaning the water is not safe to drink. In 2005, the entire

Kashechewan Reserve in northern Ontario was evacuated because of E. coli contamination of its only water supply. Housing, especially in Nunavut in the Canadian Arctic, is not only in appalling condition, but is also seriously overcrowded. The health effects of overcrowding are cumulative and include psychological problems, stress, anxiety, and aggression, as well as elevated incidence of infectious diseases, notably skin and respiratory infections.

In recent years, infant mortality rates and infectious disease incidence have fallen dramatically in the Canadian Arctic and among Indigenous people living in southern Canada. However, chronic disease rates, particularly diabetes incidence, have continued to rise. Moreover, social exclusion, poverty, and continuing poor living conditions fuel mental health problems, addictions, family violence, and suicide. Accident, violence, and suicide rates for Inuit and First Nations populations in Canada remain high; in fact, suicide rates among the Inuit are the highest in the world. In general, Table 8.2 shows physical and mental health is worst for Inuit, slightly better for First Nations, better still for Métis, and best for non-Indigenous Canadians. The largest differences are in self-reported physical and mental health. It should be noted that self-report is a robust measure that aligns well with measures by independent observers.

Understanding the Determinants of Indigenous Health

A useful way to look at the variables affecting the health of Indigenous people is to categorize them as macro, intermediate (meso), and individual-level variables. **Macro determinants** are contextual and historical. They include colonialism, social exclusion and racism, and community governance/self-determination. These macro-level variables create broader circumstances under which individuals live and come

Table 8.2 Health Indicators, First Nations,* Métis, Inuit, and Non-Indigenous, 12 Years and Older, per cent

	First Nations	Métis	Inuit	Non-Indigenous
Arthritis	18.7	10.1	14.5	16.1
Asthma	12.9	14.4	8.9	8.0
Diabetes	8.2	6.4	2.6	6.5
High blood pressure/CHD	17.7	18.3	13.7	20.1
Health "very good"	48.5	51.3	44.9	59.9
Health "fair or poor"	19.1	16.0	14.5	11.0
Mental health "very good"	61.3	63.5	59.5	71.9
Mental health "fair or poor"	10.8	8.8	6.9	5.9

*on and off reserve. On-reserve disease prevalence is much higher than shown here.
Source: Data drawn from Statistics Canada, Table CANSIM 105-0512, 2015.

to understand their social world. The key **intermediate determinants** or meso-level variables are community capacity and opportunity structure. The availability of affordable high-quality food, access to primary health care, community infrastructure, such as roads, potable water supply, garbage removal and sewage treatment, and educational opportunities all fit here. As we have seen, those intermediate-level variables profoundly affect health behaviour and have direct impacts on individual health. The familiar individual-level determinants are income, workplace quality, and level of remuneration from employment; housing conditions; exposure to environmental contaminants; and health behaviour ranging from food choices to smoking to use of alcohol to risk taking. Each level of determinant, as Krieger (2008) argues, interacts with the other levels, as well as shaping the beliefs, attitudes, behaviour, health, and well-being of the person. An example is provided by Figure 8.3. Interaction between determinants is further illustrated in the following passage from Reading and Wien (2009):

> Not only do social determinants influence diverse dimensions of health, but they also create health issues that often lead to circumstances and environments that, in turn, represent subsequent determinants of health. For instance, living in conditions of low income have been linked [directly] to increased illness and disability, which in turn represents a social determinant, which is linked to diminished opportunities to engage in gainful employment thereby aggravating poverty. (p. 2)

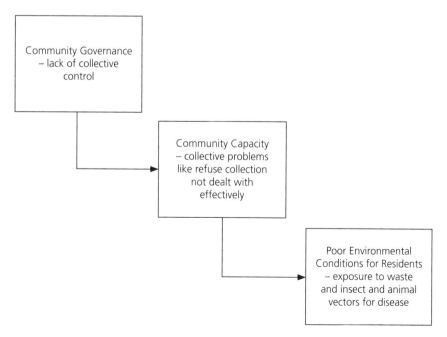

Figure 8.3 Example of Levels of Determination

Macro Determinants

The processes of conquest and colonization systematically dislocated Indigenous people from the land, their principal basis for defining themselves. Additionally, as we noted, governments in Canada aggressively pursued the assimilation and acculturation of Indigenous people, a process that many Indigenous people regard as a form of genocide. In Canada, as we noted earlier, about 20 per cent of adults living on reserve attended residential schools and, of that 20 per cent, approximately 80 per cent report they were negatively affected by isolation from their family, verbal or emotional abuse, harsh discipline, and loss of cultural identity (Reading & Wien, 2009). Individual-level outcomes ranging from a sense of alienation, pervasive depression, family and community instability, and general loss of sense of well-being have all been attributed to the colonial/assimilationist history. Perhaps even more significant is the community-level loss of self-determination which, in turn, undermines individual-level self-esteem, sense of control and belief in personal efficacy—all key determinants of individual health. Adopting healthy behaviours, for example, requires a belief in one's personal capacity to make the necessary behavioural change as well as the sense that one's quality of life will benefit from it.

Intermediate Determinants

Box 8.2	Case Study ○ Birthing Centres

The Inuit in Canada continue to have a relatively high infant mortality rate and very limited access to obstetrical services. Many pregnant women continue to be transferred by medevac to southern hospitals where they give birth alone, separated from their family and their community. To address this problem, Canada adopted in 2004 a model that had proved successful in Greenland: birthing centres. However, shortly afterward, the Nunavut centres were considered failures and were all closed. Gold, O'Neil, and Van Wagner (2007) argued that birthing centres failed because the requisite macro and intermediate variables were not appropriately addressed. The Nunavut centres could only be successful, in their view, if more attention were placed on community development, Inuit self-government, housing, and education. Gold and her colleagues called for a more integrated, community-based approach, rooted in Inuit traditions.

How and why are community development and self-government connected to the success of community health and social services?

The discussion of intermediate determinants raises the question "How important are health and social services to Indigenous health?" While not the major determinant of health, access to quality health care plays a role, especially in managing disease or trauma once it has occurred. As already noted, health care and other services on reserve are not good. Reading and Wien (2009, p. 15) aptly characterize the situation on Canadian reserves: "The federal system of health care delivery . . . resembles a collage of public health programs with limited accountability, fragmented delivery, and jurisdictional ambiguity." Historically, provincial and federal governments have fought over who is responsible for and who should pay the cost of health care for Indigenous people, typically creating enormous confusion and gaps in service. Because First Nations and Inuit are federal wards and the national government is responsible for their health care, provinces refused to extend health care insurance ("Medicare") and public health services to Indigenous communities. (This problem has now been largely solved by federal–provincial agreements.) Non-treaty Indians and off-reserve Indigenous people not infrequently found themselves *without either federal or provincial coverage for their health care needs.* Staffing health care facilities in rural and remote communities has been and remains challenging and turnover, under-qualified personnel, and closures are commonplace. Where services are available, they often are not culturally sensitive nor delivered appropriately from the perspective of the Indigenous community.

Educational programming has also been haphazard and ineffectual. The final report on the Nunavut Land Claims Agreement described the education system in Canada's Far North as "in a shambles" (Curry, 2007). Key initiatives such as the Aboriginal Head Start Program—an infant and early childhood development program—remain underdeveloped and underfunded (Reading & Wien, 2009). Lack of cultural relevance of the school curriculum and its delivery are factors in the poor high-school completion rate; nearly half of Indigenous children drop out of high school, although some return as adult learners. Approximately 36 per cent of on-reserve adults have completed high school compared with 85 per cent of adults off reserve. The situation is even worse for Inuit; in Nunavut, there is a 75 per cent school drop-out rate (Curry, 2007). Only 5 per cent of on-reserve Indigenous adults have any post-secondary education compared with 22.7 per cent for Canadian adults as a whole. In consequence, the unemployment rate on reserve is 28 per cent compared to 7 per cent for Canada as a whole (Health Canada, 2011). We have already seen that education is a major determinant of health; Chapter 9 will show the importance of steady, high-quality employment for health and well-being.

Individual-Level Determinants

Nearly one-third of Inuit and about 15 per cent of on-reserve First Nations Indigenous people report living in overcrowded dwellings (Reading & Wien, 2009). Crowding is very stressful and is implicated in anxiety, depression, family violence, substance abuse, and poor learning by children. It is also a direct cause of adverse health outcomes through factors such as poor indoor air quality, poor sanitation, and transmission of skin and respiratory diseases.

The state of housing on reserve and in the Arctic is also a major health issue. Nearly one-third of houses need substantial repairs (Reading & Wien, 2009). Poor ventilation and heating, as well as mould and unsafe electrical, cooking, and heating arrangements all take a toll on the health and safety of occupants. Fatal house fires remain common on reserve and in the Arctic, partly due to the fire dangers associated with prefabricated housing, partly due to heating by wood fires, partly due to faulty wiring, and partly due to the absence of smoke detectors and the lack of community fire-suppression capabilities, such as fire engines and hydrants.

Suicide, particularly among adolescent males, is a major social and health problem. The male rate of suicide in Nunavut in 2001 was 131.9 per 100,000, compared to a Canadian rate of 17.9 (Dobrota, 2007). Epidemics of suicide are commonplace in isolated First Nations reserves and small Arctic hamlets. For example, in a single week in the small community of Hazelton, British Columbia, seven Gitxsan youth attempted suicide ("BC Community Pleads for Help," 2007). Chandler and Lalonde (1998) show that suicide on reserves is largely a function of social disintegration and collapse of identity. Communities with stronger "cultural continuity" and a higher degree of social cohesion have lower rates of suicide (Reading & Wien, 2009). Causes are thus more macro and less individual than might first appear.

Approximately 16 per cent of on-reserve Indigenous people drink heavily compared to 8 per cent of Canadians as a whole. Heavy alcohol use, not only among Indigenous people but also in other populations, is associated with depression and loss of meaning. Young men are particularly vulnerable because, in the absence of traditional hunting roles and contemporary roles as paid workers in steady employment, they often perceive their lives as meaningless and without direction. Nearly two-thirds of First Nations on-reserve adults smoke, compared with less than one-quarter of Canadian adults as a whole (Health Canada, 2011). Smoking, like alcohol use, is associated with depression and loss of meaning. Nearly 40 per cent of Indigenous women report smoking during pregnancy and a substantial proportion also drink alcohol while pregnant, even though it is widely understood by Indigenous people themselves that smoking and drinking during pregnancy can harm the fetus (Reading & Wien, 2009). Low levels of education and expensive and hard to acquire nutrient-rich (versus energy-rich) foods contribute to high rates of obesity and consequent diabetes and renal disease. Almost three-quarters of on-reserve First Nations adults are overweight, compared to one-half of the general Canadian adult population (Health Canada, 2011).

The big differences displayed in Table 8.3 are the per cent overweight, the per cent who have a regular doctor, the per cent smoking, and the per cent getting the recommended servings of fruit and vegetables. As in disease prevalence (Table 8.2), in general,

Table 8.3 Individual-Level Factors, First Nations,* Métis, Inuit, and Non-Indigenous, 12 years and Older, per cent

Factor	First Nations	Métis	Inuit	Non-Indigenous
BMI overweight or obese	64.3	61.1	62.1	52.7
Regular doctor	78.1	80.8	43.3	85.1
Current smoker	28.7	27.3	44.7	14.1
Five or more drinks on one or more occasion per month	25.3	26.1	23.1	18.0
Fruit and vegetables five times a day	31.0	37.1	24.0	40.6
Physically active	53.1	57.2	48.2	54.1

*on and off reserve. On reserve individual-level risk factors are much greater than shown here.
Source: Data drawn from Statistics Canada, Table CANSIM 105-0512, 2015.

individual-level factors are worst for Inuit, slightly better for First Nations, better yet for Métis, and best for non-Indigenous Canadians.

Smoking, diet, and obesity play a role in the health gap between Indigenous and non-Indigenous people, but it would be a mistake to regard health disparities as arising from individual-level health behaviour and intermediate-level community resources. Garner and colleagues (2010) adjusted for known health-risk factors such as smoking, body mass index, and access to health care services. They found that controlling for those factors did little to lessen health disparities. Socio-economic conditions account for almost all of the difference seen between health of Indigenous people and health of the broader population. Risky behaviours such as smoking and substance abuse heighten or amplify, but do not create, the differences in health status. Rather, they, like the health impacts, arise from the conditions under which Indigenous people are living.

It is easy to demonstrate that the adverse health effects are primarily socio-economic. In Canada, for example, the health of Indigenous people living off reserve, even though most urban Indigenous people remain poorer than other Canadians, is much better than the health of their even poorer brothers and sisters who remain on reserve. This demonstrates that the health disadvantage of Indigenous people is not arising from genetic or biologic factors, but rather from the conditions under which they are living. Income, housing, nutrition, and education are better, on average, for off-reserve Indigenous people than they are for their on-reserve counterparts. Those better conditions are reflected in better health and longevity. Similarly, income aligns with Indigenous identity, as shown in Table 8.4, an alignment that translates into health and life expectancies.

Since 2000, the income gap between Indigenous and non-Indigenous Canadians has been shrinking, but it remains close to 30 per cent. For Indigenous Canadians with a university degree, the gap has disappeared, and incomes have become equivalent (Wilson & Macdonald, 2010). Slowly, progress has been made, mostly because educational attainment among Indigenous people has increased dramatically, although it still lags behind non-Indigenous Canadians.

Table 8.4 Income Characteristics, Canadian Population 15 Years of Age and Older, 2001

Income	Indigenous (total)	First Nations	Métis	Inuit	Non-Indigenous
Full-time employment	33,416	32,176	34,778	36,152	43,486
Part-time employment	13,795	12,837	15,386	12,866	19,383
Government transfers as % of total income	20.8	24.3	15.7	20.3	11.5
Median income	13,525	12,263	16,542	13,699	22,431
Incidence of low-income families (%)	31.2	37.3	24.5	21.9	12.4
Incidence of low-income, unattached individuals (%)	55.9	59.8	51.7	56.8	37.6

Source: Based on Statistics Canada, Topic-based Tabulations, Census topic number 97F0011XCB2001047.

Far and away the biggest factor impacting Indigenous health remains income and its correlates, education and employment. Low income and low levels of education not only severely limit the opportunities and capabilities of Indigenous people but also mean many are dependent on their band, tribal council, or the federal government for income and housing. Welfare dependency, another intermediate-level variable, undermines initiative and the sense of personal control and self-esteem. Moreover, the arbitrary character of the chronic poor governance experienced by people in Indigenous communities, whether it is capricious changes in programs, services, or beneficiaries by the federal authorities or corruption and nepotism at the level of community leadership, undermines predictability and sense of personal efficacy at the individual level.

A Story of Dramatic Improvement

In recent years, First Nations, Métis, and Canadian governments have rediscovered that the way forward is the one recommended by Virchow over 160 years ago—empowerment through recognition and enforcement of human and civil rights, combined with the economic resources required to transform living conditions. This is in fact now taking place through land-claims negotiations, devolution of authority from governments to tribal councils and economic joint ventures between tribes, other levels of government, and private investors.

Over the past 20 years, the federal government devolved many of its responsibilities for housing, social services, and health care onto First Nations. Provincial governments have similarly devolved services like child welfare. Municipalities and First Nations governments have struck agreements on fire protection, ambulance services, land use, and much else, ending decades of conflict and confusion. The federal and provincial governments have worked out arrangements to prevent Indigenous people from falling through the gaps in federal and provincial jurisdiction. Canadian forestry, mining, and pipeline companies increasingly include Indigenous people in planning, joint project management, and employment generation schemes. Examples of recent private sector–Indigenous partnerships are as diverse as diamond mines in the Far North to wineries in the south. Additionally, Indigenous organizations have, since the 1980s, increasingly looked to the judicial system to uphold their rights. In consequence of all of those related changes, living conditions for Indigenous people have improved dramatically and the health gap between them and other Canadians has finally begun to close. That positive change is to be credited mostly to the perseverance and resilience of the Indigenous peoples themselves.

Since the 2015 election, First Nations governments have found a more willing partner in the federal government. Prime Minister Justin Trudeau vowed to eliminate the income and health gaps between First Nations and other Canadians (Tasker, 2018, February 14). Unfortunately, as noted, the ambitious effort to end boil-water advisories have so far delivered less than hoped for, and some setbacks have been encountered in negotiations on pipelines, resource sharing, housing, and a number of other matters of prime importance to Indigenous people. The federal government has committed to redoubling its efforts, and in the summer of 2017 it completely restructured government departments with a view to becoming more responsive to, and more effective in meeting the needs of, Indigenous people in Canada. There is no question the relationships between First Nations and Canada's federal and provincial governments are now better than they ever have been, and real progress is being made. New landmarks are the February 2018 federal commitment to a legal framework expanding and strengthening Indigenous rights. Prime Minister Trudeau, in a speech to Parliament, emphasized the government's commitment to self-determination, affirmation of Indigenous treaty rights, and development in consultation with Indigenous peoples of a comprehensive Indigenous rights framework. While symbolic, it is also important that the federal government acknowledged, in March 2018, the injustice of prosecuting and executing the Tsilhqot'in chiefs in 1864 who were defending their land (BC was then a British crown colony) from miners and settlers (Tasker, 2018, March 26). According recognition to and bestowing value upon the experience of indigeneity are important steps toward reconciliation.

Theoretical Considerations

Chapter 8 brings to the forefront the issue of levels of analysis. It illustrates three explanatory levels: macro, intermediate, and individual level, introduced at the beginning of the book. We will encounter an application of levels of analysis again in Chapter 9, when we examine unemployment—an area where the literature makes a similar set of theoretical distinctions, in that case between effects on the individual from losing a job (e.g., loss of social network, loss of income), household effects (e.g., impact on relationship with spouse and children), and neighbourhood effects (e.g., different meanings and impacts on health depending on proportion of people in the neighbourhood who are unemployed). As we have seen in the case of Indigenous health, there are significant interactional effects across levels. The impact of factors at one level might be amplified or ameliorated by effects at another. For example, we saw that the effects of poverty, poor housing, limited job opportunities, and the like will be less when, at the community level, there is greater solidarity and more cultural continuity. Contrariwise, cultural disintegration and social disruption will amplify the health effects of poverty, poor housing, limited job availability, and so on.

Summary

The health of Indigenous peoples is a case study of social exclusion, racism, and marginalization. It well illustrates the principles of population health and, in particular, multi-level determination of health outcomes. Broader historical, political, and cultural determinants work in conjunction with intermediate-level determinants such as community organization and capacity and individual-level determinants such as health behaviour and specific exposures to risks of a variety of kinds. Indigenous people suffer ill health and shortened lives not because of smoking, alcohol consumption, and exposure to hazards associated with poor housing and water supply, but rather because of the interactions among those individual-level determinants with low socio-economic status and the quality of education, health care, and community governance in a context of social exclusion and cultural dislocation. Solutions to the problem of health disparities must, in consequence, be multi-factoral and be undertaken by and through the people affected.

The health of Indigenous peoples in the Americas and Australia also illustrates the close link between health of populations and social justice. The current ill health of Indigenous peoples arises primarily from the unjust exclusion of people from resources such as their land, their cultural legacies, employment, and the educational and health services of the broader society.

Critical Thinking Questions

1. Indigenous people have been substantially harmed by the colonization of the Americas. Not only were they exposed to diseases and products (e.g., alcohol) that have done untold damage to their well-being, but also their identity, links to the land, culture, and languages have all been undermined. Sociologists contend that all of us are now confronting "colonizing forces" of commercialism, commodification, and secularization that threaten to undermine our cultures and ways of being, contributing to mental illness and chronic disease. Is globalization a continuation of colonizing forces? Is it probable that globalization will harm our health?

2. The health and life expectancy of Indigenous women more closely resembles the health and life expectancy of non-Indigenous women than does the health and life expectancy of Indigenous men and non-Indigenous men. Why might Indigenous status have a more profound negative effect on the health of men than on the health of women?

3. Through what pathways might racism and social exclusion affect the health of a population? Thinking back to the early chapters, which pathways are psychosocial and which are material in nature? What does the chapter on Indigenous health suggest about the relative importance of psychosocial versus material factors?

Annotated Suggested Readings

The most comprehensive and well-researched book on the subject of health of Indigenous people in Canada is J. Waldram, D. Herring, and T. Young, *Aboriginal Health in Canada: Historical, Cultural and Epidemiological Perspectives* (Toronto: University of Toronto Press, 2006). As its title implies, the book covers the history and geographic distribution of Indigenous Peoples, a summary of the impacts of contact with Europeans, and the historical, political, social, and economic developments that have impacted on the health of Indigenous people.

The Globe and Mail produced a detailed profile of Nunavut and its health and social issues, history, and prospects, on 1 April 1 2011. This excellent feature is available at www.theglobeandmail.com/news/national/nunavut/the-trials-of-nunavut-lament-for-an-arctic-nation/article547265/?page=1.

The complex issues of governance, property rights, and education are outlined in the commentary available at the following link: www.theglobeandmail.com/commentary/how-first-nations-can-own-their-future/article554842/. Within the article, there are links to quality, contemporary descriptions of conditions on some of Canada's First Nation's reserves.

For a comprehensive account of residential schools in Canada, the best source is *Honouring the Truth: Summary of the Truth and Reconciliation Commission of Canada* (2015), available as an electronic document from http://www.trc.ca

Annotated Web Resources

"First Nations and Inuit Health"
www.hc-sc.gc.ca/fniah-spnia/index-eng.php
Health Canada provides a comprehensive range
of information on the health of Indigenous
people and the health care services available
to them.

Public Health Agency of Canada:
    "Aboriginal Peoples"
www.phac-aspc.gc.ca/chn-rcs/aboriginal-
    autochtones-eng.php
The Public Health Agency of Canada provides
useful information on diabetes control,
substance abuse, and suicide prevention
among Canadian Indigenous peoples.

National Inquiry into Missing and Murdered
    Indigenous Women and Girls
http://www.mmiwg-ffada.ca
While it got off to a rocky start, the work of the
National Inquiry into Missing and Murdered
Indigenous Women and Girls is an important
inquiry into violence against Indigenous women
in Canada.

"*Lancet* Series Calls on Canada for Concrete
    Action on Indigenous, Global Health"
http://www.cbc.ca/beta/news/health/
    lancet-canada-1.4548587
The Lancet published a blistering critique of
Canada's response to Indigenous health issues,
and questioned whether the federal government's commitment to change is substantive or
merely rhetoric. This article outlines the critique.

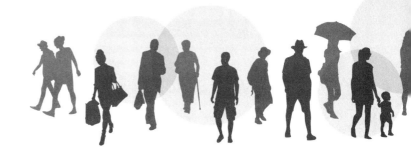

9 Employment, Working Conditions, and Health

Objectives

By the end of your study of this chapter, you should be able to
- understand how employment, unemployment, and health interrelate;
- appreciate the health implications of recent changes in the labour market;
- see how on-the-job experiences affect health and well-being;
- assess how policy responses to employment and working conditions impact on population health.

Synopsis

Chapter 9 reviews the research relating to the health effects of employment, unemployment, and working conditions. It examines the changes that have taken place in the labour market and the workplace over the past few decades as globalization and neo-liberalism have changed the employment landscape. The chapter ends with a discussion of positive changes that can be made to working conditions and employment benefits.

The Centrality of Employment to Adult Health

Pause and Reflect Employment, Health, and Well Being

What features and consequences of employment influence the health and well-being of the individual?

Employment in market societies such as ours is the principal source of personal income and, as we have seen, income is the single most important determinant of health. But employment is more than a source of income. Individuals, especially men, define who they are and their social position through their employment. One's working life is a key source of personal identity. Moreover, the workplace accords many opportunities to build social networks, garner social support, learn new skills, and exercise a sense of mastery and control. Employment shapes our non-work responses and behaviours. Whether you go to the opera after work or home to watch sports on television, or whether you go to a coffee bar or a cocktail lounge at the end of the day, depends largely on what work you do and with whom you do it. Paid work determines where and how and with whom you spend most of your waking time and significantly conditions where you live. Our employment shapes our beliefs, habits, pursuits and character, which in turn influence our health.

The workplace may not be positive and supportive. Superiors or fellow workers may subject an employee to coercion or harassment. The conditions under which the work is performed may be unsafe, impose restrictions on movement, or require physically repetitive actions, or the work environment may be too hot, too cold, or poorly ventilated. Task allocation, shift assignment, or pay and benefits may be unfairly decided. There may be a lack of opportunity to exercise meaningful control over work timing, pace, and process. The workplace might be characterized by poor communications, a lack of respect, or other conditions that undermine dignity. Some job types—unskilled labour and many positions in the service industry—combine unhealthy working conditions with low levels of control over the work, the potential for poor treatment, even abuse, by supervisors or customers, and job insecurity—creating an atmosphere of perpetual fear that the job and associated income will disappear. Workplace conditions and unstable employment are the greatest sources of stress in many people's lives.

Box 9.1	Case Study ○ Low Wages, Abuse, and Job Insecurity: The American Waitress

Chelsea Welch was a server in an Applebee's restaurant in Saint Louis. She was paid $3.25 per hour, plus tips. Welch was expected to work up until 1:30 a.m. and then return at 10:30 a.m. to open the restaurant, unless it was quiet, in which case she would be sent home and not be paid. One day, a customer wrote on the bill "I give God 10 per cent. Why do you get 18?"—presumably referring to (a) tithing to his/her religion (common among Mormons and Catholics, and tax deductible in the US) and (b) Applebee's suggested tip of 18 per cent. He or she left nothing by way of a tip. Welch took a photo of the bill and posted it online (with the customer's name blanked out). The ensuing publicity caught the attention of the customer, and he or she demanded that Applebee's fire all the employees in the Saint Louis restaurant. Applebee's investigated and promptly fired Welch, an employee about whom no complaints had been made and whose work record and reputation were solid. (Welch was not the server of the customer who left the nasty note and no tip; that was a fellow employee.)

In the US, starvation wages plus tips are accepted because it is widely believed employees will work harder and provide better customer service. In reality, employees are harassed, abused, and fired on whim, in addition to living below the poverty line, even though they are working full time. Moreover, it is difficult to contend that the work ethic and service

continued

are better in the United Kingdom (low wages plus tips) than Australia (high wages, no tips); the opposite would be closer to the truth. If service is better in America, something many would contest, it likely arises from employees' terror at being fired for annoying a customer. Only the US affords almost no job protection to its service workers, and therefore employees must continuously strive to please their supervisors and customers if they want to keep the job. No wonder service industry workers, especially in the US, have such poor health.

Health and Jobs

In general, people in stable, well-paying jobs are healthier than people in unstable or poorly paying work. Being employed promotes health (Lavis, McLeod, Mustard, & Stoddart, 2003). And as the Whitehall Studies show, the higher the quality of the job, whether measured by job status, income, or degree of control the employee has over his or her work, the better the person's mental and physical health. Life expectancy also varies by occupation, as shown in Table 9.1.

Marmot remarked that patterns of employment both reflect and reinforce the social gradient (Marmot, 2010). He was pointing out that people higher up on the socio-economic scale are those with the education and other resources to secure the highest-quality jobs. These high-quality jobs, in turn, reinforce—through high income, capacity to build social networks, and control over the work—the good health associated with education and other benefits accrued over the life course. There is a virtuous circle, a positive cumulative effect. Conversely, people lower down on the socio-economic ladder compete for lower-quality jobs. These jobs, in turn, reinforce existing and generate new health problems through low income, monotonous work, limited social interaction, adverse working conditions, and limited control over the work. There is a vicious circle, a cumulative negative effect.

Table 9.1 Occupation and Life Expectancy, England

Example Jobs*	Men	Women
Doctor, senior manager	82.5	85.2
Accountant, lawyer	80.8	84.5
Systems manager, nurse	80.4	83.9
Office administrator, senior sales	80.0	83.5
Small business owner, farmer	78.9	81.9
Tradesperson	77.9	81.7
Server, construction worker, truck or bus driver	76.6	80.8

* Example jobs from ONS occupational classification.
Source: Office for National Statistics, 2017. https://www.ons.gov.uk/peoplepopulationandcommunity/birthsdeaths andmarriages/lifeexpectancies/bulletins/trendinlifeexpectancyatbirthandage65bysocioeconomicpositionbasedon thenationalstatisticssocioeconomicclassificationenglandandwales/2015-10-21

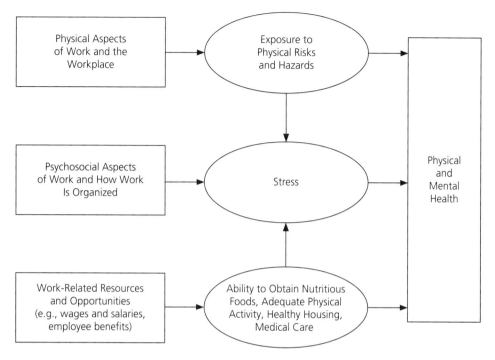

Figure 9.1 How Work Affects Health

Source: From Robert Wood Johnson Foundation, *Exploring the Social Determinants of Health: Work, Workplaces and Health*, May 2011. Reproduced with permission of the Robert Wood Johnson Foundation, Princeton, NJ.

In short, good jobs are health enhancing; bad jobs are health destroying. Hence, the gradient in health is reflected, reinforced, and magnified by employment patterns.

Figure 9.1 is a schematic showing how work affects human health.

We can readily see the health effects of higher- or lower-quality jobs. Figure 9.2 shows the odds of developing **metabolic syndrome**. Employees in the lowest-government jobs, clerical staff, are 2.7 times as likely to develop the syndrome, a precursor to heart disease and diabetes, than employees in the highest ranking government jobs (Marmot, 2010).

Unemployment and Health

In our modern market societies, people in the lowest quality, worst-paid jobs are at the greatest risk of unemployment, whereas people in the best quality, highest-paid jobs are at the least risk of unemployment. The quality of the job is largely a function of education, which in turn is largely a function of social class at birth. In recent years, pockets of highly paid jobs for workers with limited education, for example factory and manufacturing work, have almost entirely disappeared in North America and the United Kingdom. Today, the relationship between socio-economic position of origin and quality of work obtained in adulthood is stronger than ever. Thus, too, is the relationship between risk of unemployment and social class. The lower a person's socio-economic status, the higher their risk of unemployment.

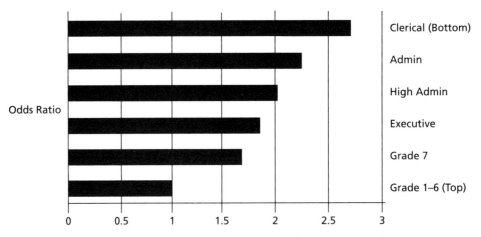

Figure 9.2 Odds of Developing Metabolic Syndrome by Occupational Position (Whitehall II)

Source: Based on Marmot, 2010.

Unemployment affects health in several ways. The most obvious is the loss of employment income. From this we would deduce that negative health effects are greatest where unemployment insurance and welfare schemes for the unemployed are weakest. And that, in fact, is true. Unemployed Swedes suffer fewer health effects than unemployed Americans because Swedish citizens receive more generous unemployment assistance in the forms of guaranteed income and publicly funded job retraining (Kim et al., 2012). But loss of employment also means loss of socialization outlets, truncation of social networks, loss of self-actualization possibilities, and potential loss of sense of personal identity and self-worth. The extent to which these are important could, at least in part, hinge on the qualities of the job lost. If the job was bad, exposed the worker to poor working conditions, and provided few positive outlets, its loss may have no more than the income effects, which may be partly offset by no longer being exposed to the poor conditions.

Unemployment may run through three levels of causality: (1) there may be individual-level effects, such as loss of personal resources and increased personal stress; (2) there may be effects at the level of the family, such as family breakdown or the effects on the family of a forced relocation (the intermediate level); (3) there may be contextual effects of living in a community where unemployment is rising, such as perceiving one's own unemployment differently, reductions in public service levels, and deterioration of the neighbourhood (macro level). All three levels—individual, intermediate, and contexual—may impact on the health of an unemployed person. Areas adversely affected by economic change such as the "rust belt" (mid-western and northeastern US) have large numbers of residents who are chronically unemployed, who belong to families who have lost their homes, and live in neighbourhoods that have degraded schools, parks, libraries, and other public services. De-industrialization has robbed many areas in central Canada, the mid-western US, and northern England of jobs. Consequently, life expectancies, general health, and well-being have declined.

Box 9.2	Case Study ○ Unemployment

Many companies in fields as diverse as textiles, shoe manufacturing, machine parts, and electronics have moved their assembly operations "offshore," mostly to Mexico, China, and South Asia. Plants involved in large-scale assembly have, consequently, closed and the many well-paying jobs in historic manufacturing centres in Canada (mostly Quebec and Ontario), the United States and the United Kingdom have vanished. In other labour-intensive industries such as automobile assembly and banking, robots have replaced assembly-line workers, and online banking and cash machines have replaced bank clerks. How might job loss affect individuals? How might extensive job loss affect communities? What health consequences ensue?

Sophisticated modelling and multi-level analyses are required to untangle the individual and contextual effects of unemployment on health. Moreover, there are direct, indirect, and buffering effects to consider. Direct effects, such as income effects, must be separated from other individual-level direct effects of unemployment. Some effects might be buffered by other factors. For example, "supportive social contexts will buffer the effect of an individual's unemployment" (Beland, Birch, & Stoddart, 2002). Being a member of tightly knit, loving family situated in a safe neighbourhood can reduce the negative effects of job loss on an unemployed person. Contrariwise, living in a community in decline like Detroit, where unemployment is widespread and neighbourhoods are decaying, will amplify individual and household (intermediate) effects of job loss. That will be manifested both directly in near-term adverse health outcomes and indirectly in unhealthy behaviour contributing to long-term adverse health outcomes.

Empirically, it has been shown that unemployment increases the risk of cardiovascular disease (Gallo et al., 2004), suicide (Voss, Nylen, Floderus, Diderichsen, & Terry, 2004), and use of prescription medication (Jin, Shaw, & Suoboda, 1997). Unemployment is associated with increased smoking and alcohol consumption (Marmot, 2010) and with the epidemics of opioid drug abuse (mostly oral prescription drugs) and the fentanyl crisis (mostly IV street drugs).

The negative effects of unemployment increase with the frequency of periods of unemployment and the duration of each period of unemployment, demonstrating a clear cumulative impact (Marmot, 2010). And, as Marmot points out, "the longer a person is unemployed, the risk of subsequent illness increases greatly, and therefore further reduces the likelihood of returning to employment" (Marmot, 2010).

Changes in the Nature of Employment

Globalization and the transition to the "knowledge economy" have had dramatic effects on work. "Globalization" refers to the complex interaction of contemporary factors that include rapid and inexpensive communications and transportation (mostly due to technological change) and the systematic removal of barriers to travel, communication, transporting goods and services, and moving money and other resources from one geographic place to another (mostly due to changes in government policies). "Knowledge economies" refers to the belief in, and pursuit by, governments and companies of economic growth by seeking to capitalize on technical innovation and providing cutting-edge goods and services (which, in theory, ought to have greater value and fetch higher prices than old-fashioned production of basic goods and services).

Commitment to economic growth, globalization, and the emphasis on building a knowledge economy create steadily growing pressure for increased productivity—doing more with less, greater work intensity, increased hours of work, and decreased wages and benefits. The push for greater product innovation at lower cost spawned just-in-time and flexible production modalities, which in turn have dramatically increased the use of part-time, temporary, casual, and contract employees. They have also increased reliance on shift work. Figure 9.3 shows how the gap between wages and productivity has grown in the United States—i.e., how low-wage workers are being paid a diminishing proportion of their actual output. Or, to put it another way, the figure shows how work has changed so that workers must work harder or longer to maintain the same earnings.

A good example of the revolution that has taken place in the past 20 years is the automobile industry, which used to introduce new models every five to seven years, making only modest and largely cosmetic changes between changeovers. Parts were ordered, manufactured, and inventoried for years; assembly lines using the same equipment and workers ran virtually unchanged. Now no manufacturer who hopes to stay in business can avoid continuous innovation, ordering only the components needed

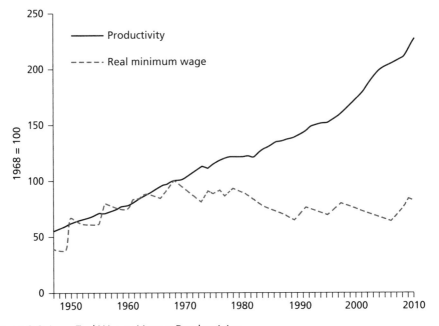

Figure 9.3 Low-End Wages Versus Productivity

Note: Productivity is measured by the US Bureau of Labor Statistics as the output per hour of all persons in the non-farm business sectors.

Source: Center for Economic and Policy Research, 2012. http://cepr.net/documents/publications/min-wage1-2012-03.pdf

in the next few days or weeks, and switching suppliers and assembly modalities to keep costs down and quality up. Today's production techniques are incompatible with large, stable workforces, and the numbers of full-time and continuing jobs have been slashed. Technological change, which introduced robotic assembly lines, has slashed jobs further.

Perhaps an even better example is consumer electronics, where even large and successful companies like Sony and Panasonic are teetering on insolvency as they shuffle their product lines, open and close new manufacturing facilities, and shed jobs. A few giants, notably Apple and Samsung, have come to dominate world markets, with their widely distributed component supply and product assembly models.

The emerging knowledge economy functions through projects, not ongoing routine work. Less continuous production means more contract work and less regular employment. Not surprisingly, globalization and the shift to a knowledge economy have been linked to degraded health (Blouin, Chopra, & van der Hoeven, 2009). While many young people like the flexibility of short-term contract work, it comes with no job or income security, no employment benefits such as health care, vacation, and sick leave, and no pension. As workers age, the flexibility becomes less and the lack of stability and benefits become more important to health and well-being.

Traditionally, both unions and companies pursued the goal of a stable workforce, albeit for different reasons. Now, in the liberal regime world of which Canada is a part, the only large-scale labour-intensive work conducted in stable environments is found in government offices, universities, schools, institutional health care, and the few remaining assembly plants, mills, and large-scale mining operations. Traditional production jobs have been replaced by service jobs, mostly low-end jobs, such as sales clerks and restaurant workers. The less skilled are increasingly competing for low-paid, unstable jobs with few or no fringe benefits.

Box 9.3   Case Study ○ Cleaners, Then and Now

In September 2017, *The New York Times* published a case study aimed at helping Americans see what has happened to US employment and how the changes have affected ordinary people (Irwin, 2017). The study follows two women, Gail Evans and Marta Ramos, each of whom worked as a cleaner for large, highly successful corporations—Evans for Kodak in the 1980s and Ramos for Apple currently. In today's money, their earnings were roughly comparable, but Evans was an employee of the company and received health, vacation, and sick leave benefits, whereas Ramos is a contract worker who receives nothing beyond her base pay. Evans also received, from Kodak, in-house training and support for further education. As an employee, she was eligible to compete for better jobs within the company. She ended up as a senior executive officer with the corporation. Ramos will remain a cleaner. Obviously not every employee in a 1980s entry-level job in a corporation ended up in the executive suite, but some did, and most made some progress up the ranks. Today's contract economy does not provide that opportunity.

We are currently experiencing the collective effects of four related trends: de-industrialization, de-unionization, de-skilling, and privatization. We already referred to de-industrialization and its impact on jobs in the old manufacturing heartlands of Canada, the United States, and the United Kingdom. The so-called post-industrial or service-economy countries of the liberal regime world now import rather than manufacture the vast majority of finished goods, from shoes and socks to mobile phones. This is because corporations have sought out lower-wage and lower-taxation places to site their manufacturing activities, a process made possible by the innovations in the communications and transportation sectors, the abundance of cheap energy for global shipping, and changes in international trade rules and tariffs. Relatively well-paid jobs for relatively low-skilled workers have vanished along with the assembly plants, forcing large numbers of people to seek work in the lower-paying service sector (e.g., retail sales, restaurants, maintenance, and cleaning).

De-unionization, employers' successful efforts to exclude unions from workplaces, is connected to manufacturing's move offshore because remaining industrial employers have demanded wage and contract concessions and new employers have pursued low-wage/no union labour practices to bring wages and benefits closer to those of the developing world. Governments in Canada, the US, and the UK have contributed to the trend by making it more difficult for unions to organize workers and easier to get unions decertified.

De-skilling is multi-dimensional and includes increased use of automated processes and routines, importation of prefabricated materials, rather than skilled construction on site, and modular construction of consumer items such as automobiles so that component assemblies are swapped rather than the vehicle repaired by a skilled mechanic. In labour-intensive areas like health care, less expensive, lower-trained nursing assistants and aides have replaced qualified nurses. The effect of de-skilling is depression of wages and replacement of higher-quality jobs with higher job satisfaction by lower-quality, more routinized work.

Finally, governments at all levels and quasi-governmental bodies like health authorities and universities have aggressively privatized. Privatization includes contracting out and changing ownership of assets. Rather than employing people directly to undertake tasks like cleaning, maintenance, grounds work, garbage removal, and the like, governmental and quasi-governmental bodies in the liberal regime world now typically contract with private companies (almost always low-bid, non-union companies) to take over the service. The reason is to achieve (short-term) cost reduction. Wages, benefits, skill levels, opportunities for training and advancement, and quality of work are all driven downward. In the case of changing ownership of assets, governments turn over a public asset (such as a publicly owned nursing home) to a private operator. The usual effect of the transfer of ownership is to have higher-paid (usually unionized), skilled workers replaced by lower-paid (usually non-unionized) employees who experience less job security, less control over the work, and lower wages and benefits. Again, the motive is reduced cost.

Apart from the damage to health done by low wages and physically challenging working conditions, diminished job security is itself a serious threat to health. Job insecurity is linked to both physical and mental health problems (Ferrie, 2001). Higher use of medical services, increased sick days, obesity, psychological problems, and elevated blood pressure and blood glucose have all been linked to job insecurity.

Working Conditions and Health

Chronic stresses and excessive demands at work that are not compensated by adequate social support constitute **isostrain**—isolated high-strain work. Many routine jobs over which the worker has little control—a server in a busy restaurant, a bus driver, a sales clerk, a junior office worker—involve high strain, limited control by the employee, and little or no support from others.

Pause and Reflect   Isostrain and the Warehouse Worker

A "picker" is a warehouse worker who receives requests for items ordered by customers via a headset, pushes a cart to the correct shelving or bin area in the warehouse, picks the item requested, puts it on the cart and proceeds to collect the next order. When the cart is full, the picker pushes it to the shipping department for unloading. Pickers work the warehouses for virtually all online companies, most famously the industry giant Amazon.

Amazon's pickers work 10.5 hours a day. They are entitled to two 15-minute and one 30-minute break. Pickers are electronically monitored to ensure they collect a minimum of 110 items per hour, two per minute. Failure to make quotas, or an error, earns demerits. A few demerits and the worker will be summarily fired. Pickers at Amazon, one of the best online companies in terms of treatment of its employees, are paid $12.40 per hour.

Isostrain is linked to **metabolic syndrome**—extra fat around the mid-section, insulin resistance, elevated blood pressure—a constellation of risk factors, which together increase the risk of diabetes and heart disease. Bus drivers, for example, have been shown to have an elevated risk of diabetes and heart disease associated with factors such as traffic congestion, time pressures, social isolation, poor passenger behaviour, lack of control over features of the work and so on (Evans & Carrere, 1991). In addition to isostrain, the physical features of the work, immobility, and the quality of seating and ergonomics, contribute to elevated levels of musculoskeletal disease, making bus drivers among the least healthy people in the affluent world.

While stress at work, and the associated psychosocial impact on health, are clearly important, we must be a bit cautious about pushing work-related stress explanations of ill health too far. A recent Canadian study found that only 27 per cent of Canadian workers reported moderate or high levels of stress, and 40 per cent of those identified the major sources of their stress to be non–work related. The researchers found no correlation between reported stress and gender nor between reported stress and education (Crompton, 2011). As one would expect, less-educated people reported more stress associated with financial matters, but this was compensated for by more-educated people expressing stress over family matters.

Box 9.4   Case Study ○ Work and Pregnancy

Working throughout pregnancy in a job that is physically demanding or involves a substantial amount of standing is associated with impaired fetal growth and reduction in head circumference of the child (Snijder et al., 2012). Women who have low incomes and limited educational attainment are much more likely to be engaged in physically demanding work or hold jobs, such as sale associates in shops, where they have to stand for sustained periods of time. They are also more likely to work throughout their pregnancies because they cannot afford to take time off. As we saw earlier, children of low socio-economic mothers are predisposed to impaired fetal growth for reasons such as maternal nutritional status. Maternal working conditions may compound the risk (cumulative risk or "pile-up" of risk factors). What are the long-term implications for the health and well-being of the mother and child? What workplace and social policy measures might mitigate risks of less-than-optimal health outcomes?

Explanatory Models of Workplace Impacts on Health

Two models have been developed to explain how work can make you sick. Those are the "demand–control" model and the "effort–reward" model. While they feature different elements, they are not mutually exclusive and both may be applied to a work situation. The **demand–control model** attempts to measure the relationship between the demands made of an employee and the capacity to meet those demands. A junior clerk in an office who works for several managers likely has an overflowing in-basket of work and superiors who all think their work is the top priority. She faces heavy, in fact impossible, demands, yet has no control over how much work comes her way. A significant discrepancy between what is demanded of the employee and what can be accomplished is associated with fatigue, headache, body aches and pains, sleep disturbances, anxiety, elevated blood pressure, and stroke (Van der Doef, 1999). The **effort–reward model** attempts to measure the relationship between the work effort of the employee and various rewards received including pay, bonuses, recognition, and workplace social support. Workers in many low-end jobs, such as labourers in the construction industry, must make maximal effort to maintain their jobs but receive little or no recognition or support from their employers. Again, a significant discrepancy between the effort the employee makes and the rewards received is predictive of emotional, psychosomatic, and chronic disease outcomes (de Jonge, Bosma, Peter, & Slegrist, 2000). Because the demand–control and effort–reward models are independently predictive of health outcomes, various efforts have been made to combine them.

Forced Inactivity in the Workplace

Many jobs today, as the bus driver example illustrates, combine high isostrain derived from demand–control and effort–reward imbalances with environmental factors inimical to good health. Commonplace is sedentary work involving long periods of sitting—office workers, drivers in the transport sector, check-out cashiers. Not only does prolonged sitting contribute to musculoskeletal problems, but lack of physical activity compounds the isostrain effects on metabolic syndrome, notably by promoting central obesity and hence the risks of heart disease and diabetes. Thus, pathways to chronic diseases such as arthritis, coronary heart disease, and diabetes can be found in the workplace.

Research has recently demonstrated links between sedentary work and many negative health outcomes, including shortened life expectancy (Thorpe, Owen, Neuhaus, & Dunstan, 2011). Sedentary lifestyle, even if the individual engages in episodic vigorous exercise, can shorten life expectancy by more than two years.

Box 9.5	Case Study ○ Different Employment Situations, Different Health Risks

Sonya is a 34-year-old woman with a 3-year-old daughter, whose neighbour babysits at a rate of $25 per day while Sonya works. Sonya has only her grade 12 and a certificate from a secretarial school. She holds two jobs currently: she works part-time for a private long-term care home as a clerk/receptionist and picks up as many shifts as she can as a server in a local restaurant. Sonya gets paid $10.25 an hour at the care home and $8.75 plus tips at the restaurant. She has no benefits on top of her pay. Rent in her one-bedroom apartment is $600 per month, plus utilities.

What health challenges confront Sonya?

Sara is a 34-year-old woman with a 3-year-old daughter. Her daughter goes to a neighbourhood play school every weekday. Sara is in a stable relationship with John, her partner, who has a law practice. Sara has a degree in business administration and runs her own small advertising company. Sara and John own their house, making mortgage payments of $1,200 per month. They both own cars.

What health challenges confront Sara?

The Workplace and Health Behaviour

The modern, high-pressure workplace also structures some of our behaviour. In addition to forcing us to be more sedentary, the workplace encourages bad eating habits—grabbing something and eating it at our workstation or behind the wheel—and bad food choices—something quick and easy that we can eat out of hand. Muffins, burgers, wraps, and snack foods are among the worst things we can eat but are the mainstays in today's work world.

Some types of workplace foster highly destructive behaviour. Long-distance transport truck driving encourages the use of stimulants. Workers in routinized employment, such as framing carpenters and miners, are vulnerable to recreational drug use. Some trades, an example being roofing, encourage high-risk lifestyles and safety violations on the job. Servers and line cooks are vulnerable to cocaine use and heavy drinking. According the US Substance Abuse and Mental Health Services Administration (2015), the food services industry has the worst substance abuse problem, with nearly 20 per cent of workers abusing alcohol or drugs or both. These workplace cultures, fostered by stressful conditions, boredom, and shift work, are very difficult to change, and get reinforced by self-selection—new employees drawn to the lifestyle.

Policies Affecting Employment, Earnings, Job Benefits, and Working Conditions

We already noted how central employment is to our adult lives. Most adults receive virtually all of their income through paid employment, and most adults spend roughly half of their waking time at work. Securing reasonably paid work with safe and healthy working conditions and benefits, such as paid leave, are among the strongest determinants of our overall health and well-being. Public policies affect employment levels, earnings, job benefits, and working conditions. Government spending determines the number of jobs in areas as diverse as construction, education, and health care. Government regulations determine maximum working hours and minimum wages. Thus, government policies that might at first glance appear "economic" are, in fact, important from a population-health standpoint. In this section, we will begin by discussing the near-universal policy commitment to full employment, and why governments, at least those in Canada, the United States, and the United Kingdom, abandoned that commitment. We will then look at policies regarding unemployment insurance, wages, benefits, and working conditions.

Keynesianism and Its Demise

Until the end of the 1970s, governments throughout the affluent Western world held a common understanding of macro-level economic principles derived from the work of the great economist John Maynard Keynes (1883–1946). Keynesian economics holds that modern governments need to intervene in order to ensure that employment remains at the highest sustainable level, as close to full employment as possible, because only under those conditions is economic growth sustainable.

Keynes pointed out that companies can expand their production, spurring economic growth, only if there is enough demand in the economy for their products. Consumer demand is highly sensitive to income, and as most people's income is derived from work, employment levels and wages determine overall (aggregate) demand. Thus, boosting employment (and wages) is the chief prerequisite for steady economic growth. That growth is also the prerequisite for governments to be able to pay down public debt and, hopefully, build up budget surpluses for a rainy day. High, stable incomes maintain consumer demand for products, and provide high, stable tax revenue, while simultaneously reducing the need for government spending on social programs. Moreover, as the economy grows and government revenues and expenditures stabilize, governments can reduce taxes. Maximizing employment is thus the key to everything we are striving to achieve.

According to Keynes, near full employment can be achieved by increasing the money supply through reducing interest rates and increasing government spending. But once near full employment is achieved, low interest rates and a tightening of the labour market together tend to drive up prices and wages, which sparks inflation. Governments should respond to accelerating inflation, according to Keynes, by gentle braking, a slow, step-wise increase in interest rates, a slow cutting back on public expenditures, accompanied by a slow, step-wise increase in taxes. Once the economy starts to "cool," taxes should be lowered, interest rates dropped, and public spending picked up, even if that requires heavy government borrowing, until the economy starts to overheat and so on into the next cycle. The aim of it all is to keep as many of those able to work working full time, thus effectively ending the "boom and bust cycle" typical of capitalist market societies. Keynes, after all, was most interested in providing the economic theory and practical advice that would prevent another devastating depression, such as the total collapse of the liberal regime economies in 1929.

From the end of the Second World War until the mid-1970s, Keynesianism seemed to work. All the affluent countries of the West enjoyed a fairly sustained period of economic growth and near full employment. But by 1975, the massive debts piled up by the United States in pursuing the Vietnam and Cold Wars put huge upward pressure on interest rates worldwide. The sudden rise in oil prices following the 1973 Arab-Israeli war put huge downward pressure on industrial production due to the sharp increase in the cost of producing and transporting goods. Suddenly rich countries had the twin problems of economic recession and rising unemployment, coupled with inflation and rising prices. That was not supposed to be possible. According to the usual reading of Keynes, an economy either grows too fast, causing inflation, or contracts, causing recession. In theory, at least in Keynesian theory, inflation and recession cannot occur together because the former, inflation, is caused by rapid economic growth whereas the latter, by definition, is a shrinking, failing economy.

Starting with the United States, countries abandoned Keynesianism and resorted to manipulation of the money supply as a means to control inflation ("monetarism"), a strategy that at once drove interest rates even higher and the economic downturn even deeper. Again, starting with the United States, governments then resorted to cutting government programs and services while lowering taxes. Typically, they had more success with the latter—cutting taxes—than the former—cutting spending—because so much of the spending was bound up politically, especially in the United States, with the military, pensions, and big, powerful lobbies like the food and agriculture industries. That meant in practice cherry-picking programs serving minorities, the poor, and other politically insignificant social groups. Out of this was born **neo-liberalism** and a new-found tolerance for high levels of unemployment. Seven to 10 per cent, numbers considered disastrous in the 1940s, '50s, and '60s, became not only thinkable, but increasingly commonplace.

High Chronic Unemployment in Canada, the United States, and the United Kingdom

From 2008, with a serious economic downturn and the Canadian federal government, US Congress, and the Conservative government in the UK firmly opposed to Keynesian economics, joblessness soared. In spite of all the evidence that it does not work, the political consensus hardened around low taxes and limited government spending as the route to economic growth and, eventually, more jobs. The employment situation was marginally better in Australia (mostly because of heavy Chinese demand for raw materials). In Canada, the unemployment situation would have been worse but it stabilized in the 7 per cent zone mostly due to high oil prices and the resultant construction boom in the Alberta oil sands. When oil prices started to fall, the Canadian economy was in real trouble. Recognition that a slowdown in the oil sands would drive Canada deep into recession recently led the Canadian government to gut environmental protection regulations and sponsor new pipeline construction, sparking conflict with First Nations and environmentalists.

The economic situation changed, beginning slowly around 2010 and picking up speed in 2016 and 2017. The US economy sharply improved, and with it, the Canadian economy began again to grow, reaching a startling 4 per cent annual growth rate in the summer of 2017. Unemployment plummeted in the US, but moved down more modestly in Canada to the 6 per cent range. Unfortunately, most job growth was low-end, service sector, and part-time, but with continuing growth, that could change. Since government policy regarding employment has not changed, the big question is whether the recent surge in economic activity can be sustained.

It is important to understand that official unemployment figures do not really reflect how many people are unemployed. To count as unemployed, you must be (a) recently out of work, (b) actively seeking work, and (c) available to take a job if one should be offered to you. The long-term unemployed and those who currently have some commitment like looking after a child or an aging parent that limits their availability, drop out of the numbers. Thus, paradoxically, the worse the employment situation, the longer it remains bad; the poorer the pay, the less secure the work; and the higher the hardships a job seeker must face, the lower the proportion of people who will count as unemployed. Or, to put the point differently, many more people in Canada, the United States, and the United Kingdom than those currently labelled "unemployed" would seek and obtain work if the jobs were available. That is why unemployment figures tend to spike when economic conditions improve—the "hidden unemployed" flood into the job market hoping for work.

Official unemployment rates for select wealthy countries are presented in Table 9.2. Since peaking following the 2008 economic crisis, unemployment rates slowly improved to reach record lows by 2018.

From a population-health perspective, the important points are that (1) governments can heavily influence levels of employment and (2) those levels of employment heavily influence health outcomes. Unemployment, insecure employment, and poorly paid employment are major determinants of poor health outcomes in affluent countries. The current hands-off attitude of Canada, the United States, and the United Kingdom (less so Australia, whose government continues to follow full-employment policies) risks consigning many of their citizens to low income, job insecurity, and unemployment. A recent study (Kim et al., 2012) shows that governments' policies regarding full-time, stable employment have profound effects on the health of their populations. Liberal regime countries with high

Table 9.2 Unemployment (December 2012 and May 2017)

Jurisdiction	Unemployment Rate 2012*	Unemployment Rate 2017**
United States	8.1	4.3
United Kingdom	8.0	4.4
Canada	7.3	6.6
Germany	5.5	3.8
Australia	5.2	5.5

*Source: US Central Intelligence Agency World Fact Book, www.cia.gov/library/publications/the-world-factbook/rankorder/2129rank-html.
**Source: OECD, 2017 http://stats.oecd.org/index.aspx?queryid=36324

unemployment and precarious work have poorer self-rated health, more musculoskeletal disorders, and higher incidence of mental illness than countries that have stuck with Keynesian economics, full employment, and progressive income tax (Northern Europe and Australia).

The liberal regime countries of the world, except Australia, have abandoned full-employment policies and now tolerate high levels of unemployment. This is justified according to their governments because it reduces inflationary pressure (employees have little bargaining power to increase their pay) and increases economic productivity (by lowering labour costs and by forcing existing workers to work longer and harder). But the hidden cost, of course, is significant hardship, reduced personal income, and diminished health.

Unemployment Insurance

Along with allowing rates of unemployment to rise, liberal regime governments also acted to tighten eligibility for unemployment insurance, turning what were once essentially social welfare mechanisms, designed to provide income support to part-time, seasonal, and casual labour, into contributory schemes. Canada "reformed" unemployment insurance, making it harder to collect and incentivizing low-paid work rather than benefits. In Canada and the United Kingdom, worker eligibility now depends on the length of employment service and the amount contributed to the insurance plan. No longer are the unemployment insurance plans backed by tax dollars, but instead rely on contributions from the currently employed to provide minimal benefits to those who lose their jobs. Most affected by these changes are women who work part-time, seasonal workers such as loggers, fishermen, and construction workers, and people in "sunset industries," failing enterprises such as the Canadian pulp and paper industry where work is sporadic. Communities where much of the work is seasonal, or where whole sectors of the local economy are in difficulty, suffer alongside the individual workers from the loss of spending power derived from unemployment-insurance sources.

As in so many matters relating to income support and employment, Australia is an exception to the liberal regime pattern. In Australia, unemployment benefits are part of the income tax system. There is no insurance fund and there are no compulsory premiums to be paid by workers. For single, unemployed people aged 21 to 60, a maximum of 535.60 AUD (530 CAD) is paid per fortnight (267.80 AUD per week) in income support. Amounts payable depend on income, assets, and actual cost of accommodation. Payments are statutory rights and there is no cut-off; benefits run indefinitely. However, people on benefits are required to enter into Activity Agreements that specify a set of obligations the person must meet to maintain eligibility for support, including training and an acceptable level of job seeking.

The high level of income security and the relative generosity of the benefits are contributory factors to the superior health of Australians compared to Canadians, Americans, and residents of the United Kingdom. However, the guaranteed income program is also controversial. Australian conservative politicians have argued against the scheme, claiming that it contributes to a "welfare mentality," and the current benefits are less than they were before 2014. As with conservatives everywhere, they believe very low or no benefits are a better approach because then the unemployed would be forced to seek work.

Education and Training for the Workforce

In most of Europe and in Japan, employers are required to provide much of the education and training needed by their employees. Often this is formal in nature, such as apprenticeships, internships, and the like. The government provides general education, numeracy, literacy, and foundational science, with the employer providing specialized knowledge and skills. In liberal regime countries, the arrangements are quite different. Employers expect their workers to be pretty much "job ready," and it is the joint responsibility of the individual and the government to ensure that the requisite training (much of it at the individual's expense in technical schools or college) has been completed. What is an employer's responsibility and cost in much of the world is a taxpayer's and individual worker's responsibility and cost in Canada, the United States, and the United Kingdom.

Commitment between worker and employer is obviously much stronger in social democratic systems because each party has a great deal invested in the other. In consequence, job security, full-time work (as opposed to casual and part-time work), and more robust rights and benefits typify the Northern European labour markets. This is reinforced by much deeper penetration by labour unions, which collaborate with employers on training, job security, and other matters in ways that are unfamiliar to the liberal regime world, where relations between unions—where they still exist—and employers are often adversarial. In Germany, for example, automobile manufacturers hire employees more or less for life, providing them with the training and retraining they need as the companies' needs change. The unions and the employers work together to ensure that layoffs do not occur, and that the fit between existing employees and the companies' production requirements remains tight. In Canada and the US, automobile industry unions and employers are adversaries, with the former trying to protect as many jobs as possible and the latter trying to lay off as many workers as possible. In the UK, those adversarial dynamics completely destroyed the British automobile industry, a loss of tens of thousands of highly paid jobs.

Because of an employer's responsibility for developing skills in their own workers, the common problem in the liberal regime world of disconnects between the training workers have and what employers are seeking is avoided in many other countries. Not so in Canada: it is common to have health care facilities desperate for health care technicians, with training slots in colleges for those self-same technicians going unfilled or students flooding into some hot new field only to discover when they graduate that there are no jobs.

Similarly, governments in Canada and the United States mount (or fund colleges and other agencies to mount) training programs to make welfare recipients and the recently unemployed more competitive in the labour market. But again, those training efforts are often misaligned with the job market or, alternatively, are aimed at low-end entry-level work where there are already more qualified applicants than positions. In Canada, the Canada Economic Action Plan, sponsored by the federal Conservative government until its defeat in 2015, and the BC Job Plan, sponsored by the right-of-centre BC provincial government before its defeat in 2017, both targeted marginalized populations and low-skill jobs. This raises an important question: Why does Canada repeatedly offer ad hoc, ineffectual job training? The answer is that training efforts of this type are cheap, easy to mount, and politically popular; further, they create the impression governments are doing something and they require nothing of the business community.

Solutions for the liberal regime problems of education and training of the workforce are not easy to come by. Employers are not at all keen to assume new costs such as a more robust role in educating and developing their workforces. The amount of coordination required among government, employers, and unions is alien to the more free-market-oriented countries, especially the United States, but also Canada. (Something akin to European coordinated labour-market approaches exists in Australia.) Unfortunately, the misalignments and lack of commitment by employers to their employees in Canada, the United States, and the United Kingdom mean wastage of human resources, underemployment, and job insecurity. This is not only inefficient, but it is also harmful to the health of the population.

Some (mostly social democratic) countries have pioneered alternative approaches to education and training. Over the past 50 years, Denmark developed a continuous vocational training program. Skill-development services geared directly to workplace opportunities are provided to both employed and unemployed people. The program is a joint government/industry venture with funding provided from government sources (Commission on Social Determinants of Health, 2008). Similar programs continue to operate throughout Scandinavia, Germany, and the Netherlands.

Wages and Benefits

As one might expect from this chapter's discussion, the minimum wage a government permits employers to pay is lowest in the United States, roughly similar in the United Kingdom and Canada, and significantly higher than other liberal regime countries in Australia. In 2017, rates were $8.80 per hour in the United States (federal), $10.76 per hour in the United Kingdom, and a range between $10.75 (Newfoundland) and $13.00 (Nunavut) per hour in Canada. The United States, Canada, and the United Kingdom allow for lower minimum wages for youth and trainees and differential (lower) wages for people who may receive tips (primarily food and beverage workers). Minimum wages for select countries and provinces are presented in Table 9.3 and Figure 9.4. Apart from Australia and Denmark, working full time would leave the employee on minimum wage well below the poverty line and incapable of acquiring the resources required for healthy living. Without some other special income supports, single parents working at or near the minimum wage in Canada, the United States, and the United Kingdom would remain unable to provide the means for a healthy life for themselves and their children.

Table 9.3 Minimum Wage (expressed in Canadian dollars)

Jurisdiction	Minimum Wage
United States (federally mandated)*	$8.80
United Kingdom	$10.76
Australia	$17.50
Denmark**	$24.50

*Applies to federal government and federal government contractors. Employees of private companies such as servers in restaurants may be paid as little as $3.00 per hour plus tips.
**Lowest government-permitted wage for private and public sector collective agreements, averaged across different sectors.

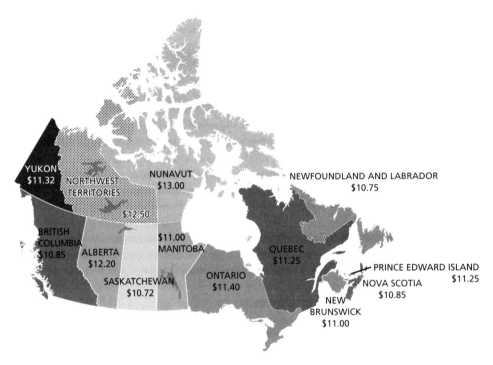

Figure 9.4 Minimum Wage in Canada, by Province
Source: Retail Council of Canada, 2017 https://www.retailcouncil.org/quickfacts/minimum-wage.

Poverty and low income are, of course, closely linked to the labour market. As Brady, Fullerton, and Cross (2010) note, "In 2000, more than 11 per cent of the US population resided in poor households with at least one employed person, while only 4.1 per cent resided in poor single-mother households and 2.6 per cent resided in poor households with no one employed." Contrary to common prejudices, *most poor people in the liberal regime world are employed, albeit in low-paid jobs.*

The exception to the liberal regime pattern is, once again, Australia. Fair Work Australia is the national workplace relations tribunal that, among other things, sets minimum wages across employment sectors. The minimum wage order is $589.30 AUD per week ($17.50 CAD per hour). Of all the liberal regime countries, Australia alone guarantees something approximating a "living wage." The approach not only solves the working-poor problem, but also eliminates the reliance of food- and beverage-sector workers on tips.

It should be noted that some US cities have implemented "living wage" legislation. Seattle's minimum wage was raised to $17 USD per hour in 2017. Some US employers, notably universities, have also implemented "living wages." In BC, the NDP government that took office in August 2017 promised to raise the province's minimum wage to $15; Alberta's NDP government raised the minimum wage to $13.60 in the autumn of 2017, and Ontario's Liberal government raised the minimum wage in that province to $14.00 effective 1 January 2018. The changes are heartening because so many workers are engaged in minimum wage employment—between 5 per cent in BC and 11 per cent in Ontario (Statistics Canada, 2018).

Guaranteed benefits such as stable, steady hours of employment, mandated rest breaks, vacation time, sick leave, and health care benefits are minimal in the liberal regime world. With the exception of gender equity in Canada, governments in the United States and Canada have deregulated employment standards, shifting policy in employers' favour over the past 25 years. Minimum wage workers are now least likely to enjoy the security of hours, consistent shifts, regular paid breaks, or any other significant employment benefits. Again, the exception is Australia, where the Fair Work Australia tribunal establishes industry-wide standards that must be followed by employers, providing greater levels of employee benefits and more consistent (and fair) treatment of workers than is typical of Canada and the United States.

Life at the bottom, then, except in Australia, has generally gotten worse over the past 25 years. The number of working poor has risen and lower-income people are working longer and harder in less and less secure employment settings. But life at the top is quite otherwise. In the United States, in 2009, while workers at the twenty-fifth percentile of the income distribution earned under $8 per hour, about the same or slightly less than they did 30 years ago, employees at the ninety-fifth percentile earned $48 per hour, a substantial increase. Chief executive officers in American companies soared from an average pay of $2 million per annum to $6 million over the same period. CEOs, earning on average about 150 times the earnings of their factory floor workers in 1980, now earn about 400 times as much (Hallock, 2011).

Improving Working Conditions and Employee Benefits

In general, fewer liberal regime workers today than in the past are exposed to the dangerous working conditions associated with mines, forestry, the fishing industry, and heavy manufacturing, mostly because these activities have been outsourced to poorer countries. But sizable pockets of dangerous work remain, such as the construction trades and vehicular transport. More common are the risks associated with sedentary work in shops and offices, repetitive strain injuries associated with keyboards, back injuries (also associated with extensive sitting), and hearing loss arising from noisy worksites and driving trucks and other heavy vehicles. Overall, regulation of worksites has greatly improved workplace safety throughout the liberal regime world, but the sedentary and repetitive nature of modern work remains a serious health threat for many. Few workplaces, unlike their Japanese counterparts, require group exercises. *Rajio taiso*, an institutionalized feature in Japanese life, involves stretches, knee bends, and arm windmills.

More problematic than lack of exercise is a lack of worker control over the work, how it is to be done, and scheduling. Few Canadian, American, and British workplaces accord meaningful input by workers into the work process, thus failing to close the gap between worker control and job demand that is known to foster mental and physical disease. Other countries such as Germany do much better, involving workers and their unions in workplace decisions. Volkswagen, for example, enables its employees to shape company plans and work processes through workplace participation in formal joint committees.

Box 9.6	Case Study ○ Health Circles

Some workplace interventions such as Health Circles, implemented in German industrial enterprises, have been shown to be effective in reducing stress and in improving worker satisfaction (Aust & Ducki, 2004). Health Circles are structured discussion groups convened at work and charged with exploring health-related problems and solutions. The goals are to improve working conditions and enhance employee health.

Do you see potential for instituting something along these lines in British or North American workplaces? What resistance might there be? How might it best be overcome?

Fairness in the allocation of tasks and even-handed payment of bonuses and perks remain important, unresolved issues. Consequently, the gap between effort and reward remains large in Canada, the United States, and the United Kingdom. But fairness extends well beyond processes used for decision making about the work. Many workplaces tolerate health-harming power imbalances ranging from gender inequity to discrimination to worker harassment by supervisors, fellow workers, or clients.

However, considerable progress has been made on a number of fronts. Canada, in particular, moved aggressively to improve gender equity in the workplace. Canada also, through provincial and federal human rights codes, imposed clear employment standards with respect to race, religion, and ethnicity. Some employers, such as universities, have attempted voluntarily to become exemplars of best practices, forbidding harassment and bullying of employees, establishing internal human rights offices and protocols, enforcing hiring guidelines intended to better represent women and minorities within the workforce, and regularizing promotion through transparent, democratic workplace processes. Other employers, notably in the information technology sector, have, in order to retain their valued employees, established health and wellness programs, provided access to recreation and created more flexible work processes that align better with their employees' wishes.

Overall, however, there has not been a stampede toward healthier workplaces, and some of the progress in the late 1990s and early 2000s was lost with the 2008–2014 economic slowdown, the political tide toward conservatism, and persistent high levels of unemployment. The liberal regime world remains well behind leading countries such as Germany, the Netherlands, and the Nordic countries in creating fairer, healthier workplaces.

Family-Friendly Policy

Other key issues in the liberal regime context are child care and maternity/paternity benefits. None of the liberal regime countries provide universally available, licensed, subsidized child care, although many European countries do. In the absence of quality, affordable child care, many parents are faced with paying for child care of uneven or unknown quality, the cost of which can challenge or even exceed their total earnings. Child care tax credits come nowhere near offsetting those costs, amounting typically to well under 10 per cent of the cost of care. Canada came close to an agreement among provincial and federal governments over a universal child care plan in 2004, but the subsequent election of a Conservative federal government put plans for such a scheme on hold. The current situation embeds a serious gender bias against women, precludes many women with younger children from working, and impacts significantly on the disposable income of women with families, especially sole-support mothers. The lack of support for women and families is unlikely to change in the United States or the United Kingdom in the foreseeable future; however, the Canadian Liberal government signed in the summer of 2017 an agreement with the provinces to create up to 40,000 new child care spaces, with a view to creating a fully inclusive child care system in Canada. In December 2017, the government further improved the situation for Canadians by expanding and increasing the flexibility of parental leave benefits.

In general, though, the liberal regime countries, in comparison with social democratic ones, are unwilling to provide significant maternal/paternal benefits, whether in terms of mandated employment leave or government-funded payments to new parents. In the United Kingdom, a woman may apply for up to 26 weeks of "ordinary maternal leave" and 26 weeks of "additional leave." In order to qualify, she must have worked 26 weeks with the same employer. In order to qualify for the maximum 39 weeks of paid leave, she must have earned at least £102 ($165 CAD) per week. If eligible for paid leave, she may receive up to 90 per cent of her earnings for the first 6 weeks and up to £128.73 ($211 CAD) per week for the next 33 weeks. In Canada, the leave provisions are governed by employment insurance rules. A woman must have worked enough hours to qualify for employment insurance, at which point either she or her spouse may apply for "parental leave" upon the birth of their child. Employment insurance pays 55 per cent of the woman's salary, up to a maximum of $468 per week, for 52 weeks (this is now being enhanced). In contrast, Sweden entitles all parents to 16 months of 100 per cent paid leave for each child, whereas the US does not mandate any form of paid parental leave (even low-income Cuba provides 18 weeks at 100 per cent of salary).

Shift Work and Commuting

Also of concern, especially in the liberal regime world, is the growth in both shift work and lengthy commuting to the workplace. Shift work is strongly associated with coronary heart disease, sleep disorders, anxiety and depression, substance abuse, and family breakdown (Scott, 2000). It has implications not only for the health of the worker, but also, especially in the case of women, negative ramifications for the emotional and intellectual development of her children. Shift work can impair emotional bonding and attachment, as well as degrade the quality and quantity of interaction between mother and young child.

Distances travelled by private vehicle to work, the time required, and the density of traffic encountered have all increased dramatically in Canada, the United States, the United Kingdom, and Australia. Commuting by car is a major contributor to sedentary lifestyles, and hence to obesity and its negative health correlates. It is also a major source of stress in many working people's lives. The average commuting time in Canada is 26 minutes—appreciably longer in larger urban centres (Turcotte, 2011). In Toronto, 29 per cent of commuters are caught in traffic jams daily. Thirty-six per cent of commuters with longer commutes (greater than 45 minutes) report being "quite" or "extremely" stressed (Turcotte, 2011).

Processes of assigning shift work and longer-term urban planning, coupled with affordable housing and public transit designed to reduce the burdens of commuting, are matters amenable to public policy. Many countries, notably those in Northern Europe, have already made significant strides in addressing both sets of issues. Norway and the Netherlands, for example, have focused on coordinating urban planning with patterns of work and commuting, encouraging more use of bicycles, public transit, pedestrian-only zones, and staggered opening times of businesses to reduce congestion.

Theoretical Considerations

Employment is the confluence of a range of material and psychosocial factors. Income, personal safety, training opportunities, and the informational and emotional support of others all derive from employment. So do dangerous exposures and physical risks. On the psychosocial side, how we feel about ourselves and others is deeply influenced by workplace conditions, especially the fit between the demands made of us and the control we feel we have over the nature and pace of the work and the congruence between how hard we feel we are working and how well we feel we are rewarded for that work. Employment and workplace studies are thus a kind of vehicle for test-driving hypotheses from both the material and psychosocial traditions. The review we conducted in Chapter 9 shows us clearly that both material and psychosocial factors are important, and complete analyses must incorporate both theoretical traditions. Moreover, employment studies neatly show how we must also attend to levels of analysis. Many factors are properly treated as individual, such as a person's experience of workplace realities, but others, such as area-level unemployment, are clearly population-level variables. As the chapter pointed out, it is important to consider individual-level, household-level (family), and community-level variables associated with paid work.

Summary

Paid employment is one of the central features of adult life in capitalist societies such as the liberal regime countries. Work experiences and the level of income derived from employment shape beliefs, values, and health behaviour; provide or undermine social support; and substantially determine the conditions under which we live. Paid employment is especially important in liberal regime countries because there is little income support outside of the labour market, little social housing, and limited unemployment insurance.

Some policy conclusions that emerge from the discussion in Chapter 9 are as follows:

- A policy that aims for adequate income for the population but does not promote full employment at fair wages cannot succeed. Rather than focusing on safety nets to support those who are excluded from work (or who cannot earn enough money through paid employment to support themselves and their families), governments must do more to ensure jobs are available, people are appropriately prepared in terms of skills and knowledge to assume those jobs, and that the jobs pay wages and provide benefits that are adequate to support healthy living. Of the liberal regime countries, only Australia comes close to recognizing these realities.

- Closer collaboration between governments at all levels and employers is required to improve the fit between education and training and available work.
- For the health of the majority of the population to improve, minimum wages and minimum benefits must be raised in Canada, the United States, and the United Kingdom. Evidence does not support the right-wing contention that higher minimum wages and improved benefits "kill jobs," making the less well-off even worse. In fact, economic recessions are so intractable in the liberal regime world precisely because lower-income people cannot afford to buy the things they need, even when they go deeply into debt.
- Governments should structure tax and employment policy to discourage insecure forms of employment and incentivize long-term employer commitment to employees. Many social democratic countries already do this (e.g., the Netherlands, Germany, Finland).
- Adequate child care and maternity/paternity leave should be mandated everywhere. Without such policies, we cannot achieve the healthy start for every child that is the cornerstone for improved population health.
- Healthy workplaces and healthy communities go hand-in-glove, and policy and planning must be coordinated to ensure both move ahead together.

Critical Thinking Questions

1. In Chapter 5 we discussed some of the determinants of health associated with infancy, and in Case Study 9.4 we looked at one aspect of work's impact on fetal development. More broadly, how might employment and workplace policies support early childhood development? Alternatively, how might employment policies and workplace practices harm children and young families?

2. The effort–reward model depends on our sense of fairness. In particular, it assumes that a sense of unfairness will cause considerable distress, which in turn will affect our emotional, mental, and physical health. The demand–control model depends on our sense of self-efficacy. In particular, it assumes that we will experience our work life as "out of control" if other people or mechanical processes determine the amount and pace of work. A sense of lack of control over what we must respond to, in turn, will generate stress-causing emotional difficulties and illness. How adequate are these psychosocial models? What other assumptions about health-relevant mechanisms do they incorporate?

3. How do gender and employment interact? Which employment conditions typically affect mostly women? Men? How might working conditions be experienced differently by women than men?

Annotated Suggested Readings

The best resource on employment and health is the publication *Work, Stress, Health: The Whitehall II Study*. Written for an educated lay audience, the short report covers the background to and findings of this seminal prospective cohort study. The document may be acquired at www.ucl. ac.uk/whitehallII/pdf/Whitehallbooklet_1_.pdf.

An excellent book on the health effects of stress in the workplace is Jennie Grimshaw's *Employment and Health: Psychosocial Stress in the Workplace* (London: British Library, 1999). While somewhat dated and focused on Europe, the book does a good job of exploring the relationships among the changing nature of work, government policies, and employee health.

For a more recent and comprehensive overview of employment conditions and health, consult *Employment Conditions and Health Inequalities* (Geneva: World Health Organization Commission on the Social Determinants of Health, 2007), available at www.who.int/social_determinants/ resources/articles/emconet_who_report.pdf.

Annotated Web Resources

"Work Matters for Health"
www.commissiononhealth.org/PDF/0e8ca13d-6fb8-451d-bac8-7d15343aacff/Issue%20 Brief%204%20Dec%2008%20-%20 Work%20and%20Health.pdf
The Robert Wood Johnson Foundation produced "Issue Brief 4: Work and Health" in 2008. While relying on US experience and data, the brief is highly relevant to Canada, as well as the United States and the United Kingdom. It provides a comprehensive overview of the relationships among work, unemployment, working conditions, and health, as well as providing policy recommendations and a blueprint for creating a healthier workplace.

"Fair Society, Healthy Lives"
www.youtube.com/watch?v=FF2SV-VfaC0
While covering a number of topics related to the social determinants of health, Sir Michael Marmot also speaks about his work on employment. Along the way, he draws out a large number of policy recommendations flowing from his analysis. This video is an excellent review of the subjects covered up to this point.

Institute for Work and Health
www.iwh.on.ca
For specifically Canadian content (although the site provides articles of an international and scientific nature as well), the Institute for Work and Health is an especially rich resource. Articles range from workplace safety to issues of gender in the workplace to fair compensation.

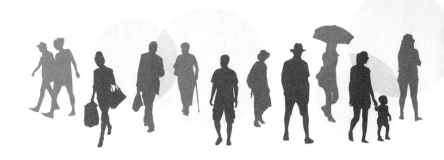

10 Housing and Neighbourhood

Objectives

By the end of your study of this chapter, you should be able to
- distinguish between housing and neighbourhood effects on health;
- understand how and why urban design and the built environment influence health outcomes;
- appreciate how public policies and government programs modify the health effects of housing and neighbourhood variables.

Where people live affects their health and chances of leading flourishing lives. Communities and neighbourhoods that ensure access to basic goods, that are socially cohesive, that are designed to promote good physical and psychological well-being, and that are protective of the natural environment are essential for health equity. (Commission on Social Determinants of Health, 2008)

Synopsis

Chapter 10 reviews the impact of housing quality and homelessness on health, before turning to a discussion of healthy and unhealthy neighbourhood characteristics. Policy implications for improving population health, including healthy urban design and housing policy, complete the chapter.

Homes and Health

Being appropriately housed is an obvious determinant of good health. Appropriate housing—homes with good ventilation, well-regulated heating and cooling, low-density occupancy, ample and well-designed food storage, and adequate toilets and washing facilities—supports the health of the occupants.

Bad housing is associated with a host of ill health effects. Poor ventilation, especially if combined with heating or cooking with wood- or coal-burning appliances (or smoking indoors), contributes significantly to respiratory diseases ranging from asthma in children to chronic bronchitis in adults to risk of lung cancer in older adults. Poor ventilation is also associated with poor control of humidity. High humidity levels foster the growth of harmful moulds, mildews, and bacteria, which in turn increase risk of respiratory disease. Overcrowding in housing, particularly if combined with inadequate garbage disposal and toilet facilities, increases the risk of communicable disease, especially the risk of respiratory and food-borne illnesses. Overcrowding also fosters, as Engels pointed out 150 years ago, stress, depression, family violence, and substance abuse.

Housing may also be dangerous in other ways. Low-income housing often does not meet safety standards. Smoke detectors and hand railings may be missing or damaged. Wiring might be unsafe. Consequently, the preponderance of home injuries and fatalities from house fires, from children falling on stairs or from balconies, or from other causes occur in low-income contexts.

Inadequate food storage and refuse disposal create insect and animal vectors for disease, such as cockroaches and rodents. Additionally, improper food storage and waste disposal can lead directly to food poisoning. Environmental hazards in older houses, such as lead paint and asbestos fibre, pose serious health threats to occupants, particularly toddlers and young children who are most often indoors and most likely to ingest substances like paint residues.

Lead-based paints were used until the 1970s. Degraded paint yields chips and dust heavily contaminated with lead. Lead poisoning irreversibly damages the brain, and small children can suffer large effects at low doses. An estimated 310,000 mostly poor, inner-city American children between the ages of one and five, in consequence of lead paint in older homes, have elevated blood-lead levels (Jacobs et al., 2002). Almost 35 per cent of all low-cost housing in the United States is contaminated with lead.

Inadequate regulation of heating and cooling can literally kill people, as happens both in hot spells and cold snaps to people who are disabled and face mobility issues. "Fuel poverty," the inability of poorer people to pay for adequate electricity, gas, or oil to heat their homes, is a significant health risk. Cold housing is associated with stress and mental illness, especially among children. It is also associated with elevated incidence of viral infection and with exacerbation of symptoms of arthritis. In the UK, up to 27,000 additional deaths each winter are associated with fuel poverty (BBC, 2011). Death rates in the summertime in the US are 42 per cent lower among people whose houses are air conditioned (Rogot, Sorlie, & Backlund, 1992).

Housing also has psychological and psychosocial effects. Physical and mental well-being require a degree of privacy and the possibility of the home serving as a refuge from the pressures of the outside world. Crowding, noise, and lack of privacy are major stressors for lower-income people.

Homelessness and Health

Pause and Reflect   Causal Pathways and Homelessness

A disproportionate number of homeless people have a health problem such as a mental disorder or an addiction. Does homelessness lead to those health problems or, alternatively, do the health problems lead to homelessness?

Homelessness would be expected to negatively affect health, but the relationship between ill health and homelessness is complicated by the fact that people who are not well, especially those with substance abuse or mental health issues, are most at risk of becoming homeless. Poor health, substance abuse, or disability may lead to low income, which in turn leads to homelessness. But it is also true that being without a home creates stress, disrupts the person's capacity to lead a stable life, and thus leads to mental illness, especially depression and anxiety. It is also true that being on the street, partly through stress and partly through exposure to "street culture," can lead to substance abuse. It can also lead to becoming a victim of violence.

It is wrong to think that people are homeless because of pre-existing mental illness or substance abuse. Surveys show that a larger proportion of people who are homeless than the general population have serious mental illness such as schizophrenia, but the seriously mentally ill still make up only 6 per cent of the total homeless population in Canada (Frankish, Hwang, & Quantz, 2005).

For obvious reasons, homeless people have significantly worse health than the general population. Mortality rates in Canada are approximately eight times higher for homeless men and 30 times higher for homeless women than for their housed counterparts. In the US, being homeless will reduce life expectancy by 20 years. The situation is worse in the United Kingdom, where the average life expectancy of a homeless person is 42 years.

Exposure to the elements can lead to heat stroke or hypothermia and frostbite. The lack of a secure place to stay also makes homeless people victims of violence. In Canada, approximately 40 per cent of homeless people are assaulted each and every year, and 25 per cent of homeless women report being raped (Hwang, 2001). Homeless shelters are often unsafe and overcrowded. Prolonged walking and sitting on the pavement, combined with inadequate hygiene, lead to foot infections and pressure ulcers.

The stress of living on the street contributes to high rates of smoking and alcohol and drug abuse. Poor nutrition, elevated stress, lack of sleep, and alcohol abuse compromise immune status, making homeless people more susceptible to infectious diseases such as TB. Moreover, homeless people face substantial barriers in accessing health and social services and, when they do, frequently fail to comply with treatment. Life on the streets is not conducive to following a treatment plan. Homeless people may also be barred from use of food banks; the policies of some food banks allow only people with a fixed address to seek support.

Table 10.1 Variables Associated with Homelessness

Individual	Macro
Lack of job skills	Income inequality
Low educational attainment	Economy/unemployment
Mental illness	High housing costs
Substance abuse	Lack of social assistance and income support
Family breakdown	Discrimination
Adverse childhood experience (abuse)	
Chronic illness or disability	

Scope of the Problem of Homelessness

Homelessness is not a trivial health problem in wealthy countries such as Canada, the United States, and the United Kingdom. An estimated 250,000 to 300,000 people experience homelessness each year in Canada; approximately 30,000 Canadians are homeless on any given night. About 3.5 million people, 1.35 million of them children, are estimated to experience homelessness every year in the United States. Rates of homelessness for families and women have been steadily rising (National Coalition for the Homeless, 2011; Picard, 2016).

A significant factor driving up rates of homelessness is the housing boom—rapidly rising housing prices and associated increases in rent. Vacancy rates in many Canadian housing markets have been steadily falling and now average around 1 per cent. (They are substantially lower in the "hot" property markets of Toronto and Vancouver. For example, assuming a person was lucky enough to find one, the rent he or she would pay for an average two-bedroom apartment in Toronto rose from $984 to $1426 between 2000 and 2017 [Myles, 2017].)

Housing Costs and Health

By 2016, more than 3.3 million Canadian households were spending in excess of 30 per cent of their total household incomes on housing (Statistics Canada, 2017). And as of 2017, in the expensive housing markets of Vancouver and Toronto, a third of households spend above the 30 per cent threshold (Statistics Canada, 2017). Spending at 30 or more per cent places a family at risk of **food insecurity** and of being unable to meet their basic needs for healthy living. In Vancouver, by 2017, nearly 10 per cent of renters were paying between 50 and 100 per cent of their total household incomes on housing (City of Vancouver, 2017). Households cannot withhold rents, so they economize by skipping meals and buying lower-cost, lower-quality foods (see Chapter 11). At current housing prices and rents, a third of Canadians cannot afford appropriate levels of recreation and leisure or good-quality diets.

Neighbourhood and Health

In general, the patterning of health status in a population is determined, in part, by the contexts, places, and locations where people spend their lives. Extensive systematic review of high-quality research literature found consistent effects of places on human health, independent of individual level attributes (Pickett & Pearl, 2001). Area-level socio-economic variables are strongly associated with individual-level health outcomes, and strong associations have been demonstrated between area of residence, health behaviour, and self-rated health (Blaxter, 1990). Differential access to services and amenities afforded by neighbourhoods affect health behaviour, mental-health status, body size and shape, and activity level (Ellaway & Macintyre, 1996, 1997; Robert & Reither, 2004; Seliske, Pickett, & Janssen, 2012). The degree of social cohesion in a neighbourhood is predictive of rates of schizophrenia (Van Os, Driessen, Gunther, & Delespaul, 2000). Collective efficacy, community capacity, and social cohesion affect health outcomes and the developmental trajectories of children (Kawachi, Kennedy, & Glass, 1999; Hertzman and Power, 2006). Hertzman and Power (2006) showed that neighbourhood characteristics influence child readiness for school and a range of child-development outcomes independently of family of origin variables (although those remain the most important). Kohen, Brooks-Gunn, Leventhal, & Hertzman (2002) showed that safer and more cohesive neighbourhoods have better child-development outcomes. Neighbourhood-level measures of deprivation are predictive of both the rates of uptake of smoking and the amount of tobacco smoked (Duncan, Jones, & Moon, 1996). There is more than a three-fold difference in coronary heart disease between rich and poor neighbourhoods after controlling for individual-level income (Diez Roux et al., 2001).

In many ways, it is not surprising that characteristics of neighbourhoods can exert a strong influence on health. Neighbourhoods differ in the degree of personal security and sense of safety; the quality of housing; access to good-quality shops; the availability of transportation; the proximity and character of green spaces, parks, and recreational facilities; access to social services and health care; and the quality of schools and other services.

Neighbourhoods, Community Resources, and Opportunity Structures

From a materialist perspective, most neighbourhood characteristics can be regarded as resources or opportunities for the residents. The range of shops and what they stock at what price point, amenities like parks, recreation facilities, and public libraries, schools and health care, public transit, and so on are all part of the opportunity structure afforded by the neighbourhood. Those opportunity structures follow a pattern of **deprivation amplification** (Macintyre & Ellaway, 2000), meaning that there is generally a direct relationship between the opportunities a community has on offer and the income and education of its residents. Poorer and less-educated people, in other words, often end up, not by choice but by necessity, living in neighbourhoods with impoverished opportunity structures, whereas those already privileged usually end up in neighbourhoods with rich amenities. Hence, we find the amplification effect. However, it is important to note that "pouring resources into" troubled or deprived neighbourhoods does not automatically improve opportunities and hence health of residents. For example, for years, a million dollars a day have been spent by 260 agencies on community services in Vancouver's Downtown Eastside, yet problems of homelessness, drug use and impaired health remain (McMartin, 2016). Proper program design and effective community engagement are critical for success, which might well take many years if not decades.

Levels of health and well-being vary by Canadian city. Figure 10.1 provides some data on self-reported health and stress at the municipal level.

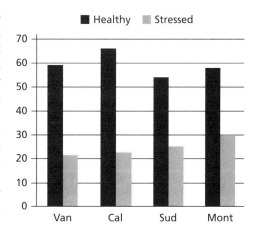

Figure 10.1 Self-Reported Health and Stress Levels by Select Canadian Cities (Per Cent)

Source: Based on Gandhi, 2006.

A well-known example is the so-called food desert. Poor people, particularly in the United States (which has significant neighbourhood segregation by income and race), end up in neighbourhoods where there aren't any quality grocery stores offering reasonably priced fruit and vegetables, nor any readily accessible and affordable transit to stores that do. Poor neighbourhoods are riddled with convenience stores, tobacco shops, liquor stores, and fast-food outlets, but are wastelands when it comes to vendors of healthy foods. Products such as fresh food, when they can be found, are paradoxically more expensive than the same products in more affluent areas. The reasons for this are not fully understood but likely include lack of competition, a "captive market" due to the lack of ready access to affordable transportation, the lower educational level of the clientele, and straightforward exploitation of vulnerable people.

The pattern of what shops are available, what they offer for sale, and what they charge shapes the choices residents make regarding their purchases. That is true not only for food but for other health-relevant choices as well. For example, Frohlich, Potvin, Chabut, & Lorin (2002) explored opportunity structures for smoking in Quebec. The researchers sought out community variables that might facilitate or discourage smoking, such as locations where tobacco was sold. They found that 51 per cent of smoking behaviour in Quebec could be attributed to community-level variables. Alcohol consumption has also been shown to vary depending on the number of bars and liquor retail outlets within a neighbourhood.

Pause and Reflect   Effect on Poorer People of Living in Richer Neighbourhoods

Poorer parents sometimes move from low-income to higher-income neighbourhoods, believing their children will have better opportunities and consequently do better over their life course. Often, lower-class children face discrimination, teasing, and bullying because they do not have the latest clothes, bikes, gadgets, etc. Overall, do you think parents who move into more affluent neighbourhoods are doing something positive or negative for their children? Why?

We know that more-affluent neighbourhoods, in terms of median income, generate better health outcomes for both their rich and their less-rich inhabitants, whereas the opposite is true for less-affluent neighbourhoods. The lower the degree of neighbourhood segregation, the more mixing there is at the neighbourhood level of richer and poorer people, and the greater the health of the average resident. This appears to be a key reason why Canada has a better overall health profile than the United States. It also helps explain why income inequality in Canada does not have the same devastating health effects typically found in the United States (Ross, 2004; Ross et al., 2000).

Merkin and colleagues (2009) established that Americans living in poorer neighbourhoods, regardless of their personal incomes, suffered adverse health effects. The negative health results of living in a deprived neighbourhood are worse for blacks than for Hispanics and whites, illustrating the cumulative effects of social segregation and negative neighbourhood characteristics and the ability of those population-level effects to amplify individual-level impacts such as personal income.

Comparing Canada to the US offers an interesting test of the psychosocial hypothesis. Based on psychosocial thinking, one might assume a neighbourhood made up of people all of similar income level might have a better health profile than a more mixed neighbourhood. Certainly the stress of everyday interpersonal comparisons of status would be reduced by mixing only with people with a similar socio-economic status. But recent research shows exactly the opposite is true (Hou & Miles, 2005). Poorer people do better when mixed with richer ones, presumably because they benefit from an improved opportunity structure at the neighbourhood level—better schools, better shops, better public services, and so on. Poorer people are well aware of this and many try to move to better neighbourhoods precisely so their children might benefit from better schools or so that they may feel safer.

A worrying recent trend is the growing segregation within Canadian cities. Shifting from the situation just 35 years ago when Canadian cities were quite homogeneous, with few rich or poor enclaves, cities are polarizing. The once ubiquitous "middle-class neighbourhood" composed of mixed incomes is disappearing (McMartin, 2012). The outcome is called "socio-spatial income polarization" (Ley & Lynch, 2012) and marks a potentially dangerous divide between income and racial groups. Should the trend continue, the large health disparities associated with US cities are likely to emerge in Canada.

The US situation is extreme. In the case of Detroit, outmigration of richer residents means the city of Detroit is now 85 per cent black, whereas the suburbs are more than 70 per cent white. Figure 10.2 illustrates neighbourhood effects on life expectancy. The data has been

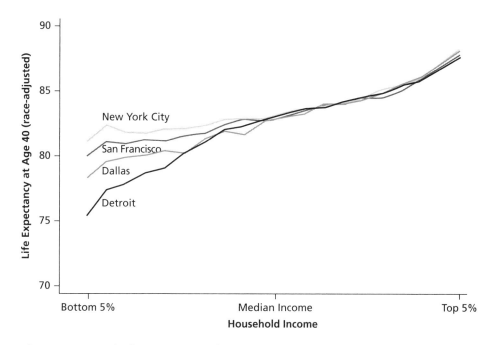

Figure 10.2 Local Life Expectancies by Income

Source: Health Inequality Project, 2016 https://healthinequality.org

adjusted for race, and thus reflects mostly the opportunity structures of the neighbourhoods in the cities compared on the graph. Detroit and Dallas are highly segregated cities, not only by race, but also by income and education, whereas San Francisco and New York City are less so (by US standards, but highly segregated by Canadian ones). The effect of the individual-level variable *income* is amplified by neighbourhood *variables associated with the opportunities each city's neighbourhoods afford their residents*, creating up to a 10-year loss of life.

Neighbourhood Order, Disorder, and Stress

Ross and colleagues (2000) ranked US and Canadian neighbourhoods based on order/disorder. People in **disordered neighbourhoods**—defined as having poorly functioning public services, graffiti, and crime—feel powerless to enact positive change, experience elevated stress, and engage in more risky behaviour (Brody, Ge, Conger, Gibbons, & Murray, 2001). Klinenburg (2002) added to Ross's findings of stress and powerlessness the idea of "**dangerous ecology**." Disordered neighbourhoods are less likely settings for individuals to be watchful over the vulnerable (children, the elderly, the disabled) or to offer assistance to those in need. Thus, we find deaths of the elderly during heat waves or cold snaps to be much more common in disordered neighbourhoods. The observed effects stem from disorder, not poverty. Even in poor neighbourhoods, those that are less disordered (vibrant ethnic enclaves, for example) have higher levels of health and safety, largely due to better social integration.

Box 10.1   Case Study ○ The Urban Environment and Health

Urban health is complex because the solutions to health challenges in towns and cities do not lie with the health sector alone but with decisions made by others: in local government, education, urban planners, engineers, and those who determine physical infrastructure to social and health services. These professionals have to face the challenges of overloaded water and sanitation systems, polluting traffic and factories, lack of space to walk or cycle, inadequate waste disposal, crime, and injury.

Nevertheless, solutions exist to tackle the root causes of urban health challenges. Urban planning can promote healthy behaviour and safety through investment in active transport, designing areas to promote physical activity and passing regulatory controls on tobacco and food safety. Improving urban living conditions in the areas of housing, water, and sanitation will go a long way to mitigating health risks. Building green, inclusive cities that are accessible and age-friendly benefits all urban residents and their health. The Healthy Cities movement emphasizes the need for community participation in the decisions that affect people's lives.

Source: World Health Organization, 2011. Urban Health at http://www.euro.who.int/en/what-we-do/health-topics/environment-and-health/urban-health.

How might the characteristics of the urban environment impact health? Given your analysis, why is it a common finding that residents living in or near the city centre enjoy better health and fitness than residents with a similar income living in the suburbs? What message(s) should that send to municipal planners and local governments?

There are some important psychosocial health effects of neighbourhood character-istics in addition to the materialist ones just discussed. Stress over personal safety has been linked to emotional disorders and destructive Health behaviours such as overeating. Access to green spaces and parks has been shown to reduce stress, blood pressure, anxiety, and depression. High levels of neighbourhood stability provide a buffer to the otherwise damaging effects of excess stress (Boardman, 2004). Neighbourhoods can also provide psychosocial benefits in terms of personal identity and sense of belonging (Omariba, 2010).

Urban Design, the Built Environment, and Physical Activity

Access to recreational facilities, parks, and urban design features such as bike paths, sidewalks, and adequate lighting at night deeply influence the physical activity level of people living in the area. So do transport policies such as rules for road use and availability and affordability of public transportation (Heath et al., 2012). The installation of fitness equipment in outdoor parks, now fairly commonplace in British Columbia communities (and standard practice in countries as diverse as China and Turkey for decades), increases the activity levels among children, adults, and the elderly (Cohen, Marsh, Williamson, Golinelli, & McKenzie, 2012). Heath and colleagues (2006) showed, for Canada and the US, that road patterns, whether grid or cul-de-sac, influenced walking, jogging, and cyc-ling. *Ciclovia* ("open streets"), the practice of closing streets to motor vehicles, has been a feature of life in Bogota, Colombia, since 1976. Every Sunday, streets are closed to cars and trucks from 8:00 a.m. to 2:00 p.m., not only in Bogota, but also in Cali and Medellin. Some Canadian cities have conducted limited experiments in creating space for pedestrians and cyclists, notably Winnipeg, Calgary, Vancouver, Hamilton, and Ottawa.

Inactivity and Health

Much of the current interest in urban design is focused on increasing the activity level of the population, based on the premise that better health will inevitably follow. Inactivity is associated with a number of adverse health outcomes, whereas regular physical activity is associated with lower incidence of heart disease, diabetes, hypertension, and obesity (Lee et al., 2012). However, the relationship between population-level inactivity and population-level health outcomes is imperfect, to say the least. Consider Table 10.2 below.

Japan is the healthiest of the countries listed in the table, and has an obesity rate of only 3.2 per cent in spite of having one of world's least active populations. France, a middle-ranking country in terms of activity levels, has excellent health and a relatively low rate of obesity (9 per cent). The United Kingdom and the United States have high rates of obesity (23 per cent and 30 per cent respectively), as well as high rates of heart disease and diabetes, but the (more inactive) British have better health than the (heavier and sicker but much more active) Americans. Obesity and health, then, do not track well with ac-tivity levels, demonstrating that diet and other factors are overall of greater import than physical activity. Nevertheless, physical activity is an important determinant of health, and it, like eating patterns and food choices, is heavily influenced by characteristics of the community in which a person resides.

Table 10.2 Per Cent of Population Inactive,* by Gender and Country (2012)

Country	Men and Women	Men	Women
Argentina	68.3	65.8	70.9
United Kingdom	63.3	58	68.6
Japan	60.2	58.9	61.6
United States	40.5	33.5	47.4
Australia	37.9	35.9	39.9
Canada	33.9	32.3	35.4
France	32.5	27.7	37.2
Netherlands	18.2	21.3	15.2

* Inactivity is defined as not meeting any of the following criteria: (1) 5 x 30 minutes of moderate-intensity exercise per week; (2) 3 x 20 minutes of vigorous-intensity exercise per week; (3) a combination of 1 and 2, achieving 600 metabolic equivalent minutes per week.
Source: Adapted from Guardian Datablog, 2012, "Which are the laziest countries on earth?" www.theguardian.com/news/datablog/2012/jul/18/physical-inactivity-country-laziest.

Housing Policy and Health

We learned earlier that housing is a significant determinant of health. The quality of housing refers to ventilation, heating and cooling, food storage and preparation capabilities, presence of toxins, washing and toilet facilities, and the number of rooms/amount of space for the number of occupants. Quality of housing also refers to neighbourhood variables, the opportunity structure of the area, security, and the standard of living of neighbours.

The cost of housing—its affordability—is also important. From the point of view of family budgets, housing is a relatively fixed cost and people must pay the rent or mortgage before they pay for other things. Otherwise, they will be homeless. If reasonable-quality housing is relatively expensive, downward pressure is put on other discretionary family budget items, especially food, causing food insecurity, another important contributor to poor health. Lower-income families may be confronted with poor-quality housing in bad neighbourhoods that is nevertheless expensive and thus crowds out other health-related budget items.

After the Second World War, governments in Canada, the United States, the United Kingdom, and Australia all busied themselves with funding affordable housing. This had much to do with their experience earlier with demobilization of millions of armed forces personnel after the First World War. Governments failed to ensure that housing and jobs were available in 1918 at the end of hostilities, leading to a period of riots, social unrest, and potential civil insurrection by ex–military personnel. No one wanted a repeat of that in 1945.

By 1975, several things had changed. First, liberal regime economies faced the first post-war credit crunch. Second, government deficits soared to record peacetime levels. Third, the economic slowdown reduced government revenues. In short, there was something of a perfect storm. As noted earlier, Keynesian economics was a victim of these remarkable circumstances. Related to this was government's withdrawal from the housing market. First came a cutback on funding for social housing, then a transfer of responsibilities for backing mortgages from government to quasi-private agencies, and then, in the

1980s, an effort to sell off public housing and return it to the private property market. In short, after 1975, housing in the liberal regime world was increasingly turned over to private market forces.

Private property developers and house builders share an interest in building large homes packed with as many luxury items as possible because those properties generate the most profit, just as big luxury cars are far more profitable to manufacturers and dealers than basic small cars. In the absence of regulation through building codes and local government zoning, the market will increasingly skew toward more expensive, larger houses even as average family size decreases. Rising prices in the new-build sub-sector will put upward pressure on prices of existing houses. That in turn creates incentives to renovate and render more modern and luxurious old housing stock, especially when the location is desirable. By and large, governments are supportive of those trends because a lot of money and jobs are generated through the commercial supply chain. The jobs and income associated with home construction range from the forest industry to lumber mills, from building supply and home improvement stores to the construction trades, and from home furnishings and appliance manufacture to furniture and appliance retailing. All of this related economic activity depends on sustaining the housing construction boom.

But the unfettered housing-market forces increase all housing prices. Along with higher costs of buying homes, the process both reduces the number of places to rent (because it is more profitable to renovate and sell than have tenants) and increases the cost of rent (because the alternative for landlords, selling, becomes more lucrative). Also, areas of modest housing become "gentrified" and put out of the reach of modest income earners, but areas with very poor housing—bad locations or bad reputations—are ignored by developers, becoming blighted yet increasingly the only places low-income people can afford.

Middle- and low-income earners are thus confronted with fewer housing choices and higher prices. Some are driven into poor-quality neighbourhoods, others into homelessness. All of this was made worse by deregulation, which lessened tenants' rights and reduced the obligations on developers to produce low-cost and multiple-family residences in addition to the lucrative single-family luxury houses and condominiums they prefer to build.

Once housing costs comprise more than 30 per cent of a household's disposable income, that household is both housing and food insecure—in other words, at risk of not being able to maintain their home and unable to afford adequate amounts of healthy food. Rising housing costs, for lower-income people, are thus a serious threat to their health.

The collapse of the US housing boom in 2008 brought some reason back into housing markets and led American and Canadian governments back into more regulation of the sector. But the response by governments has been modest and halting. Liberal regime governments appear to be waiting, hoping markets will find their own equilibrium. Small measures like tiny interest rate hikes and stricter eligibility rules for mortgage lending in Canada have done nothing to dampen hot markets like Vancouver's. More robust policy interventions have been avoided because of governments' fears of blowing the bottom out of the housing market. Vancouver and the BC provincial government have imposed punitive taxes on property speculation and foreign buyers of BC real estate, but those have not, at least at time of writing, had any discernable impact on housing affordability (Alini, 2017). It is likely that only a big jump in interest rates or a big drop in prosperity will force major decreases in housing prices (but these may well not improve affordability).

Some municipalities, however, have shown leadership in terms of support for social housing, a more aggressive stance with developers on multiple family and affordable housing, stricter zoning, and better town planning. Portland, Oregon, stands out with its robust effort to house homeless people through a "housing first" initiative, which recognizes that a person is unlikely to get control over his or her life or find secure work unless they are safely and appropriately housed. The approach was pioneered by Dr Tsemberis at the New York University School of Medicine in the 1990s and has been thoroughly evaluated since (Larimer et al., 2009). Seattle, Washington, and Vancouver, along with many other American and Canadian cities and British local authorities, have adopted a "housing first" policy, with promising results. Not only have clients' lives been stabilized by being housed, but their health and social function has also significantly improved. The British Columbia provincial government recently committed substantially more money to social housing.

Theoretical Considerations

Chapter 10 once again demonstrates the importance and power of multi-level analysis. At the individual level, risks to health arise from housing conditions; at the community level, the neighbourhood and the built environment support or undermine the health of residents. As Boardman (2004) showed, neighbourhood attributes can mediate and moderate (or amplify) effects arising from individual-level variables. Bad housing in a bad neighbourhood, the usual case, is substantially worse for health than bad housing in a good neighbourhood. Contrariwise, a good neighbourhood amplifies the positive effects of good housing. These effects have been empirically demonstrated in studies of childhood development, infectious disease, chronic disease, coronary heart disease, health behaviour, and mental health.

In the US in the 1990s, the federal government sponsored an experiment, Moving to Opportunity, a program that relocated nearly 5,000 families from bad to good neighbourhoods. The experiment had mixed results. Incomes and employment did not change as expected, but health measures, notably mental health measures, improved, especially for girls and women (Gennetian et al., 2012). The intervention provides experimental evidence that changing neighbourhood variables can change individual health ones.

Summary

The quality of housing and the capacity to heat and cool residential accommodation are significant determinants of health, especially for infants, children, and the frail elderly. Housing quality is primarily a function of income. Exposure to poor indoor air quality, inadequate food storage, mould, poor ventilation, overcrowding, indoor contaminants such as lead, asbestos, and radon gas, all rise as income falls. This is a key reason why respiratory disease tracks so closely with income.

Very low income, in the absence of robust social assistance and social housing, results in homelessness. Homelessness is associated with infectious and chronic disease, elevated stress, anxiety and depression, exposure to violence, substance abuse, and premature death.

Rising house prices in the context of flat or declining earnings among the lower-middle and lower classes decrease the quality of housing available to less well-off people and push up rates of homelessness.

Characteristics of residential neighbourhoods have profound health effects ranging from conditioning the type and amount of exercise undertaken by residents, to influencing the type and amounts of food consumed, to the levels of stress or emotional well-being experienced by residents. Neighbourhood characteristics also shape social networks and health behaviour, ranging from the amount people smoke or drink to the degree people engage in risky behaviour such as criminal activity or unsafe sex.

Urban design and the built environment heavily influence how people use spaces. Sidewalks and bicycle paths can encourage non-vehicular travel. Parks and green spaces can encourage active recreation. Road design and public transport can influence automobile use. All of these may have health impacts.

Some key policy directions emerging from Chapter 10 are listed below.

- We need enhanced co-operation among all levels of government to fund an appropriate level of social housing. Talks on affordable housing began in Canada in 2017 between the federal and provincial governments. Many Canadian municipalities are experimenting, often with support from their respective provincial government, on low-cost housing options such as prefabricated stacked housing units on vacant land.
- Local governments and citizen coalitions must work together to ensure that municipal planning, approvals for property development, and zoning by-laws are consistent with the principles of population health. For example, provincial health authorities in British Columbia have developed liaison mechanisms with community coalitions and city planners designed to foster healthy communities. Initiatives range from community gardens to block parties to cycle paths and cluster parks.
- National and sub-national levels of government must act in co-operation with local authorities in support of affordable housing, healthy neighbourhoods, and housing those who are homeless. In this regard, the Canadian federal government announced in 2017 a new national housing strategy and in March 2018 began talks on legislating a right to housing.
- National governments need to regulate credit and mortgage lending as well as tax law respecting capital gains to prevent property speculation, profiteering, and housing market "bubbles." Here again, mortgage rules were tightened up in 2017, and municipal governments (e.g., Vancouver in 2017) and provincial governments (e.g., Ontario in 2017 and BC in 2018) announced new measures to curtail speculation.

Critical Thinking Questions

1. In what ways did your housing situation and neighbourhood influence your childhood development, health, and overall well-being? Which factors do you consider most significant?

2. Examining your current housing situation, how might your home influence your health?

3. Examining your current neighbourhood, how might the built environment and "opportunity structure" influence your health and well-being?

Annotated Suggested Readings

An excellent resource on the topic of neighbourhoods and health is I. Kawachi and L. Berkman (eds.), *Neighborhood and Health* (New York: Oxford University Press, 2003). The chapter by Sally Macintyre and Anne Ellaway, "Neighbourhoods and Health, An Overview" (pp. 20–42) is clear and comprehensive. The chapter "Multi-level Methods for Public Health Research" (S. Subramanin, K. Jones and C. Duncan, pp. 65–112) provides an accessible overview of the theoretical importance of multi-level research.

Elsevier publishes the excellent academic journal *Health and Place*. The journal includes a wide range of international articles on subjects ranging from obesity and the local environment to alcohol consumption and the location of retail sales outlets.

A lot of attention has gone into planning for healthier cities, especially in Europe. *Healthy Urban Planning in Practice: Experience of European Cities* (World Health Organization) outlines European experience in planning urban spaces that will improve population health. The electronic book (available at www.euro.who.int/__data/assets/pdf_file/0003/98400/E82657.pdf) discusses how we may best promote healthy exercise; social cohesion; equity; and environmental, economic, and social sustainability.

In 2001, Ana Diez Roux published what is now a classic work in the field: "Investigating Neighborhood and Area Effects in Health," available at www.ncbi.nlm.nih.gov/pmc/articles/PMC1446876/. The article summarizes the literature to date, and explores the conceptual, theoretical, and methodological issues that arise.

Annotated Web Resources

"Exploring the Social Determinants of Health"
www.rwjf.org/content/dam/farm/reports/issue_briefs/2011/rwjf70451
The Robert Wood Johnson Foundation developed two excellent briefing papers on housing and neighbourhoods, available at the link above. While the analysis and data are American, the principles and policy considerations transfer well to Canada, the United Kingdom, and Australia.

Neighbourhood Change & Building Inclusive Communities from Within
neighbourhoodchange.ca/cities/vancouver
Canada Research Chair David Ley heads a project on neighbourhood change and building inclusive cities. The project's website has a wealth of resources for Vancouver.

WHO European Healthy Cities Network
www.euro.who.int/en/health-topics/environment-and-health/urban-health/activities/healthy-cities
The World Health Organization hosts a portal into urban health and healthy cities where a large number of policy-related resources may be found.

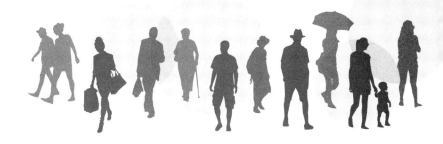

11   Food, Food Insecurity, Nutrition, Obesity, and Health

Objectives

By the end of your study of this chapter, you should be able to
- determine which factors influence food choices and eating behaviour;
- understand the causes and significance of food insecurity;
- appreciate the complexity of issues associated with obesity;
- estimate the probable impact of public policies relating to food on population health.

Synopsis

Chapter 11 opens with a consideration of factors that influence diet, and then moves to discussions of food security and obesity. Following an overview of diet and health, the chapter concludes with a review of policy and program options that could influence eating behaviour, nutrition, and health.

Diet and the Health of Populations

We have known since McKeown's work on the modern rise of populations that the availability, quality, and affordability of food are major determinants of the health of populations. Just as a strong link exists between income and housing, there is an equally strong link between income and food. People with lower income, both in the past and in the present, rely on low-cost, high-energy, but nutrient-poor foods. The potato played this role in nineteenth-century Ireland; processed foods with their high levels of sugar, refined carbohydrates, and fat play that role today.

What Determines Diet?

Pause and Reflect   Influences on Diet

What individual and community factors influence people's eating behaviour?

Many factors impact on people's choice and use of foods. These include

- the amount and stability of income and the cost of other necessities, such as housing, utilities, and basic clothing;
- the capacity to plan and to budget, which in turn depends on a person's level of education and mental health;
- the features of the person's home: the adequacy of food storage and the means to prepare healthy food;
- the knowledge and skills a person has: the ability to cook, to understand food preparation and the nutritional values of different foods;
- the relative availability and affordability of foods: the accessibility of shops/supermarkets/superstores and what they stock;
- the pervasive and persuasive marketing of food choices; marketing targeting children, who in turn insist on certain products;
- a person's ethnic, cultural, religious, and family background: cultural and social factors shape perceptions of acceptable food and acceptable uses of that food;
- peer pressure, norms, and the behavioural impact of the person's social network;
- the constraints on the person's time and energy, the time they have for shopping, food preparation, sitting down to eat a proper meal, etc.

The relationship between family income and diet is illustrated in Figure 11.1.

In general, all of the factors listed above will vary by income, education, and quality of housing and neighbourhood. All will tend toward a gradient with capacity to choose and use more healthy foods rising with income. In short, diet shows a quality gradient just like income and health. More affluent people eat a more diverse, nutritionally sound diet than poorer ones (Shohaimi et al., 2004; Tarasuk, Fitzpatrick, & Ward, 2010).

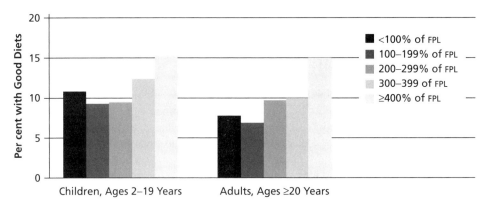

Figure 11.1 Family Income and Diet: United States

*The mean healthy eating index (HEI) score measures intake of 10 key diet components (grains, vegetables, fruits, milk, meat, total fat, saturated fat, sodium, cholesterol, and variety), each ranging from 0–10, with higher scores indicating healthier eating. A good diet is defined as a having an HEI score above 80. FPL stands for Federal Poverty Line, currently (2014) standing at $23,859 US for a family of four. Notice those below the poverty line have better diets than the working poor earning up to 2 x the poverty line. This is due to the Food Stamps program available to only the poorest Americans.

Source: Robert Wood Johnson Foundation, 2011. www.rwjf.org/content/dam/farm/reports/issue_briefs/2011/rwjf70442, p. 3. Reproduced with permission of the Robert Wood Johnson Foundation, Princeton, NJ.

What Is a Healthy Diet? Canada's Food Guide

During wartime, the Canadian federal government worried about the nutritional status of civilians deteriorating due to shortages, rationing, and rising prices. It requested that the Canadian Nutrition Council, a body formed during the 1930s Great Depression, develop a set of guidelines for a nutritious diet. Canada's Official Food Rules, published in 1942, were the result (see Figure 11.2).

The food rules were regularly revised and broadened to include meal planning. In 1961 they became less prescriptive and more advisory in nature. The name was changed to reflect the idea that the government was providing informed guidance and not prescribing how much of what Canadians must eat. Ever since, the federal government food rules have been referred to as *Canada's Food Guide* (see Figure 11.3).

The *Guide* has been criticized over the years for supporting the consumption of meat and dairy products and emphasizing grains over fruits, vegetables, and nuts. In recent years, alternatives to animal sourced foods have appeared in the *Guide*, and more stress has been laid on fish, fruits, and vegetables. Health Canada recently produced a version of the *Food Guide* for Indigenous people. The new guide, *Eating Well with Canada's Food Guide: Inuit, First Nations and Métis*, includes traditional foods and is available in several Indigenous languages.

An entirely new *Food Guide* is expected in 2018. The process of developing it has been controversial, with critics saying food interest groups have had too big a say, especially the

CANADA'S OFFICIAL FOOD RULES

These are the Health-Protective Foods

Be sure you eat them every day in at least these amounts.

(Use more if you can)

MILK—Adults–1/2 pint. Children–more than 1 pint. And some CHEESE, as available.

FRUITS—One serving of tomatoes daily, or of a citrus fruit, or of tomato or citrus fruit juices, and one serving of other fruits, fresh, canned or dried.

VEGETABLES (In addition to potatoes of which you need one serving daily)—Two servings daily of vegetables, preferably leafy green, or yellow, and frequently raw.

CEREALS AND BREAD—One serving of a whole-grain cereal and 4 to 6 slices of Canada Approved Bread, brown or white.

MEAT, FISH, etc.—One serving a day of meat, fish, or meat substitutes. Liver, heart or kidney once a week.

EGGS—At least 3 or 4 eggs weekly.

Eat these foods first, then add these and other foods you wish.

Some sources of Vitamin D such as fish liver oils, is essential for children, and may be advisable for adults.

Figure 11.2 Canada's Official Food Rules, 1942

Recommended Number of Food Guide Servings per Day

	Children			Teens		Adults			
	2–3	**4–8**	**9–13**	**14–18 Years**		**19–50 Years**		**51+ Years**	
	Girls and Boys			**Female**	**Male**	**Female**	**Male**	**Female**	**Male**
Vegetables and Fruit	4	5	6	7	8	7–8	8–10	7	7
Grain Products	3	4	6	6	7	6–7	8	6	7
Milk and Alternatives	2	2	3–4	3–4	3–4	2	2	3	3
Meat Alternatives	1	1	1–2	2	3	2	3	2	3

For example:

If you are a 35-year-old woman you should aim to have:

- 7–8 vegetables and fruit
- 6–7 grain products
- 2 milk and alternatives
- 2 meat and alternatives
- 30–45 mL (2 to 3 Tbsp) of unsaturated oils and fats

Figure 11.3 Canada's Current *Food Guide*

Source: Health Canada www.hc-sc.gc.ca/fn-an/food-guide-aliment/basics-base/quantit-eng.php. © All rights reserved. *Eating Well with Canada's Food Guide*. Health Canada, 2011. Reproduced with permission from the Minister of Health, 2014

dairy industry. The new guide is expected to put more emphasis on fruits and vegetables, discourage eating large amounts of meat, provide more information on nutritional science, and make recommendations on shopping for, and preparing, nutrient-dense meals.

The Relative Cost of Healthy Foods

In British Columbia, the 2009 monthly cost of a nutritious diet for a family of four was $872. For low-income families, the combined cost of nutritious food and housing exceeded total income, leaving nothing (in fact, resulting in a budget deficit of over $100) for other necessary expenditures (Cost of Eating, 2010). A more recent estimate places the monthly average cost of a nutritious diet for a family of four at close to $1000 (BC Provincial Health Services Authority, 2016). In Canada, housing costs are rising, very rapidly in some markets, food costs are increasing, and low- and middle-income earners' disposable incomes are falling. Thus, the majority of people are experiencing a worsening squeeze on their food budget.

The United Kingdom, faced with the worst economic prospects in the liberal regime world, is experiencing a "nutritional recession." Rising food prices combined with falling incomes since 2008 have driven up consumption of cheap, fatty, and salty foods, and driven down consumption of fruit and vegetables. It is estimated that, as of 2010, nearly a million more people in the UK are eating high-fat processed foods and failing to meet the government guideline of five daily fruit and vegetable servings (Butler, 2012). The consumption of instant noodles, baked beans, pasta, pizza, and fried food has gone up dramatically in poorer families because those foods are more affordable and are perceived to be more "filling." The effects are mostly the results of an increase of one-third in the cost of food in the past five years, supermarket promotions of processed food, and the decline in home cooking associated with the time constraints on poorer families (Butler, 2012).

Box 11.1	Case Study ○ Rising Food Commodity Prices

Extreme weather events, global warming, and reduced food stocks due to the conversion of agricultural land from food crops to bio-energy crops have, since 2007, dramatically driven up the prices of basic food commodities such as corn, rice, wheat, and soya. Widespread drought and destructive storms devastated American food production in the summer of 2012, a situation that drove up world prices for basic food commodities and meat. With heavy flooding in the Indian subcontinent and a wet, cold spring in Europe and parts of the Americas, 2013 was worse. Droughts, floods, fires, and extreme winds wreaked havoc with agriculture in 2017, and North America experienced heavy spring flooding in 2018. What are the probable impacts on population health in affluent countries like Canada? How will those impacts differ for poorer countries such as those of sub-Saharan Africa?

Food and Nutrition Insecurity

Food insecurity is defined as "the inability to acquire or consume an adequate diet quality or sufficient quantity of food in socially acceptable ways, or the uncertainty that one will be able to do so" (Health Canada, 2008). Especially vulnerable to food insecurity are low-income people, single mothers, rural residents, Canadian and Australian Indigenous people and, in the United States, African Americans. **Nutrition insecurity** may be defined as the inability to access at all the times the nutrients needed for a healthy and active life. Statistics Canada (2015) reported that more than 1.1 million Canadian households cannot afford a healthy diet. In Nunavut, two-thirds of children are living in food-insecure households ("Food Insecurity in Nunavut," 2017).

Episodes of food and nutrition insecurity have been linked to poorer self-reported health, obesity in children and women, diabetes, heart disease, depression, and anxiety (Vozoris & Tarasuk, 2003; Kirkpatrick & Tarasuk, 2008). Moreover, inadequately fed children do worse in school. Their cognitive, general academic, and psychosocial development are all significantly impaired (Alaimo, Olson, & Frongillo, 2001). Rose-Jacobs and colleagues (2008) showed a strong association between household food insecurity and compromised toddler development. Four- to 36-month-old children from food-insecure households are at elevated risk of developmental delays and impaired school readiness. In Canada, 23 per cent of single-parent households are food insecure (Health Canada, 2011).

Food insecurity is mostly a problem of low household income. Figure 11.4 shows food insecurity by income decile in Canada.

Food Insecurity and Canada's Indigenous People

Access to safe, nutritious, and culturally appropriate foods is an especially serious problem for many of Canada's Indigenous people (see Figure 11.5). Low income, high prices, lack of fresh produce in the Far North (and on isolated reserves), and disruption of traditional food sources all play a role. Consequently, Indigenous people are at high risk of poor nutritional status and poor health outcomes.

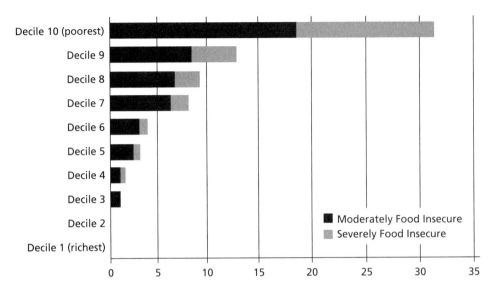

Figure 11.4 Food Insecurity by Income Decile, Canada, 2007–08 (per cent)

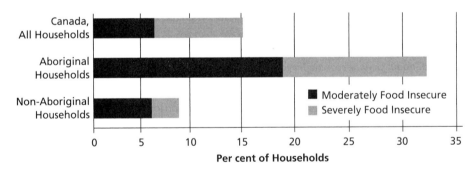

Figure 11.5 Food Insecurity and Canada's Indigenous People

Food Banks

In Canada, over two million households are food and nutrition insecure. In Nova Scotia, nearly 15 per cent of households are food insecure. Approximately 25 per cent of single-parent, woman-headed households and over one-third of Indigenous households face food insecurity (Health Canada, 2008). Food banks and charity-run community kitchens have become features of Canadian towns and cities.

Whereas in the social democratic countries of Europe there is a recognized right to food, and good nutrition for all citizens is considered a public obligation, food and nutrition are considered private matters in liberal regime countries such as Canada. Hence, the response to food insecurity, in spite of Canada being a signatory to the Universal Declaration of Human Rights (which included food as a fundamental human right), is a mix of targeted children's feeding programs, private commercial ventures such as farmers' markets, voluntary community action such as community gardening ventures, and charities such as food banks and community kitchens.

Food banks were introduced as a short-term stop-gap measure to deal with the fallout from the economic downturn in the early 1980s. Now there are over 670 food banks in Canada supporting over 750,000 people. They lack demonstrated effectiveness because food banks provide a limited amount of food to people whose real problems are low income and expensive housing.

Food banks have also been criticized for creating the pretense of a solution to a serious problem. Governments can "look the other way" and continue to ignore the health and social effects of a low-wage, insecure employment market, the high costs of housing, and an inadequate diet. Food banks obscure the existence of a complex social justice issue demanding a public response.

Obesity

There is some evidence that people facing moderate food insecurity are at risk of becoming obese. This seems particularly true of women because for women, but not so clearly for men, obesity follows the familiar health gradient. The lower a woman's income and education, the higher the probability that she will become obese. This may have to do with disordered eating patterns. For example, repeated dieting has been linked to eating disorders and obesity in women (Neumark-Sztainer et al., 2006). Periods with limited amounts of food may also promote overeating when food is available. Dieting and bingeing can also induce epigenetic changes, as well as cause profound shifts in the balance of intestinal flora; both sets of changes increase the propensity to gain weight.

Box 11.2   Case Study ○ Rising Incidence of Obesity

Over the past 30 years, obesity prevalence rose sharply around the world, even in some relatively poor countries. Currently, about one-third of Americans are obese—that is, they score over 30 when you divide their weight in kilograms by their height in metres squared (kg/m^2 = BMI). That compares with just over 20 per cent of residents of the United Kingdom and Canada and around 3 per cent in Japan (OECD, 2010).

In 2009, 55 per cent of the populations in Canada and the United Kingdom were overweight compared with 64 per cent in Australia and 65 per cent in the United States. The rate of increase in obesity has slowed in Canada, but the trend toward obesity has remained strong in the United States and Australia (OECD, 2011).

What factors lie behind these statistics?

In addition to individual-level factors influencing food choice and eating habits, there are some important contextual variables as well. Poorer neighbourhoods in the United States have less diversity of foodstuffs available for residents, greater concentrations of processed foods and fast foods, and higher food prices than richer neighbourhoods (Morland, Wing, Diez Roux, & Poole, 2002; Morland & Filomena, 2007; Powell, Slater, Mirtcheva, Bao, & Chaloupka, 2007). These features help concentrate food purchases on high-energy but low-nutrition items.

As noted earlier, obesity follows a consistent gradient like many other health attributes, but only for women. In Canada (but not in the United States or the United Kingdom), affluent men are almost as likely to be obese as poor men. Presumably the stronger gradient effects for women reflect the enormous social pressure on more affluent women to stay slim (which may partly account for the prevalence of anorexia among more privileged women). As Christakis and Fowler (2009) have shown, whom you know and whom you are associated with will have an enormous influence on your BMI, due to transmission of norms, group disciplining effects, and other macro-level considerations. The social network effects act to amplify the social gradient because most people's associations are with others of similar class, income, and educational backgrounds to themselves.

There are large regional variations in obesity rates in Canada. Rural areas have larger concentrations of overweight and obese people than do urban ones; suburbs generally have higher rates of obesity than city centres. Provincial variations are also significant (Public Health Agency of Canada, 2011).

Neighbourhood characteristics play a role in the obesity epidemic in the United States. Healthy foods are harder to find and cost more in less-affluent neighbourhoods, whereas fast-food outlets and convenience stores with highly processed energy-rich foods are commonplace in deprived neighbourhoods. That pattern, however, is almost uniquely American. Canadian, British, and Australian neighbourhoods do not exhibit "food deserts" to the same extent as US cities. In other words, access to foods and pricing are more equal across social classes and races in countries other than the United States, because of less extreme neighbourhood segregation. Some comparisons between affluent OECD countries are provided in Figure 11.6.

Pause and Reflect   Is Obesity a Disease?

In June 2013, the American Medical Association declared obesity a "disease," rendering one-third of mostly well Americans sick. The decision is highly controversial. Some hold that overweight people are being stigmatized. Others contend calling obesity a disease discounts the behavioural aspects of overeating, removing responsibility from the overweight person. Some claim this is a further example of abuse by doctors, medicalizing a social problem and failing to appreciate the cultural, economic, and political dimensions of disordered eating in America. Others see it as a money grab by the medical and pharmaceutical industries seeking to cash in on the fear, frustration, and unhappiness of people distressed by their appearance. Medical experts in other countries are divided.

Obesity may raise the risk of some diseases, but can it be considered itself to be a disease? Is smoking a disease? Failing to wear a seatbelt? Alcohol abuse?

In what sense is obesity a health condition or a disease? What are the implications of the American Medical Association decision?

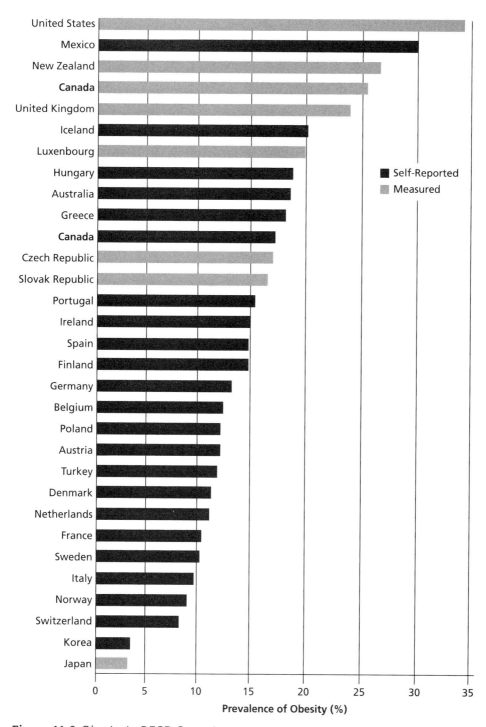

Figure 11.6 Obesity in OECD Countries

Why obesity rates rose so rapidly is not well understood. Suspects are as follows:

- Some foods, in real price terms, have become (until recently) progressively cheaper and, in general, take up less of most people's disposable income. These include red meat, pork, and highly processed, packaged foods.
- Processed foods are now readily available, cheap, and convenient, but energy dense and nutritionally poor.
- Eating in fast-food and conventional restaurants has increased dramatically. About a third of meals consumed by Canadians, Americans, Britons, and Australians are eaten in restaurants (Mooney, Haw, & Frank, 2011). Food consumed in full-service restaurants can be as high, or even higher, in fats, sugar, and salt than fast-food meals.
- Portion sizes have skyrocketed since the 1970s. Bigger portion sizes have been linked to increased food consumption and obesity (Ello-Martin, Ledikwe, & Rolls, 2005).
- Disordered eating. Rather than regular sit-down meals, people in Canada, the United States, the United Kingdom, and Australia are often eating on the fly. Snacking and grabbing something to eat and drink whenever an opportunity affords itself have become common. Under such conditions, people consume more calories than they need (and many more than they realize). If people do not clearly remember how much they have eaten, their appetite and propensity to keep on eating are enhanced (Brunstrom et al., 2012).
- Soft drinks. The sale of sugared beverages doubled in the United States between 1977 and 2002 (Brownell et al., 2009) but now is declining in Canada, which has seen a 28 per cent decrease in non-diet soda pop consumption between 2004 and 2017, along with a partially offsetting rise in other sugary drinks, notably sports drinks (Jones, Veerman, & Hammond, 2017).
- Public policies such as farm subsidies have distorted markets and created gluts of cheap corn, corn derivatives such as high-fructose corn syrup, and other cheap ingredients for the processed food industry.
- Increased car ownership, reduced walking, and the effects of built environments (absence of bike lanes or safe footpaths and other urban features that reduce opportunities for walking and cycling) have lowered physical activity levels.

Whatever the causes, the outcomes of severe obesity are serious. A morbidly obese person (BMI greater than 40) can expect to live 11 years less than someone with a BMI in the 20–25 range (Mooney, Haw, & Frank, 2011). They can also expect health issues such as problems with joints, diabetes, high blood pressure, and heart disease. Back pain, gallbladder disease, and several types of cancer have also been linked to obesity (Public Health Agency of Canada, 2011). However, recent systematic reviews suggest people who are overweight (but not obese) may be healthier and live longer than either normal weight or obese people (Flegal, Kit, Orpana, & Graubard, 2013). And, paradoxically, obese people who have developed heart disease have a higher probability of survival than non-obese people in spite of the facts that their self-reported health, risk factors for disease, and physical activity levels are all worse than those of non-obese people (Hamer & Stamatakis, 2013). Why this should be so is not understood.

Box 11.3	Case Study ○ Is Being Fat the Person's Own Fault?

What do you think of overweight individuals? How much are they to blame for their situation? Watch the video "Weight Prejudice: Myths and Facts," prepared by Yale University's Rudd Center, at https://www.youtube.com/watch?v=92rWQ-Olb1Y. Have any of your ideas changed as a result of viewing this video?

Obesity provides a nice case study of the tendency for being judgmental and victim blaming. Historically, "portly" middle-aged men were esteemed as wearing their wealth and social position well, although the very fat have, in Christian cultures, always been tagged as "gluttons," and hence guilty of sinful overindulgence. In general, it was expected, even socially encouraged, for both affluent men and women from ancient Romans to modern times to gain considerable weight after the age of 40, in keeping with their social station. Brutus was regarded with suspicion in Shakespeare's play because he was thin; Judas is portrayed as the skinny "hungry man" in medieval and Renaissance art. Renaissance Venetians, as everyone who has seen Titian's (d. 1576) *Venus of Urbino* knows, thought fleshy, curvy women were attractive. Something changed in our culture. Slimness and well-defined muscles have become identified with vigour and virtue; overweight with sloth and sin.

Fat shaming and blaming overweight people for any poor health outcomes that befall them are not consistent with obesity as a risk factor for ill health. If we learn a friend has high blood pressure, for example, we are more likely to be sympathetic and to commiserate over his or her bad fortune, even though that blood pressure is partly a result of behavioural factors like exercise and diet. But with a risk factor that is visible, something we can all see, like how large a person is, blame comes first and commiseration last: "It's plainly their fault; they should have noticed their weight gain and arrested it by exercise or diet." Why this should be so is puzzling. There is no moral link to body size and composition, and very little direct health implication for weight gain. And who exactly is harmed by someone else gaining weight?

The reason for shaming must lie partly in the modern Western obsession with control, combined with the sense that our health is our own personal responsibility. Both of these ideas, we should see clearly by now, are mistaken. Neither you nor I can exercise control over our health (or much of anything else in our lives). So much depends on extraneous variables, context, and just plain luck. And our health in a very real sense is everyone's responsibility—so many population factors and variables associated with our interactions with others determine how our biology plays out. And our choices, as we will see in more detail in Chapter 13, are not freely made but are heavily conditioned by time, place, and social variables. No one chooses to be obese, any more than one chooses to have high blood pressure. And both of those individual-level attributes, obesity and blood pressure, have complex histories, from pre-conception, through fetal development, and on through the life course.

Diet and Health

Overall, diets in Canada, the United States, the United Kingdom, and Australia are not very healthy. In all four countries people consume too much red meat, refined carbohydrates, and saturated fat, and too few vegetables and fresh fruit. Sugar and salt intake are excessive, and diets are insufficiently rich in folates and a number of trace elements. There is also a lack of vitamin D in diets and from available sunlight in Canada and the United Kingdom. Thirty-five per cent of sugar consumed by Canadians comes from things that are not recognizable "foods"—soft drinks, salad dressings, and candy (Langlois & Garriguet, 2011). And people in general consume too many calories, causing progressive weight gain.

Like so much that is health relevant, the quality of diets is at least partly a function of income and education. Table 11.1 and Figure 11.7 illustrate the relationship between healthy eating and educational attainment.

Some of the best data on diet in affluent liberal regime countries come from Scotland. There, on average, women eat 3.4 portions of fruit and vegetables a day, 1.6 portions per day less than the recommended minimum. Men eat even less fruit and vegetables, 3.1 portions. Only about one-fifth of men and one-quarter of women eat the recommended amount of fresh produce (ScottishGovernment, 2008). The quality of diet shows a very marked social gradient. Twenty-six per cent of the best-educated, most affluent men eat a diet close to current recommendations; only 14 per cent of the least-educated, least affluent men eat a reasonably healthy diet. For women, the figures are not much better—31 per cent of affluent women eat adequate amounts of fruit and vegetables and only 17 per cent of the least-affluent women do so (Scottish Health Survey, 2008).

The gradient is similar to education level for household income; in other words, the lower the family income, the worse the average healthy index score.

Can Supplements Compensate for Poor Diet?

Clinical trials and other high-quality studies have shown that dietary supplements and health foods are not even part of the answer to the problem of poor quality diets. With the exceptions of folate, iron and vitamin D in pregnancy and during lactation, mineral, vitamin, and amino acid supplements have been shown to be either ineffectual or potentially harmful to health (Bausell, 2007; Singh, 2008). Health food marketing and dietary supplementation are big businesses in North America and thus influential with government. Consequently, their lobbyists have succeeded in convincing governments to regulate less and allow manufacturers to make more (unsubstantiated) health-related claims—more on this later in the chapter.

Table 11.1   Healthy Eating Index Scores,* Canada, 2004

Highest Level of Education in the Household	Average Score (out of 100) on the Healthy Eating Index
Less than high-school completion	59.5
High-school diploma	62.1
Some post-secondary education	63.0
Completion of a post-secondary degree	64.8

*The Healthy Eating Index (HEI) is a standard measure of the extent to which a given diet meets federal dietary guidelines (100 signifies the diet meets or exceeds the current dietary guidelines).
Source: Adapted from Garriguet, 2009.

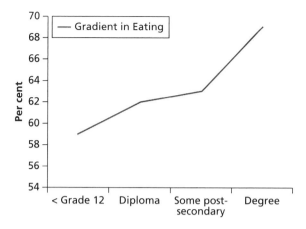

Figure 11.7 Gradient in Healthy Eating: Per Cent Eating Healthy Diet by Education, Canada

Healthier Eating

The answer to better nutrition lies in greater diet diversity—fruit, nuts, cereals, a wide range of vegetables, fish, eggs, meat, and dairy products (the last four in moderation). While conceptually simple, actually achieving balance and diversity in food consumption is not easy, particularly when eating in our contemporary context is mostly ad hoc, on the run, and increasingly dependent on restaurants, fast-food outlets, supermarket heat-and-eats, and take-out. Difficulties in making changes are especially evident in the liberal regime world, given the enormous political clout of the commercial food industry, the intensity of marketing, and the light touch of government regulators.

Promotion of the Unhealthy

In Canada, the dairy and meat industries are important to the economy and are influential politically. Controversially, public health food advice has been based on consultations with industry, and consequently, food guides in Canada have promoted both dairy and meat, even though epidemiologic studies have shown for decades that North Americans consume too much of both. Dairy and meat are not *unhealthy*; the scientific literature in no way supports that, despite the claims of some celebrities and social media health gurus. But eating large quantities of them, especially if that means eating less fruit and vegetables, does compromise health. Most heavily promoted of all, though, are convenience foods: packaged, processed products ranging from breakfast cereals, to multi-course heat-and-eat-meals, to bags of potato chips, to energy bars and candy. These are plainly unhealthy *as dietary mainstays* because they are energy rich, nutrient poor, loaded with salt and sugar, and contain chemicals such as bisphenol A, preservatives, stabilizers, artificial colours, and flavour enhancers. But they are part of a multi-billion-dollar industry and are thus massively promoted. The industry has enormous clout in the liberal regime world. For example, in 2018 US food convenience food, snack food and sweetened beverage manufacturers pressured the American government to threaten the imposition of tariffs on Canadian industrial products such as cars if the Canadian government proceeded with requiring better-quality nutrition and calorie content information on labels for US-manufactured food products sold in Canada (Ahmed, Richtel & Jacobs, 2018).

Figure 11.8 illustrates the proportion of energy intake represented by packaged and fresh foods by country. Processed, ready-packaged foods dominate diets in the United Kingdom and the United States (Canada is not included in the analysis), but so too do processed foods dominate diets in Japan. The latter, Japan, has much less obesity and much better health than the former, the United Kingdom and the United States.

Canada would slot in very closely with the US on the data presented in Figure 11.8: Canadians eat far too much packaged/processed food and not enough fresh meats, fish, poultry, vegetables, and fruits. Again it is important to emphasize that the scientific literature does not support the contention that packaged and processed foods are unhealthy, at least not in the sense that including some in our diet will harm us. Instead, the evidence supports the contention that *eating too much processed food and not enough fresh is detrimental to health and well-being.*

The skewed food purchasing in Figure 11.8—far too much packaged/processed food—isn't a consequence of individual consumer choice, but rather of availability, marketing, pricing, and a host of other food production system variables, combined with pressures on people's time and other exigencies that structure our behaviour. Enjoining Canadians to "eat fresh," as the new *Food Guide* is expected to do, is not likely to change much. We will all still be under the same pressures that lead to our current diets. Change, then, must be addressed in a different way, looking at multi-level determinants and multi-factoral interventions.

How Much Does Our Diet Matter to Our Health?

Surprisingly, we have very little evidence suggesting that diet is directly linked to either positive health outcomes or to disease, apart from obvious conditions like scurvy or goitre that are related to nutritional deficiencies, and folate and iron deficiencies in pregnancy. Ideas that gained traction in the 1960s through the 1980s regarding heart disease and fats in general (and cholesterol in the diet in particular), the importance of fibre in the diet for cancer

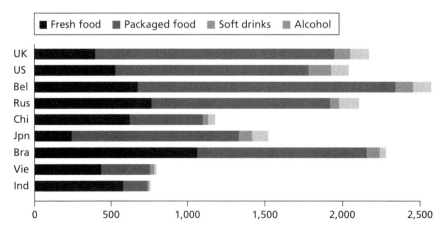

Figure 11.8 Calories Purchased Per Capita Per Day, by Country

Source: https://www.theguardian.com/society/2017/apr/07/uk-eats-almost-four-times-more-packaged-food-than-fresh

prevention, the role of antioxidants in the diet in slowing aging or reducing the risk of cancer, and the value of vitamins, especially vitamin C, in reducing the risk of infection have all failed to garner scientific support. A careful look at the literature shows that the evidence never was persuasive. Instead, promotion in the media and by the food, health food, and drug industries influenced our understanding of food, and, in particular, popularized the idea that specific foods or their components are either "neutraceuticals" or poisons, akin to drugs. More recent ideas regarding "wonder foods"—from fish oil to kale, quinoa to goji berries, cranberries to carrot juice, spelt to spinach—have proved no more defensible, and again reflect media and business hype as opposed to science.

Unfortunately, the failure of nutritional science to provide definitive dietary advice opened the way for celebrities and commercial enterprises to do so. And that has proved very dangerous to health. Following such diets is both caused by, and causes, orthorexia— the neurosis of believing some foods are "good" and some "bad," some healthy and some toxic. Because reactions to food are heavily emotionally mediated, and because digestion and the brain are so tightly wired together, emotional reactions to food engender very real symptoms. Many cases of "gluten insensitivity" (*not* celiac disease, which is a serious allergy to wheat) are, in fact, psychosomatic. Bloating, feeling "low" or having "brain fog" after eating certain foods, irritable bowel, and headache are emotionally mediated responses. The epidemic of adverse food reactions, pretty much limited to the liberal regime countries, is a social epidemic, driven by anxiety, celebrities, commerce, and culture. The genesis of orthorexia is the reductionism inherent in agent–host risk factor thinking, which leads to the entirely false hypothesis that food components are either medicines (good for us, support our biology) or poisons (toxic, make us ill). They are neither.

Foods and our emotional and physiologic responses to them are highly complex, with myriad interactions, and almost any diet, providing it is varied and includes substantial fresh components, will keep us well. The world's longest-living, healthiest people may eat a lot of dairy products and wheat (Scandinavians) or almost none (Japanese), a lot of meat (the Dutch) or very little (Hong Kong).

A varied diet, *however composed*, is essential to human health. What won't improve health or longevity is any restrictive diet that eliminates foods necessary to support us either directly or our microbial biome, which supports us indirectly. (A broad-based, non-restrictive diet that limits total calorie intake, however, might improve health and longevity. Animal studies show that some laboratory animals such as mice live longer when their food supply is reduced (Swindell, 2012). It is not clear if this applies to humans. For example, slightly overweight older adults are likely to be healthier and more resilient to disease and death than underweight ones (Flegal et al., 2013)).

Many North Americans are on a variety of restrictive diets, from "Atkins" to "paleo" to "gluten free" to a host of "juicing and cleansing" regimes, none of which is supported by evidence and all of which can contribute to malnutrition and even deadly renal and liver conditions. Going on any such diet or "cleanse" (a dubious term because the body must effectively cleanse itself of toxins 24 hours a day in order to function) may alter the body's microbial biome, the bacterial colonies in our gut. The alteration might not be reversible, and thus can induce permanent changes in our immune response, emotions, and cognitive ability. This is so because there is powerful symbiosis between the flora in our colon and us; the bacteria are essential not only to digestion but also to the rate of uptake of nutrients, the synthesis of hormones and neurotransmitters, regulation of blood sugar, and much else. A healthy microbial biome requires proper feeding, and that proper feeding includes lots of carbohydrates and soluble fibre (from grains, fruits, vegetables, nuts, and legumes). Restrictive diets upset the balance, and in the case of severe orthorexia/anorexia they recalibrate the body and brain *against* eating the foods required for good health. "Clean eating" is dangerous hokum. And so are weight-loss diets that radically restrict energy intake; they are implicated as a cause of obesity because of the damage they do to the microbial balance in our bodies.

Today's sound, scientifically backed diet advice is very simple. Eat widely, incorporating as many foods as possible into the diet, but not too much. Don't binge on any food type. Evidence supports a need for complex carbohydrates and soluble fibre, which means eating fruit, vegetables, grains, nuts, and legumes. Refined, processed foods are not "poisons," but they are high in calories, low in nutrients, and low in quality fibre, and thus should not form a major portion of the diet. Salt and sugar are not "poisons" either, but too much of them can cause health problems. Saturated fat does not constitute a health risk either. In fact, people eating diets higher in saturated fats are healthier than those eating lower-fat diets. "Organic" is not demonstrably better nutritionally than conventional food (though it may be fresher and contain fewer residual pesticides). Dairy and plants from the nightshade family (potatoes, eggplants, tomatoes) are not "toxic," and neither is wheat (which for the record, is not genetically different from the wheat of the past). These and many similar contentions by celebrities and self-styled experts are simply false. Meat is a healthy part of a balanced diet, though too much, like too many carrots, is a bad thing. But vegetarians can be perfectly healthy, too, provided they eat broadly and understand the need for diversity in their diet. Given their accumulated health advantages, it doesn't matter if the rich buy kale, juicers, coconut water, and almond milk (referred to by dietitians as "expensive water"), but deaths would ensue if less-affluent parents gave their infants juiced kale or coconut water or almond "milk" instead of real milk from humans, cows, or goats. Thus, bad, heavily promoted, and unregulated food advice can cause real population health harm.

Box 11.4   Case Study ○ Bad Nutritional Advice from the Media

The media disseminates a lot of misleading and even false information regarding nutrition. One route is the media practice of "mining" the academic literature (assigning someone to go through abstracts, not the whole studies) looking for findings that might interest or amuse their readership. Items that can be hyped as miracles or are highly counterintuitive, like the alleged health benefits of chocolate and alcohol, are popular. The result is the publication of "nutrifluff": "sensational research findings about a single food or nutrient" (Nestle, 2007). German journalists neatly demonstrated this in 2015. They conducted a three-week study (purposively designed to be too short to prove anything) involving two small groups (again too small to produce a meaningful result) in a "clinical trial" of chocolate. Both the control and experimental groups were told to reduce their calorie intake, and the experimental group was told to add a chocolate bar a day to their diet. The "researchers" found that the chocolate-eating group lost more weight than the controls. An obliging (supposedly peer-reviewed) journal, *Archives of Internal Medicine*, published the "study," the results of which appeared within days in media outlets in over 20 countries (Benedictus, 2016).

It is important to remember that there is no magic correlation between what we eat and how well we are. Shifting our own diet toward less salt, or less saturated fat, or more broccoli and fewer fried potatoes is not going to substantially change our risk of disease (the individual level). Remember Rose and the important recent studies on salt and fat intake cited earlier (e.g., Hooper et al., 2011). But, as a society, if we lower our consumption of processed foods, sugar, and fats and increase our consumption of vegetables, nuts, and fruits, non-trivial improvements in population health are possible. And that is why food and nutritional policy is so central to population health—a theme we shall now build on.

Policies and Programs

Obesity was very much in the news from 2005 to 2015. Pressure mounted on public authorities to take action to reduce weight gain in the population. In the United States, the Obama administration decided to tackle obesity with something analogous to previous administrations' "wars" on drugs and crime. First Lady Michelle Obama worked with policy advisors, celebrity chefs, and sports figures to profile the "obesity epidemic." Tellingly, and consistent with what we would expect in a liberal regime country, Obama's *Let's Move* campaign emphasized physical activity and downplayed convenience food, fast food, and the soft drinks industry—potentially important sources of presidential campaign funds and powerful corporate interests in the US Congress. The *Let's Move* campaign was deliberately non-prescriptive and avoided suggesting regulation of the US food and drinks industry. As Michelle Obama put it in a May 2012 interview on *Good Morning America*, "What we know we need to do is give parents, community, families the tools and information they need to make choices that are right for them" ("Michelle Obama on New Book," 2012). "Tools and information" are unlikely to change American's eating habits, the real culprit in terms of obesity.

Before its decided turn rightwards in 2016, US Congress considered more prescriptive measures than envisioned by Michelle Obama. Ideas that were floated included regulation of retail food and restaurant menu labelling and the imposition of taxes and other disincentives on the production and sale of unhealthy food products. Some US cities and states had already made moves in those directions—for example, New York attempted to regulate against "super-sized" containers of soda pop, but those regulations were overturned by the courts in March 2013. Food corporations pushed back, adopting voluntary codes, sponsoring amateur sport and school-based programs, and saturating television with advertisements touting their concern with health, fitness, and rising BMIs. McDonalds and Coca-Cola invested millions in 2012, 2016, and 2018 Olympic sponsorships. All this corporate activity dissuades lawmakers from enacting regulations that might put a crimp in the multi-billion-dollar interlocking fast food, convenience food, and soft drink industries. Republican control of Congress and the 2016 election of Donald Trump put an end to all talk at the federal level in the US of regulating the food and food industry. In fact, at time of writing, the US administration is rolling back restrictions on food advertising, additives, labelling, and so on, and as noted earlier, is threatening Mexico and Canada with retaliation if either country demands labelling on products high in salt, sugar, and fat or low in nutritional value.

Canada's approach has been very similar to that of the United States. The government seeks to collaborate with, not impose rules on, the food production industry. The federal government reprised the 1970s health education initiative ParticipACTION in 2007, this time turning physical activity promotion over to a private company (funded in substantial part by grants from Coca-Cola). The new federal government (as of 2015) floated a few ideas about strengthening food labelling regulations and restricting advertising of food products to children (as the province of Quebec already has), but at the time of writing, nothing substantive has happened. As noted earlier, the government has been criticized for being too cozy with the meat and dairy industries.

Voluntary Industry Codes

In Canada and the United Kingdom, corporations struck deals with governments to adopt a variety of voluntary measures, again with a view to preclude regulation, much as the tobacco industry adopted a host of voluntary (and ineffectual) measures to stall governmental action on smoking in the 1970s and 1980s. Favoured approaches include colour coding food products. An example much debated in Australia and the UK is the "traffic-light model" of green for low fat, salt, or sugar; amber for medium levels; and red for high levels of fat, salt, or sugar. The label would be affixed to the front of the package, making it easy for consumers to identify the health characteristics of the products they buy. Unfortunately, studies of traffic-light schemes predict results from none to small (Sacks, Rayner, & Swinburn, 2009; Sacks, Veerman, Moodie, & Swinburn, 2010). Even if the traffic-light scheme could moderate the rate of weight gain in the population, overall BMIs would continue to rise, especially if the aggressive marketing of high-sugar, high-salt, and high-fat items continues unabated.

In its favour, the traffic-light scheme at least addresses the fatal flaw of current nutrition labelling. Not only is such labelling inconsistent, it is largely incoherent. Consumers, even well-educated ones, cannot readily translate portion sizes, daily allowances, caloric content, and a long list of chemicals into how much of the product he or she should eat, let alone decipher the language (or, in the case of seniors, read the small print).

Food product labelling is unlikely to improve, at least not by very much, because liberal regime governments in Canada, the United States, the United Kingdom, and Australia negotiate the form and content with the corporations producing and marketing the products. Moreover, merely providing nutritional data on the package is unlikely to lead to behavioural change, especially in light of marketing pressure, price incentives, product placement in stores, and broader social norms.

Menu labelling, with such details as calorie and salt content per serving, might be expected to be more effective than product labelling because the relevant details are prominently displayed to the consumer at point of sale. However, a recent study of the impact of menu labelling on parental and child choice in fast-food franchises shows that parents quickly learn the information and fully understand it, but their children end up with food orders containing the same number of calories as they would without the menu labels (Tandon et al., 2011).

Voluntary industry codes have not been effective. For example, in 2018, Health Canada reported that voluntary food codes negotiated with manufacturers to reduce sodium in processed foods yielded reductions "much lower than anticipated" (Health Canada, 2018).

Deterrent Taxes on Unhealthy Foods

In October 2011, Denmark (a social democratic country) introduced the first "fat tax," a surtax on all foods containing more the 2.5 per cent fat. The idea is to put a disincentive in place, discouraging people from buying as much high-fat product as they might under lower prices. Presumably, people would consume, with the tax in place, a lower-fat diet and that would reduce the rate of weight gain within, and thus improve the overall health of, the population.

This sounds simple and effective. But the matter is more complex than it first appears. Price/demand for high-fat products like butter, whole milk, and cheese is quite inelastic. That is, people buy much the same amounts irrespective of whether the price goes up or down. Because of this, price increases must be very large in order to induce even small changes in consumption—well over 20 per cent (Chouninard Davis, LaFrance, & Perloff, 2006). Moreover, how consumers will actually behave is very difficult to predict because they will adjust their purchases across a range of goods, including equally or even more unhealthy substitutes. Additionally, a tax-induced change in a person's fat intake will not bring about a significant change in their weight. A gram of fat yields 9 calories, and even a 50 per cent tax will change consumption by only 30 calories (Chouninard et al., 2006). A 100-calorie-per-day change is needed to reduce body weight. Finally, a fat tax is highly regressive; almost the entire burden falls on poorer families. Denmark, finally recognizing the "fat tax" to be bad public policy, withdrew it in 2012.

It is also worth noting that while Denmark was first with a fat tax, a number of US states have taxes on soft drinks and/or the syrups used to make them. None of those measures appears to have any effect on consumption patterns or obesity, but arguably the taxes are too low to influence consumer behaviour. It remains possible that carefully targeted, sufficiently high taxes aimed at refined carbohydrates, salt, sugar, and fat could have small health effects. But the problems of regressiveness and cross-elasticity of demand (unpredictable substitution effects) remain (Mytton, Gray, Rayner, & Rutter, 2007). Mexico's very high tax on soft drinks has brought down consumption, but public health advocates aren't sure of the effect. It was mostly the poor who bought a lot of soft drinks, frequently as a substitute for unsafe drinking water. Apart from the increased cost to them of buying soft drinks (and possible substitution effects like buying less fruit in order to save the money for the soft drinks), more poor people may be drinking contaminated water, incurring worse health risks than excessive calories. In sum, combining high taxes on unhealthy foods and providing incentives to purchase healthy ones through subsidies on fruits and vegetables have potential to shift consumer behaviour, but the impact on population health is unpredictable, and likely would be small (Tiffin & Arnoult, 2011).

Other Regulatory Strategies

While there is little evidence supporting good outcomes from special consumer taxes, harder, more prescriptive regulatory measures can and do work. Recent examples include bans on the use of hydrogenated fats in food processing (due to links to heart disease) and local initiatives to remove junk food from schools. However, their scope and overall impact is limited. For example, healthy foods programs within schools do not and cannot reach out beyond the school to the community and the child's home environment. The total impact on a child's overall intake of salt, fat, refined carbohy-drate, and sugar is bound to be small. That is not to say that such initiatives are worth-less; clearly they make some difference. Moreover, failing to take such measures makes a bad situation worse.

Under industry pressure in the 1990s, liberal regime governments in the UK, the US, and then in Canada deregulated the health food and supplements industries. Deregulation is the root cause of the increasingly unfounded and extravagant health claims made by supplement manufacturers, health food stores, and naturopaths. Celebrities like Gwyneth Paltrow promote with impunity ideas and products known to be dangerous. Social media is rife with terrible dietary advice, mostly with trails leading back to the multi-billion-dollar natural food, supplement, and alternative medicine industries. Fad diet books have replaced conventional cookbooks. With mounting evidence of major harms like liver and renal failure associated with use of herbal and protein supplements, and commun-ity mental health clinics reporting rising incidence of orthorexia and anorexia, Health Canada is reviewing regulations, labelling requirements, and advertising. Unfortunately, the horses have left the barn and it's rather late for securing the door. As noted, the good news, to the extent there is any, is that health foods, supplements, and restrictive diets do not extend very far below the richest strata of society, and hence cause far much less harm than they would otherwise do.

Population Health and Food Policy

It is clear that a multi-level, multi-pronged approach is required for policy-makers to get a handle on nutritionally poor diets. Improved food and menu labelling, combined with a simple system of graphics like a traffic-light system can improve consumer awareness. Prudent, targeted application of taxes and incentives can act in support of those infor-mational strategies. But neither an informational nor a pricing strategy alone, nor both strategies in combination, will make much difference unless the food production and dis-tribution system is overhauled in the light of a thorough re-examination of current agri-cultural and food industry subsidies, taxes, and marketing practices. And that is bound to be stoutly resisted by agri-business, the food retail sector, and the restaurant industry.

Community Action and Advocacy

Initiatives to remove sugary soft drinks and junk food from schools arose through parent advisory committees, not government policy. Likewise, movements as diverse as the 100-Mile Diet (source your foods locally, preferably from organic growers), community gardens, the urban agriculture movement, neighbourhood kitchens, and farmers' markets are slowly raising consciousness and creating healthier eating opportunities for people. Some communities (Toronto, Kelowna, and Vancouver are Canadian examples) have formed advocacy coalitions (sometimes referred to as Food Policy Councils) aimed at reducing food insecurity and improving the diet of residents within their communities. In the United Kingdom, celebrity chef Jamie Oliver reprised a government program from the Second World War, the "Ministry of Food." Oliver encourages planting community gar-dens; sourcing local fresh produce; and providing high-quality school meals, community kitchens, and cooking and shopping workshops for lower-income people. Chefs in Canada have followed Oliver's lead, and a growing number advocate for reform of food production and preparation. Some churches and voluntary organizations in Canada sponsor community kitchens for new immigrants and low-income Canadians, teaching cooking and shopping skills, basic nutrition, and how to enjoy food with friends in neighbourhoods in a socially supportive and inclusive environment. In time, this plethora of recent, community-based activity will make a difference, especially for those who will most benefit—lower-income, socially excluded Canadians.

Theoretical Considerations

Discussion of food and nutrition neatly shows how causes are multi-factoral and operate on several levels. People do not adopt eating patterns or choose specific foods in abstraction from their social context and the economic system in which they are embedded. Income, education, social class, features of housing (cooking and food storage facilities), cultural background, social network, neighbourhood opportunity structure, and features of agri-business, food production, and distribution systems all play roles in shaping when, how, where, what, and how much people eat. Individual-level factors like information, incentives, and disincentives will inevitably play a smaller part in outcomes than the broader determinants.

Summary

Overall, compared with other populations around the globe, people in the liberal regime world are well nourished, in fact "over-nourished" in terms of energy intake. People have grown increasingly taller and more robust, but also fatter. Typical diets are far from ideal. Fruit, vegetable, whole grain, and nut consumption are low even for affluent people and very low for poorer ones. Meat, saturated fat, sugar, and salt consumption are high for all social classes. Refined carbohydrate, sugar, and fat consumption are very high among less-affluent people. Meanwhile, dietary levels of folate and soluble fibre are generally low. These dietary patterns play a role in diabetes, heart disease, cancer, and birth defects.

A significant portion of the population, an estimated 6 per cent in Canada, is food insecure. While few of these people suffer chronic hunger, many consume nutritionally poor diets and depend on charities such as food banks to supplement their food supplies. Food insecurity is not so much about food as it is about disposable income, minimum wage, and the cost of housing and utilities, although the price of food obviously plays a role. Areas where incomes are low, food prices are high, and availability of highly nutritious items is constrained (rural northern Canadian communities are an example) will have high levels of food insecurity and consequently will suffer negative population-health impacts.

The rising rates of obesity have been styled "an epidemic." Certainly the proportion of the population that is overweight or obese has ballooned over the past 20 years. The problem is worse in the United States, Australia, and the United Kingdom, but it is nevertheless substantial in Canada. Among women, incidence of overweight and obesity follows the usual health/education gradient. But among men, at least in Canada, there is no clear relationship between socio-economic variables and large BMI. Current estimates are that 21.8 per cent of Canadian men and 18.7 per cent of Canadian women are obese.

The causes of rising rates of obesity are contested. Cheap, readily accessible, energy-dense processed foods are certainly part of the story. Changes in eating practices and norms are also clearly implicated.

Policies aimed at improving the food choices and eating habits of liberal regime populations include information campaigns, product and menu labelling, punitive taxes on products deemed unhealthy, subsidies on products deemed healthy, regulations mandating food additives such as folate and vitamin D, and recommended or legislated limits on ingredients, food production, and sales practices.

Some examples of food-related policies follow.

- Education and exhortation go back decades, to the Second World War and earlier, in the form of government-sponsored food guides.
- A mix of voluntary and mandatory food labelling has been in place from the 1970s.
- Taxes on sugar and sweetened beverages have been applied on and off since the 1920s. Outside the liberal regime world, Denmark fuelled the current interest in "fat taxes" with its 2011 punitive taxes on saturated fats (abandoned in autumn 2012). France imposed a "Nutella tax," a punitive tax on palm oil because of its link to heart disease and obesity (Willsher, 2012). Under pressure from Malaysia and Indonesia, major palm oil producers, it reduced the tax in 2016. Mexico's "soda tax"—in its first two years—did bring down soft drink consumption among poor people, but did not appear to change daily calorie consumption or incidence of obesity.
- Food fortification in Canada is regulated by Health Canada and includes adding vitamins C and D and folate to a variety of foods, either because the vitamins are lost in processing or because there is a scientific consensus regarding dietary deficiency. From a population health standpoint, the practice of fortification is controversial. While folate supplementation drives down rates of birth defects, people who do not need the extra folate may be harmed by its (invisible) inclusion in food products.
- Regulatory limits have been imposed on the use of hydrogenated vegetable oils.

The overall impact of these measures on population health in general and on obesity in particular (both real to date and projected by modelling the probable effects of more labelling, taxes, and subsidies) is unfortunately small. The effects are overwhelmed by the shifts in social norms regarding eating and the related changes that have occurred within contemporary agri-business, food processing, food distribution, and marketing. Deeper, more sophisticated public policy targeting the fundamental determinants is required to move populations' eating habits in a healthier direction. The prospects for this are not good, given the political power and the amount of money associated with food production and distribution in liberal regime countries.

Small-scale, incremental change, however, is possible and can, in the long run, make a difference. Community pressure to control foods sold or served in schools; support for local food initiatives such as farmers' markets, community gardens, and local food purchasing; the "eat fresh" movement in higher-end restaurants; interventions like Jamie Oliver's Ministry of Food; and community kitchens that teach people how to shop and prepare wholesome food are all making a dent in the problem. Combined with well-targeted tax and incentive policies and nutrition education programming, real progress can be made, at least over the long haul. It may be that we are already into a significant dietary change. Fruit and vegetable sales, despite higher prices, are up and rising. Soft drink sales in Canada have been falling dramatically (unfortunately prompting soft drink makers to aggressively promote energy drinks, vitamin drinks, and fruit juices, all as high or higher in sugar than traditional soft drinks).

Critical Thinking Questions

1. Food policy is an area where values and ideology become evident. Many people object to government or public health authorities telling them what or how much they should eat. Ironically, the same people seem comfortable with corporations doing precisely that. Where should responsibilities lie with respect to food choices and eating behaviour? What is the proper role of governments and public health authorities with respect to food and eating behaviour?

2. Many companies, notably cereal manufacturers and fast-food outlets, advertise heavily on children's television programs. What do you see to be the ethical ins and outs of advertising foods to children? Should industry practices be regulated and, if so, to what degree and why?

3. Eating in the liberal regime world has become disordered. People rarely eat sit-down meals, apart from visits to fast-food restaurants. Snacking throughout the day has become normal. Fewer and fewer people eat breakfast. Missing the most important meal of the day destabilizes blood sugar and appetite regulation. Can order be restored to eating? If so, how? What changes need to occur in our society?

4. Manufactured foods are the major sources of excess sugar and salt in our diets. Producers use massive amounts of salt and sugar (and fats) because their studies show people will consume more of their product. Low-salt- and low-sugar-content products generally fail in the marketplace because consumers have come to expect the taste and "mouth feel" of conventional processed food. Voluntary codes aiming at reductions in sugar, salt, and fat are bound to fail. What are the alternatives? How can processed foods be made safer for the consumer?

Annotated Suggested Readings

An excellent Canadian resource on food insecurity is the 2007 *Income-Related Household Food Security in Canada* report from Health Canada, available at www.hc-sc.gc.ca/fn-an/surveill/nutrition/commun/income_food_sec-sec_alim-eng.php.

The Cost of Eating in B.C., 2011 (available at www.dietitians.ca/Downloadable-Content/Public/CostofEatingBC2011_FINAL.aspx) clearly shows the relationship between nutritious diet, income, and other claims on that income, such as housing expenses.

For advice on what to eat, it is difficult to beat Marion Nestle's book *What to Eat: An Aisle by Aisle Guide to Savvy Food Choices and Good Eating* (New York: North Point Press, 2006).

Highly regarded dietitian Leslie Beck has joined many others in advocating a diet that contains few or no animal products. Her latest book, *Plant-Based Power Diet* (Toronto: Penguin, 2013), explains why processed foods and meats are poor choices and how human dietary needs can be better met by a diet based entirely on plants.

Annotated Web Resources

"Nutrition and Healthy Eating"
www.hc-sc.gc.ca/fn-an/nutrition/index-eng.php
A wealth of useful information about nutrition and health is available on Health Canada's website.

Vancouver Food Policy Council
www.vancouverfoodpolicycouncil.ca
Food Policy Councils have sprung up in a number of North American regions and municipalities. The Councils promote grassroots changes in our approach to producing and using food. They usually involve building coalitions of food producers, farmers' markets, community garden organizers, and food insecurity charities such as food banks and community kitchens. An example is the Vancouver Food Policy Council.

Jamie's Ministry of Food
www.jamieoliver.com/jamies-ministry-of-food/
news.php
Jamie Oliver's campaign to reduce food insecurity, improve less-advantaged people's diets, and reduce obesity is outlined, and a host of associated resources are provided at his Ministry of Food website.

Food Politics
www.foodpolitics.com
The Food Politics website is an excellent resource for information on politics and public policy relating to food and health. The site is eclectic and controversial, but also well researched.

PROOF: Food Insecurity Policy Research
http://www.proof.utoronto.ca/food-insecurity
Food Insecurity Policy Research, website of the PROOF interdisciplinary research team, is a University of Toronto–based research portal into the issue of food insecurity in Canada.

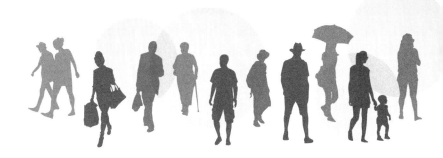

12 The Environment and Health

Objectives

By the end of your study of this chapter, you should be able to
- understand that the health effects of environmental factors may be substantially modified, either negatively through poor planning and weak regulation, or positively through effective public policy and collaborative action;
- appreciate how environmental variables interact with biologic ones to affect health outcomes;
- reflect on the interactions among economic activity, government regulation, and the health of populations.

Synopsis

Chapter 12 provides an overview of some important environmental health factors. The field of health and the environment is vast, and the term "environment" includes not only the natural environment but also the environment as modified by people, both outdoors and in. Some environmental factors central to health outcomes, such as the workplace and housing and neighbourhood, were dealt with separately in Chapters 9 and 10. Chapter 12 focuses on climate change (global warming), natural disasters, environmental and health implications of modern food production, pollution, and everyday exposures to potentially toxic compounds.

Climate Change

Over the past century, the average temperature of the land and sea has risen about one degree, with the rate of change roughly doubling since 1950. This is a clear trend and not a feature of climate variation. Scientists agree that the change is at least partly a consequence of human activities—namely, the release of carbon dioxide from burning fossil fuels; the release of methane and other "greenhouse gases" (gases that trap the heat from the sun in the atmosphere) from industry and agriculture; and deforestation, trees being important for removing CO_2 from the atmosphere and sequestering it in their tissues. The rate of warming is accelerating, and even if the world achieves strict controls on CO_2 emissions from vehicles, power plants, aircraft, heating residential and commercial buildings, and industrial processes, average temperatures are expected to rise another two degrees in the next few decades.

The temperature changes are not uniform. The northern polar region has seen the greatest and most sustained increase in temperature, as well as warming polar seas and melting Greenland's glaciers and sea ice. Warming has had, partly in consequence of the effects in the Arctic, an enormous impact on the oceans, raising sea levels and decreasing ocean salinity. That, in turn, affects the ecology of the oceans, making the seas much less hospitable to marine life, and forcing the migration of colder-water fish farther and farther north. Ocean temperature change also affects the weather, by altering the El Niño and La Niña cyclical weather events that bring precipitation or drought to the western Americas; changing the predictability, timing, and intensity of the monsoons in Asia and Africa; and creating conditions for tropical storms and hurricanes. Higher sea levels threaten low-lying land, much of it heavily populated, with flooding. Higher sea levels also mean the infiltration of salt into low-lying agricultural land, contaminating the soil and groundwater, making growing food and obtaining irrigation and drinking water difficult.

Weather patterns have become much more erratic. Extreme weather events from torrential rains, to drought, to heat waves, to prolonged periods of extreme cold are increasingly common. Weather systems that used to move relatively freely in the atmosphere now have a tendency to become "blocked"—an intense high-pressure system can keep an intense low-pressure system in place for weeks, with extreme heat and drought occurring under the high and persistent rain causing serious flooding under the low. This situation arose in 2017, leading to a protracted heat wave, drought, and widespread forest fires in western North America; hurricanes and flooding in the southeast; and cyclones and massive hailstorms in the centre. Concurrently, extreme monsoons flooded parts of India and Bangladesh, whereas parts of Africa and Europe experienced a heat wave and drought, while northwest Europe experienced rain and cold temperatures from April to September. Such unpredictable weather wreaks havoc on agriculture, natural vegetation, and wildlife, and extreme weather events constitute deadly disasters for the people experiencing them.

Warming and a CO_2-laden atmosphere have lowered the pH of the oceans, a process of *acidification* as the carbon dioxide converts to carbonic acid. Warmer acidic water is inimical to the life of any shelled sea creature because maintaining a calciferous shell is dependent on a pH of 7 or higher. Some creatures such as corals are exquisitely temperature sensitive, as well as sensitive to acidification, and thus climate change has threatened reefs. In response to acidification and rising temperatures, corals "bleach," turn white, die, then crumble. Because reefs are a major fish habitat, and protect many coastlines from erosion and flooding from the sea, their decline is calamitous.

Droughts and flooding affect the food supply and the price of food. Poorer people are worst affected because they are most sensitive to food prices. Prices of food, which had been dropping for over a century, are now increasing, very rapidly for some foods such as fruit. Food insecurity, a major topic discussed in Chapter 11, has been made much worse by climate change, threatening the health of people worldwide, particularly in poorer countries. Less well-off people substitute cheaper, energy-rich but nutrient-poor foods, particularly refined carbohydrates, for protein and the complex carbohydrates found in fruits, vegetables, and legumes.

The dramatic declines in ocean fish stocks and shellfish associated with ocean warming, reef collapse, and over-fishing further threaten food security worldwide. Warmer water means remaining major food-stock fish have migrated north toward the pole, and less desirable (from a fishing point of view) species such as jellyfish and cuttlefish have replaced them. "In a few decades the temperature of our seas is likely to be roughly the same as those found in the waters around Portugal at the turn of the last century—so we can expect to find the kind of marine life that existed there in British seas in the near future," said marine biologist Professor Stephen Simpson of Exeter University. "Apart from cuttlefish and sardines—which are already moving into our waters—we can expect fish like red mullet and John Dory to be more common. By contrast the haddock is already disappearing from the southern North Sea, while plaice and sole are also becoming less and less prevalent" (*The Guardian*, 2017). Meanwhile, "millions of non-native creatures known as pyrosomes [drawn northward by warm water] are 'blooming' off the coast of British Columbia and have the potential to devastate an already fragile food chain" (Kelly, 2017).

Climate change has also led to a spike in communicable diseases, particularly those that have an insect vector. West Nile virus (mosquito borne), Lyme disease (tick borne), dengue fever, yellow fever, and Zika virus (all mosquito borne) have become epidemic, even in countries where they previously did not exist. Recently, Italy recorded three cases of malaria contracted within the country. *Aedes aegypti*, the mosquito that spreads yellow fever, Zika, dengue, and chikungunya virus, is now resident in California, Nevada, Florida, and (probably) Texas and Louisiana. Cases of chikungunya have been reported in Italy and France. Biting insects are well adapted to the changes in rainfall and temperature, and many that would not survive and thrive at higher latitudes can now do so. Plants, too, are subjected to new disease threats because insects that were once killed off in winter now survive. The destruction of vast expanses of Canada's boreal forest by pine beetles is an example.

Natural Disasters

Disasters such as earthquakes, hurricanes, flooding events, and landslides are natural, environmental phenomena, although human changes to the landscape can change their frequency and severity. Less well-off people are disproportionately harmed by such catastrophes. Television news footage of homes smashed by cyclones almost always features mobile homes; flood scenes are mostly low-lying, poor neighbourhoods; and desperate refugees from US hurricanes are mainly poor (and frequently black) Americans.

Low-quality housing is subject to collapse in heavy winds or when stressed by the forces of an earthquake. Poorer neighbourhoods are situated either in low-lying land (a common situation in North America) or (in the case of developing countries) on steep slopes avoided by property developers because of the expense of installing infrastructure, as well as safety concerns about stability. The former, low-lying neighbourhoods, are inundated by heavy rains; the latter, hillside shantytowns, are crushed by mudslides. Low-lying, mostly poor, neighbourhoods in cities like Houston and New Orleans lack storm drainage systems that can deal with rain events, in spite of the fact that such events are commonplace on the Gulf of Mexico. Some neighbourhoods are below sea level, even though they are close to the ocean and therefore susceptible not only to flooding by rain but also to tidal surges.

When major weather events are predicted, affluent people have the ability to stock up on provisions and buy portable electric generators. They have cars and can purchase extra fuel to ensure they can leave if the situation becomes threatening. They also have friends with whom they can stay, in neighbourhoods safe from the pending disaster. Additionally, better-off people have adequate cash and credit to relocate temporarily to hotels. Poor people have none of these things. They lack private transportation and accommodation options, have no ready cash or credit, and cannot take time away from their low-wage jobs, first because they can't afford to, and second because it's likely they would be fired. Moreover, homes in poor neighbourhoods are more likely to be looted if the residents evacuate, and those homes are less likely than the homes in more affluent areas to receive adequate protection from emergency officials. Consequently, in the event of an expected disaster, it is poorer people who disproportionately remain in their homes, and those homes are disproportionately prone to the worst effects of that disaster (Kelman, 2017).

Pause and Reflect   Hurricane Katrina

In the case of Hurricane Katrina, which struck Louisiana in August 2005, approximately 2000 mostly poor people died. Flood protection infrastructure in New Orleans was inadequate, improperly maintained, and subject to widespread failure. The emergency response was slow and poorly coordinated, leading to claims of racism because the worst-affected neighbourhoods were predominantly black. More than half of the black survivors had no health care insurance and, in the aftermath of the flood, encountered difficulties filling prescriptions or obtaining health care. Many still suffer from depression and post-traumatic stress syndrome as a result of the disaster (Huelskoetter, 2015).

As Hurricane Harvey approached the Louisiana coast on August 30, 2017, New Orleans' flood protection remained inadequate, nearly half of the pumps needed to drain the storm sewers in the lowest parts of the city weren't working, and housing for residents displaced in the 2005 disaster still hadn't been completely replaced.

The effects of Hurricane Harvey on Houston, eerily occurring on the twelfth anniversary of Hurricane Katrina, are similar, but fortunately not as catastrophic.

At the time of writing, approximately 100 people are known to have died in Houston. As was the case with Katrina, the bodies of many of those who perished in Hurricane Harvey will never be found. During the disaster, sewage and chemicals from the oil refineries and chemical processing plants that are heavily concentrated in the Houston area mingled with the floodwaters, creating a highly toxic mix. That heavily polluted water was almost half a metre deep on the floor of the main refugee centre; there was no way the flood's evacuees, the city's poorest, could stay dry or clean. The long-term health implications are unknown.

Pause and Reflect   **City Planning, Regulation, and Environmental Disaster**

. . . "Houston is the most flood-prone city in the United States," said Rice University environmental engineering professor Phil Bedient. "No one is even a close second—not even New Orleans, because at least they have pumps there."

The entire system is designed to clear out only 30 centimetres of rain per 24-hour period, said Jim Blackburn, an environmental law professor at Rice University: "That's so obsolete it's just unbelievable." . . .

But mostly the problem comes down to helter-skelter development in a county with no zoning, leaving lots of concrete where water doesn't drain, and little green space to absorb it, Bedient said.

Local politicians are simply unwilling to insist in the local code that developers, who are among their biggest campaign donors, create no adverse effects, said Ed Browne, chairman of the non-profit Residents Against Flooding.

"In general, developers run this city and whatever developers want they get," Browne said. His group sued Houston last year in federal court, demanding more holding ponds and better drainage. (Borenstein & Bajak, 2017)

In the first week of September 2017, US newspapers and cable TV reported that a giant chemical plant in Houston was on fire and at risk of exploding. Highly toxic smoke was blanketing the immediate area. The plant, which required continuous cooling, had no electrical backup system. The power outage associated with Hurricane Harvey caused chain chemical reactions, leading to a series of small explosions and a fire, and fear of a massive detonation of highly poisonous chemicals.

The plant had previously been identified as possibly the most dangerous in America, one of a suite of highly polluting petrochemical and refining plants in the metro Houston area. Questions immediately arose regarding the approval process for building and operating these plants, and whether safety and public health officials had been inspecting them (Irwin, 2017).

Box 12.1   **Case Study ○ The Tale of Two Irmas**

In 2017, *The Guardian* newspaper published the case study "The Tale of Two Irmas." Hurricane Irma (August–September 2017) was one of the most powerful hurricanes to ever make landfall in the United States.

As the paper reported, one Florida resident, an affluent business owner with a home in Miami Beach, checked to ensure he was well stocked with supplies and that his private generator was in good working order, and then left his storm-fortified home to practise his golf swing. Another, a Latino man living in the predominantly African-American suburb of Miami, Liberty City (where the film *Moonlight* was shot), went to a local hardware store to get plywood to cover his windows, but the store was completely sold out. His car was out of gas and he couldn't evacuate from the vicinity, despite the fact that he had very few supplies and no electrical generator.

Many features similar to the hurricane disasters in the US apply to disasters in Canada. In the record 2017 forest fire season, First Nations people were disproportionately harmed, not only because their communities were close to some of the major fires, but because (unlike many of their non-Indigenous neighbours) they either didn't or couldn't evacuate. Government response to the evacuation of the isolated Manitoba communities of Wasagamack, Garden Hill, and St Theresa Point First Nations in late August 2017 has been widely criticized as too late and poorly organized. In BC alone, more than a million hectares of forest burned between June and September, and thousands of residents remained under evacuation orders, in some cases for months.

Governments concerned about the welfare of their citizens can be proactive, anticipate disaster, and implement effective disaster plans. Cuba, a poor country and, like New Orleans and Houston, subject to hurricanes, has had for many years a sophisticated evacuation plan and well-trained disaster responders. In the same hurricane season as Katrina, Cuba had several massive tropical storms but only five deaths. In September 2017, Cuba was devastated by a direct hit from Hurricane Irma, then the strongest hurricane on record, and at its peak velocity when it made Cuban landfall. Ten people were killed, out of a population of 11.2 million. All 20,000 tourists in the country at the time were evacuated without a single injury. Later in September 2017, Puerto Rico was hit by Hurricane Maria. Over 60 people were killed and six months later nearly a quarter of a million remained without electricity, despite being American citizens. The response by US emergency officials, Congress, and the president has been widely criticized. It plainly differed from the US government response to the mostly white, mostly non-Latino, mostly more affluent residents of Texas.

British Columbia, which has had several terrible wildfire seasons since the huge fires in 2003, improved preparedness, implemented a much more sophisticated and rapid response, and consequently lost substantially less property and life in the unprecedented 2017 fire season. Likewise, in 2017, Florida sustained fewer deaths than in previous massive tropical storms, about 30, due to much-improved planning and emergency preparedness. Nevertheless, government agencies in both Canada and Florida were widely criticized, and emergency planning and preparedness are once again under review.

A society that ensures earthquake, fire, hurricane, tsunami, and flood preparedness; designs proper infrastructure and maintains it; prevents deforestation; and regulates what gets built where and to what standard, can mitigate the risk of bad health outcomes from natural disasters. We now know what needs to be done to protect the health of populations from disasters; it's a matter of making the effort and mobilizing the resources to achieve it. Similarly, the response mustered by government when disasters occur determines how bad the outcomes will be for the population affected. The shambolic and underfunded response to the needs of poor Latino people in Puerto Rico, despite their being US citizens, contrasts sharply with the mobilization of resources on behalf of Texans in the same hurricane season.

Modern Food Production: Factory Farming

A different kind of environmental disaster is linked to factory farming. Intensive farming by large-scale commercial agri-business is associated with widespread pollution, and the production of novel pathogens, particularly **swine and avian influenzas**, but also the brain-wasting disease bovine spongiform encephalopathy, or BSE ("mad cow" disease). It is also associated with elevated risks of human infections of E. coli, listeriosis, and salmonella.

Intensive, Large-Scale Agriculture

Intensive industrial farming of corn and soya beans, encouraged by US government farm subsidies, involves monocropping, the practice of planting vast areas with only one variety of plant. Monocropping rapidly degrades the soil, requiring ever-increasing amounts of artificial fertilizer. Monocropped plants also become vulnerable to disease and depend on heavier use of pesticides. Intensive cultivation requires control of competing plants ("weeds"), and thus the application of large amounts of herbicide. All of these chemicals seep into the environment, contaminating rivers, lakes, underground aquifers, and the ocean. They are also taken up by plants and enter the food chain.

Intensive cropping of corn and soya beans requires extensive irrigation. Irrigation degrades the soil and, over time, increases its alkalinity and reduces its capacity to nourish plants, leading again to increased application of chemicals to the land. In Pakistan and Bangladesh, heavy irrigation of rice crops has brought substantial amounts of arsenic to the surface and into the plants. Much of the world's rice is now contaminated with arsenic, leading to health recommendations to limit consumption of one of the world's most important dietary staples.

The Production of Chicken, Pork, and Beef

The enormous US surpluses of corn and soy encourage their use as animal feeds, which makes possible the factory farming of chickens, pigs, and cattle. Corn and soy do not form part of the natural diet of any of these farmed animals, raising concerns not only about the health of the animals, but also about the health-relevant properties of the animal-derived food products. For example, grain- and corn-fed cattle produce beef that is higher in saturated fats than pasture-fed animals (Pighin, et.al 2016). Some epidemiologic studies claim that European dairy products are quite different from, and healthier than, North American ones because milk cows in North America are fed a variety of grains and manufactured feeds as opposed to the primarily grass diet used in Europe. The chemical composition of cow's milk and the balance of fats, proteins, and sugars vary enormously depending on the breed of the cow, the stage of lactation, whether the animal has been treated with drugs and hormones (commonplace in the US), and especially its diet (Looper, n.d.).

Factory farming of animals, from cattle feed lots, to sheds housing thousands of pigs, to factories housing tens of thousands of chickens, produces a prodigious amount of animal excrement. Mostly, it is liquefied and then spread on agricultural land as fertilizer. Unfortunately, that practice leads to surface water contamination and, worse, to nitrites percolating down through the soil to poison the freshwater aquifers that people depend on for drinking water and irrigation. Heavy spreading of manure on the land also raises the risk of produce becoming contaminated with potentially deadly E. coli bacteria. In Canada, factory farming of cattle led to the Walkerton disaster in 2000, in which at least 7 people died and over 2300 were rendered seriously ill, some of them never recovering. E. coli-laden manure percolated down from feedlots into one of the city's drinking-water wells (Salvadori, 2009).

Crowding animals together in meat production operations exponentially increases the risk of viruses in circulation among pigs, chickens, and ducks mutating into novel pathogens. Those pathogens may be communicable to people. Swine flu epidemics originating in factory farms in Mexico, the deadly Hong Kong avian flu arising from poultry, and the SARS pandemic arising from factory farming of ducks are examples.

BSE, bovine spongiform encephalopathy, is a disease that affected British and Canadian beef cattle that arose through the factory farming practice of increasing the protein content of artificial animal feeds through adding slaughterhouse waste. Prions, infectious proteins, were inadvertently transferred from the neural tissue of dead animals to ones being raised for human consumption. Consuming prion-infected meat can lead to fatal brain disease in humans.

Fish Farming

Factory farming of fish, widespread on the Canadian Pacific coast, generates massive amounts of waste that is toxic to natural marine life. It also has been implicated in the transmission of disease from the penned farmed fish to wild fish stocks. Moreover, the fish are fed artificial food (the sourcing of which creates other environmental problems) and then fed other chemicals to change their flesh colour, grey, to the bright red consumers expect. In August 2017, as many as 300,000 factory fish escaped their containment nets in the Pacific Ocean. They are an alien species to the Pacific (being Atlantic rather than Pacific salmon) and no one has any idea what environmental impact this foreign population might have on wild fish (Johnson, 2017).

The Impact of Modern Agri-Business

The quest for cheap, plentiful food has been a success. Never has there been such a variety of food at such a low price. But making food cheap has come at an enormous environmental cost. The health results are decidedly mixed. In general, people are better fed and have more food choices, but all the cheap carbohydrate from corn and wheat production is implicated in low-quality diets, too many calories, and obesity. Surplus corn provides many of the base stock chemicals for processed foods and for products like soft drinks (high-fructose corn syrup). Corn is the mainstay of the convenience food industry (Pollan, 2006). Factory farming of meat is the principal cause of its overconsumption in Canada and the US.

The world now has to stay on high alert for novel pathogens, particularly swine and avian influenzas. E. coli and parasitic infections from raw fruits and vegetables are a significant health hazard, necessitating more careful food monitoring by public health authorities and government-ordered recalls of contaminated products. The massive scale and vast numbers of animals passing through modern slaughterhouses and meat packing plants increases the risks of contamination of chicken by salmonella and beef by E. coli, particularly in the case of ground meat products. (Hamburger, sausages, and ground chicken and turkey are problematic, because those are manufactured mixes of meat sourced from multiple carcasses.) Modern industrial food practices involve risks that necessitate more public health vigilance, better regulation of the industry, robust recall systems, and much else in order to protect public health.

Factory farming also has adverse large-scale environmental impacts. Agricultural pollution of the oceans via run-off into rivers is creating extensive "dead zones," many in areas that had productive food fisheries. Large ones exist at the mouths of the Mississippi and Fraser Rivers. Methane from farm animals, particularly beef and dairy cattle, is a potent greenhouse gas and contributes to global warming.

Air Pollution

Air pollution in Canada contributes to 7700 avoidable deaths each year (International Institute for Sustainable Development, 2017). The main sources are electricity generation in coal- and oil-fired plants, motor vehicles, and emissions from domestic and factory heating. Especially dangerous are fine particles (2.5 microns or smaller) from vehicle emissions and coal and wood smoke, which not only are drawn very deeply into the lung, but migrate from the lung into the bloodstream. Consequently, beyond irritating the respiratory tract, fine particulates have systemic health effects. Gaseous emissions such as carbon monoxide, nitrogen dioxide, and sulfur dioxide are highly toxic. Tetraethyl lead additives, introduced into gasoline supplies by the major oil companies from the 1920s in order to boost the octane of low-quality gasoline and to provide extra lubrication to valves and rings in engines, was not phased out entirely until 1996, despite it having been known from *before* its use began that the lead emissions were toxic. Tens of thousands of children suffered needless neurological damage from lead pollution in the atmosphere. Especially hard hit were poor children whose homes tended to be close to busy roads and freeways.

Lead, Mercury, and Arsenic

Heavy metals are extraordinarily toxic and very difficult to metabolize and excrete. They accumulate in the body, each small dose adding to previous amounts, until a poisonous threshold is crossed and substantial physiologic damage ensues.

Ancient civilizations used a lot of lead for things like pipes and even drinking vessels because the metal is abundant, very soft, and easy to work into shapes. But by the time of the Romans, doctors recognized that lead was poisonous. The Roman civil engineer Marcus Vitruvius Pollio (born around 80 BCE) recommended getting drinking water from clay rather than lead pipes. Unfortunately, "easy and cheap" meant that cities in Canada and the US used lead pipes (and still do in some places) to connect houses to the water mains. This didn't seem to cause major problems until Flint, Michigan, tried to save even more money in 2014 by changing the source of the city's water to the Flint River without checking on the water chemistry. The low pH of the water, its acidity, reacted with the lead pipes, poisoning the community. Because lead pipes are ubiquitous in North American cities, it is critically important that municipal authorities exercise extreme caution over where drinking water is sourced and carefully monitor and correct the pH of that water.

Lead in supply lines to houses and other buildings is not the only problem with this substance. Solder used to join copper pipes and connect valves to pipes, until the late 1980s, contained lead. Consequently, houses, hospitals, schools, care homes and offices built before 1990 all have some level of lead in the water, the amount depending on the age of the piping, its condition, and the flow rates through the pipes. For this reason, it is important—especially in older buildings—to let the cold water run for a few minutes before using it for drinking or cooking. In Canada, municipalities, school districts, and hospital authorities are replacing (or removing) drinking fountains (albeit not very systematically). Business offices and universities have mostly converted to drinking water that has been treated by reverse osmosis.

Poor families are especially impacted by environmental lead, not only because of older plumbing but because their houses are often contaminated by lead dust. The reason for this is that lead was used as an additive in paint. In older, less well-maintained homes, paint is sloughing off and turning to dust that is then ingested by small children, especially toddlers crawling on the floor. Lead from paint combines in small children with lead from vehicle exhausts, and with lead from lead water pipes, until major irreversible neurological damage occurs (see Chapter 10 for more on this).

Lead is also dumped into the environment by refining and smelting operations. The Teck Resources smelter in Trail, BC, is responsible for lead pollution of both the atmosphere and the Colombia River.

Mercury is a by-product of many industrial processes, as well as from refining minerals. Like lead, it is a potent neuro-toxin that accumulates in the body. When discharged into water, or carried by rain from the atmosphere into waterways, mercury can convert from a dangerous inorganic form to an even more dangerous organic form (methyl mercury) that is readily absorbed by aquatic life. It works its way up the food chain, becoming especially concentrated in apex ocean predators like tuna, swordfish, and salmon—much-prized human foods. Consuming seafood can thus lead to mercury poisoning, first noticed in Japan (Minamata disease). In Canada, some First Nations communities (e.g., Grassy Narrows, Ontario) are particularly vulnerable because of industrial activity near their settlements and the community's historic reliance on fish for food. Because of this, public health authorities recommend limiting consumption of fish, especially tuna, and all fish caught in the waters near Grassy Meadows or harvested from Lake Winnipeg.

Arsenic, like lead, is widespread in the natural environment. It is dangerous, however, only when distributed by human activity. Well digging for irrigation in Pakistan and mining operations worldwide mobilize a lot of arsenic, spreading it through the environment and into the food chain. Arsenic contamination of drinking water is common in poorer parts of the world, leading to gastrointestinal distress, and at higher or repeated doses, nausea, headache, heart complications, and cancer. Arsenic now appears in significant amounts in important foods such as rice.

The Household Environment

High humidity or water infiltration creates ideal growing conditions for moulds and mildews, the spores of which are irritating to the respiratory tract and capable of inducing serious immune responses such as asthma. Poorer people are most at risk because older, less well-maintained homes and basement suites are ideal habitats for mould.

Indoor air particulate from cooking and heating appliances is as dangerous as outdoor air pollution. Amount is a function of the age and quality of household appliances and the quality of ventilation. Typically, only newer, more expensive homes have adequate, forced ventilation.

Products used in the domestic environment may also be environmental hazards, though it is very difficult to tell because of lax regulation. For example, all Canadians absorb an estimated 2 kilograms of chemicals into their bodies from shampoos, conditioners, creams and lotions, perfumes and deodorants, sunscreen, lip-care products, and other cosmetics. Products are tested for topical safety—that is, application on the skin—not for long-term effects *inside* the body in combination with chemicals from dozens of other products. Likewise, small amounts of household cleanser, dish soap, air fragrance, etc., are absorbed directly into the body, with unknown effects. Clearly, this is a case where less is more, at least from a health standpoint.

The home environment is also contaminated with formaldehyde off-gassed from carpets; resilient flooring and laminates; and flame retardants added to mattresses, pillows, and furnishings. The latter, flame retardants, are becoming a special cause for concern because the chemicals are hormone mimickers, and are implicated in health-related issues such as falling human fertility (Harvard School of Public Health, 2017). Many plastics, including ones used in storing food and beverages, contain bisphenol A, another hormone mimicker. Government regulation forced the removal of bisphenol from items like baby bottles, but the chemical remains in many other plastic items, including ones used for food and beverage storage (Health Canada, 2014). The plastic liners of food and beverage cans, and the packaging of processed foods such as breakfast cereals and snacks contain bisphenol A. The long-term health implications of all of these contaminants from formaldehyde to flame retardants to bisphenol A are contested; industry and government regulators currently contend that the existing levels are safe, but some epidemiologists are concerned about the cumulative impact of all of these chemical exposures, particularly when combined with residual pesticides, environmental contaminants in food and water, and increasing exposure to plastic micro-particles and -fibres.

Contaminants do not need to be concentrated to wreak biologic havoc. Environmental contaminants are especially worrying in terms of impacts on the endocrine system. Even barely measureable amounts of some hormones and hormone mimics—for example, estrogen entering sewage systems when excreted in urine by women taking birth control pills—is potent enough (even in dilution in rivers and lakes) to disrupt the normal development of fish and amphibians. Likewise, excreted metabolites of antidepressant medications are building up in the brains of fish. Tiny amounts of neonicotinoids, widely used in agriculture and previously thought to be harmless, have been implicated in honeybee "colony collapse," the sudden death of entire colonies of bees (Chensheng, Warchel, & Callahan, 2014). Because honeybees are the most effective pollinators of our food crops, their disappearance would be catastrophic for the food supply. The long-term effect of human exposure to neonicotinoids and other pesticides, now spread widely through the environment, is unknown.

Plastics

Plastics of all kinds are ubiquitous in the environment. Rather than breaking down into harmless compounds, plastics are highly durable. They don't decompose but instead fragment into smaller and smaller pieces. Micro-particles of plastic and strands of plastic fibre are readily incorporated into living things, from plants to people. Plastics are toxic, and many kinds of plastic are hormone disruptors. Moreover, the surfaces of plastic micro-particles accumulate other environmental toxins (which adhere to them), and serve as growing media for pathogenic bacteria. Those micro-particles are now incorporated into the tissues of algae, plankton, and hence shellfish and fish further up the food chain, and have found their way into the cells of terrestrial animals, including humans.

The seas, lakes and rivers, and the atmosphere are all heavily contaminated with plastic particles and fibres. Discarded plastic items, from bags, to disposable diapers, to toothbrushes, to water bottles and pop containers are sources of some particles. Others come from more surprising sources, such as micro-beads of plastic that were widely used in cosmetics until being banned in 2016, clothing (which is now made mostly synthetic fibres) when washed or put into driers (which exhaust 700,000 plastic fibres *per load* into the air, from whence they are breathed or washed by rain into waterways), and sewage sludge, one-half of which is removed from treatment plants and spread on the land, despite being heavily contaminated with plastic particles (from sources such as laundry), human pharmaceuticals, and heavy metals. Tiny particles of plastic are rubbed off vehicle tires as they roll down roads, particles that then get blown into the air or washed into rivers, lakes, and oceans. Of the 300 million tonnes of plastic produced each year, less than 20 per cent is effectively recycled (Carrington, 2017); the rest finds its way into the environment.

In 2017, it was discovered that plastic micro-particles and fibres contaminate drinking water. In North America, 94 per cent of samples, including samples of bottled water and even bottled beer, are contaminated (Carrington, 2017). It is not known how so much plastic has found its way into such unlikely places as deep freshwater aquifers; presumably the particles are so tiny they can percolate through soils. The effects on human health are also, as of yet, unknown, but they certainly are not good. Brain neurons, in particular, are highly vulnerable to damage from micro-particles of all kinds crossing the cell wall.

Theoretical Considerations

Environmental exposures highlight the importance of life course analysis and the concept of cumulative risk. Small one-off exposures to contaminants are very unlikely to lead to any health difficulty, but repeated or continuous exposure over time can have profound health effects. Dose response and the timing, frequency, duration, and amounts of exposures are important variables in assessing health risk. Moreover, environmental contaminants interact synergistically. Smoking, air pollution, exposure to dust and pollens, and exposure to fine fibres and micro-particles are *cumulative risks*; each additional exposure multiplies the risk of an adverse health outcome. Modern people are exposed to an unprecedented range of environmental factors, many of them poorly understood and subject to rapid change. Understanding how those factors impact on health is a major challenge.

Macro-level events such as weather and earthquakes can have individual-level effects through affecting food supply, availability of drinking water, sanitation, and housing. They may also have direct effects. Extreme cold kills people, especially those who are *fuel insecure* (cannot afford electricity or gas bills for heating). Extreme heat also kills; again, those who do not have air conditioning or who cannot afford the power bills to operate it are the most vulnerable. Macro-level events can also directly cause extreme stress. Forest fires, protracted extreme weather events, floods, and violent windstorms cause anxiety, fear of loss, and uncertainty. Again, those with fewer resources are most vulnerable to emotional stress associated with such events, and the adverse health consequences that flow from that stress.

Summary

Climate change, natural disasters, modern food production, and toxic environmental exposures all raise precisely the same issues: planning, regulation, monitoring, and science-informed action are required to mitigate their effects on health. Those responsibilities fall mostly to governments and their public health authorities, but also to communities of scientists and advocacy organizations whose role is critical for raising awareness and applying political pressure to ensure appropriate action.

Progress should not be underestimated. In China, the government is serious about combatting air pollution, and has moved quickly to phase out coal-fired electricity plants and gasoline-powered motor scooters. Automobile use is now restricted in Beijing and Shanghai, and the country promises to be all-electric by 2040 (as do France and the United Kingdom). Alberta, like China, is phasing out coal-fired electricity generation. Neonicotinoids and plastic micro-beads were banned in record time in the European Union; so too were plastic bags. Oslo is in the process of banning street parking for cars, as it moves aggressively to an all-cycling/walking/public transit model. Progress has been slower in North America, but if we look back 60 years we can see how far we have come. Alberta used to spread crude oil on gravel roads to reduce dust, and on ponds and swamplands to kill mosquito larvae. Edmonton and Winnipeg used to fog their cities with DDT—from trucks and low-flying aircraft—to control mosquitoes. Pesticides and herbicides were not regulated, and the use of dangerous chemicals in ways dangerous to workers and the public alike, was widespread around the world. Today, most North American and European municipalities ban herbicides and pesticides, and some even ban lawn fertilizer. Sixty years ago, America was conducting above-ground nuclear weapons tests, and winds carried enormous clouds of radioactive material into western Canada. Milk was contaminated with radioactive isotopes, necessitating, from time to time, the issuance of iodine pills to reduce thyroid uptake of radionuclides. Consumer products and food were weakly regulated, if at all. There is no doubt, despite contemporary risks and challenges, that we are in much better shape in terms of environmental contaminants today than in the past. And, as noted earlier in the chapter, our disaster-response capabilities have grown with the risks. Perhaps our greatest unaddressed environmental problem is the agricultural industry—a massive polluter, a glutton for fresh water, and a source of novel pathogens. And the slow pace of addressing climate change is a real concern. But even in the United States, despite opposition federally, states and municipalities are taking concrete steps to mitigate the production of CO_2 and other greenhouse gases. Hopefully more will be done following the record drought, forest fire, and hurricane year of 2017. That will depend on how citizens and scientists organize to apply pressure on politicians.

Critical Thinking Questions

1. If we were to pursue more sustainable agricultural practices such as limiting irrigation and the use of chemical fertilizers and pesticides, could we still feed the world's population? What might be the impact of such changes on food security?

2. How might citizens better mobilize to reduce the use of plastics, micro-beads in cosmetics, and toxic chemicals in household products, all demonstrated threats to the environment and human health?

3. Property developers in Canadian cities (and elsewhere) continue to lobby, often successfully, to drain wetlands, divert waterways, build on floodplains, and otherwise get approvals for housing projects on land subject to flooding. What may be done to counteract the pressure of developers? How might success in forcing construction to occur in safer locations affect the cost of housing, and the long-term health and well-being of the population?

Annotated Suggested Readings

Colin Butler's book *Climate Change and Global Health* (Wallingford: CABI, 2014) includes a comprehensive set of essays on the effects of climate change, from heat wave–related deaths, to changes in infectious disease rates, to impact on food security.

Disaster Management and Human Health Risk, edited by K. Duncan and C. Brebbia (Boston: WIT Press, 2009), is a reader comprising recent conference papers covering every conceivable type of disaster and explaining how action can be taken to reduce the risk on health.

David Kirby's highly readable *Animal Factory: The Looming Threat of Industrial Pig, Dairy and Poultry Farms to the Environment* (New York: St Martin's Press, 2010) was a *New York Times* bestseller.

Annotated Web Resources

"Climate Change and Human Health"
https://health2016.globalchange.gov/
climate-change-and-human-health
"Climate Change and Human Health" (2016), by the US Global Change Research Program, provides an excellent overview of how climate change may affect the health of Americans.

World Health Organization
http://www.who.int/globalchange/en
The World Health Organization offers a set of resources on climate change and health. The webpage serves as a portal into a range of related resources on this topic.

UCL Institute for Risk & Disaster Reduction
https://www.ucl.ac.uk/rdr
University College London's Institute for Risk and Disaster Reduction maintains an up-to-date website on disasters and health.

Costs of Pollution in Canada
https://www.iisd.org/sites/default/files/
publications/costs-of-pollution-in-canada.
pdf
Costs of Pollution in Canada (2017) provides an excellent overview of the financial, social, environmental, and health (Chapter 3) impacts of environmental contamination in Canada.

Invisibles: The Plastic Inside Us
https://orbmedia.org/stories/
Invisibles_plastics
The Plastic Inside Us, by Chris Tyree and Dan Morrison (2017), is a comprehensive web resource on plastic micro-particles and fibres.

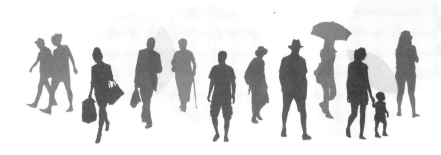

13 Social Patterning of Behaviour

Objectives

By the end of your study of this chapter, you should be able to
- understand why it is a mistake to regard health-related behaviour as freely chosen by the individual;
- provide reasons as to why much of human behaviour is context dependent;
- appreciate that health-promotion initiatives that target individual behaviour will be of limited impact if contextual variables are ignored;
- understand why the idea of "healthy lifestyles" is problematic, and therefore not a sound basis for health policy.

Synopsis

Chapter 13 returns to the question of how we should understand variables relevant to human health: in a way that is methodologically individualist (and thus concerns itself with individual-level variables) or, alternatively, in a way that is more holistic (and thus incorporates contextual features into the analysis)? The chapter argues that it is a serious mistake to construe health-relevant behaviour as "individual" in the sense that it is chosen, albeit shaped by external factors. Instead, the chapter contends, behaviour is properly understood as embedded in its social context. The example of smoking is explored before the chapter turns to examining "lifestyles." The conclusion draws out implications for health promotion and health policy.

Human Behaviour and Its Context

Health-related behaviours, like other human activities, cluster. They are not evenly distributed through the population. Most "risky behaviour" is more common among less well-off people—people with lower incomes and less education—or among the socially marginalized. Important examples include smoking, leading a sedentary lifestyle, having multiple sexual partners, and engaging in a host of dangerous activities ranging from speeding, drinking and driving, driving without use of a seatbelt, illicit drug use, and binge drinking. There are a few exceptions such as extreme sports, horse riding, boating, and skiing—all dangerous yet more common among affluent people. But risky recreation involves only a small minority and accounts overall for very little population-health impact. In contrast, smoking and inactivity, due to their prevalence, have enormous population-health implications.

We saw earlier in the book that smoking prevalence decreases as income rises. Similarly, as income and education increase, so do levels of physical activity. As we have also noted earlier in the book, diets and eating habits improve as income grows. Furthermore, violent crimes (participation in and being a victim of) also decrease as income and education increase. Risky behaviour, activity level, nutrition, and exposure to violence are all important determinants of health and all are closely associated with social position, which in turn is largely a function of income and education.

If we take physical activity levels as an example, only about 17 per cent of poorer Americans are physically active in their leisure time, compared to nearly 40 per cent of more affluent Americans. Note that this is not a poverty effect, but a gradient; activity levels rise as income rises (Braveman, Egerter, & Barclay, 2011). Education level yields very similar results. Only 16 per cent of Americans with less than high-school completion are physically active; 24 per cent of US high-school graduates are physically active; and 42 per cent of Americans with college degrees are physically active.

Smoking statistics are similar. Approximately 35 per cent of adults at or below the US federal poverty rate smoke, compared to only 21 per cent of adults earning three or more times the US federal poverty rate. Thirty per cent of Americans without a high-school diploma smoke, whereas only 8 per cent of college graduates smoke (Braveman, Egerter, & Barclay, 2011).

The series of figures below show that smoking prevalence is associated with soco-economic status of family of origin (Figure 13.1), level of education (Figure 13.2), and

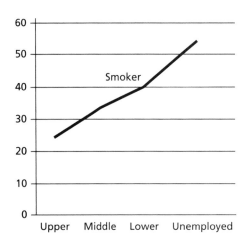

Figure 13.1 Smoking Prevalence by Economic Status of Family of Origin

Per cent smoking, young women, England, by father's employment status at birth.

Source: Graham et al., 2010.

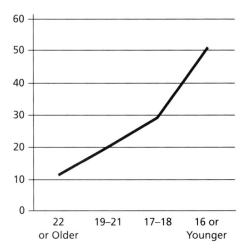

Figure 13.2 Smoking Prevalence by Numbers of Years of Education

Per cent smoking, young women, England, by age of leaving school

Source: Graham et al., 2010.

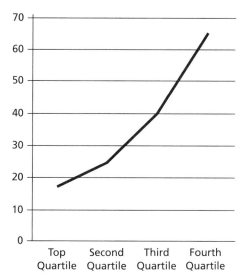

Figure 13.3 Prevalence of Smoking by Current Household Income

Per cent smoking, young women, England, by current household income.

Source: Graham et al., 2010.

current income (Figure 13.3). The strongest relationship is between smoking and current income. All figures demonstrate that smoking is very closely linked to social variables and does not arise as an individual behaviour in isolation from a person's context.

Behaviour like eating habits, physical activities, and smoking corresponds not only to an individual's income, education, and gender but also to the characteristics of his or her surroundings (Chuang, Cubbin, Ahn, & Winkleby, 2005). As we have already seen, income, education, gender, and neighbourhood characteristics strongly condition individual behaviour. At the individual level, more education means greater health knowledge, better problem-solving and planning skills, and a stronger sense of personal efficacy. At the social level, more education means a job context that reinforces health promotion and discourages health-damaging behaviour, better social support, and a broader, richer social network. More income means more access to personal, as well as community, resources supportive of healthy choices. It also means living in a better, safer, well-resourced neighbourhood among other more affluent, better-educated people. Gender roles directly affect a broad range of activities and influence behavioural determinants, such as competitiveness.

Stress, both during childhood and later in life due to workplace, neighbourhood, and other social contextual factors, is strongly linked to adult smoking, compulsive eating, binge drinking, and drug abuse. Growing up in more affluent circumstances reduces those stresses and health-behavioural outcomes.

As social animals, we humans take our cues about what is possible for us and the appropriate way to act from those with whom we associate—our social network of family, friends, co-workers, and neighbours (Christakis & Fowler, 2009). Our behaviour, ranging from the choices we make regarding our clothes and hairstyle, to the television programs we watch, to the foods we eat, to the amounts of alcohol we drink, is heavily influenced by the people with whom we interact, social trends, the pervasive advertising to which we are exposed, and the discipline imposed on our behaviour by the opinions and reactions of the people surrounding us.

Health Behaviour as "Socially Influenced"

Pause and Reflect	Are We Independent, Autonomous Actors, or Social Creatures?

The Canadian researcher Andrée Demers showed that the amount of alcohol university students drink depends on the situation. The critical variables are which friends they happen to be with, how much those friends drink, and when and where the drinking is taking place. She concludes: "It is apparent that the individual cannot be conceptualized as an autonomous actor" (Demers et al., 2002).

What does it mean to interpret behaviour as socially structured as opposed to freely chosen? Is Demers's conclusion counterintuitive? What implications does it have for designing a program to reduce dangerous drinking behaviour on campus?

Everything that has been said thus far is consistent with an individual level of analysis and the underlying belief that our actions (including our health-relevant behaviours of smoking, drinking, diet, and exercise) are socially *influenced*. By embracing the idea of **social influence**, we recognize that information available to individuals, and the content of their beliefs, may be modified by exogenous variables such as education, advertising, or information sharing within networks. Moreover, we are recognizing that people's choices may be modified by altering the mix of incentives and disincentives (changing perceived costs and benefits). If people learn that increasing their daily minutes of moderate to vigorous exercise will strengthen their hearts, and if the disincentive to jogging presented by lack of safe sidewalks is removed, they may be more inclined to choose activity over inactivity. Thus, their health might benefit. Or if advertisers are blocked from encouraging people to believe that smoking will enhance their quality of life and the public is exposed to ongoing information about the health risks of tobacco, more people may be inclined to quit smoking (or not take it up in the first place). Again, health might be improved. From a philosophical point of view, this way of framing things is **methodologically individualist** and assumes *free will*—a capacity on the part of the person to choose. Persons, as philosophers like to say, are construed as *agents*. From a health promotion point of view, this way of framing things leads to programs and initiatives that rely on education and changing the incentive structure/opportunity structure facing the individual. Such *behaviourist* interventions aim to change people's choices through health advice and education; via regulated labelling of products and services; by building sidewalks and cycling paths; by manipulating the availability and pricing of alcohol, tobacco, and food products; and by subsidizing public swimming pools and gym memberships. Policy-makers concerned with health also aim to create more opportunities for healthy living for less well-off people by enhancing public transit, supporting urban renewal, improving security by suppressing crime, and spending public funds on universal schooling.

The Health Belief Model

An especially influential model of health behaviour is the Health Belief Model, developed by Rosenstock and colleagues in the 1960s (see Figure 13.4). According to Rosenstock (1974), the model relies on four key variables:

1. self-perceived personal risk;
2. self-perceived severity of the outcomes associated with unhealthy behaviour;
3. self-perceived barriers to and costs of behavioural change; and
4. self-perceived benefits of making the behavioural change.

Mediating variables (individual and social influences) include factors such as age, gender, personality characteristics, sense of personal efficacy, and the cues, nudges, and reminders the person receives from his or her environment. So, for example, if we can get people to believe that being overweight poses a serious risk *and* to believe highly undesirable outcomes ranging from diabetes to premature death will follow from their current behaviour *and* we can make it easier for them to be more active and buy less calorie-dense foods *and* we can get them to see that those behavioural changes will benefit them directly, we may, especially if we continue to nudge them with reminders and cues, get them to exercise more and consume fewer calories. But success in modifying behaviour will be at least partly contingent on age, sex, gender, and personality attributes of the people targeted by the health promotion intervention.

All of this sounds obvious, but unfortunately is only weakly predictive of behavioural change, mostly because it fails to incorporate a robust sense of social context. In the Pause and Reflect box above, Demers is talking about something quite different. The drinking example is not about a student with a set of personal attributes being influenced by perceptions, threats, barriers, and benefits, although those influences are part of the

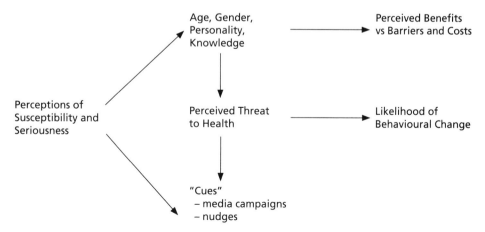

Figure 13.4 Health Belief Model
Source: Adapted from Champion & Skinner, 2008, p. 49.

picture. Instead, Demers is talking about **social patterning of behaviour**. In other words, rather than a reductionist, individual-level analysis, her conception is inherently social and contextual.

Health Behaviour as Socially Patterned

We have already seen that health behaviour is socially patterned in the sense that individual behaviour is associated with the population to which that individual belongs (income group, education level, gender, place of residence). The observed patterns may exist due to patterns of individual-level attributes and influences such as we have just discussed. But Demers and most social epidemiologists mean something quite different from this. We observe social patterning because behaviour is *socially structured*. The individual does what he or she does not as a function of individual choice influenced by some exogenous variables, but because of his or her social context. The meaning is the same one Durkheim pioneered in his classic study of suicide. As discussed earlier, Durkheim contended that social structures and processes give rise to the observed patterns of behaviour.

This more fundamental sense of social patterning of behaviour raises some deep philosophical and ethical issues, ranging from the complex problem of *structure and agency* in sociology to *choice determination* in psychology to *free will* in philosophy and ethics. While far beyond our scope and purposes in this book, a few foundational points need to be made. Before we do so, it is worth noting some of shortcomings of the behaviourist approach to choice and behaviour outlined earlier in the chapter. This is of fundamental importance because behaviourism underlies traditional health promotion and accounts for its weakness.

"Rational Behaviour" and Incentives

Recent research (Bourdieu, 1984; Unger, 1987; Giddens, 1984, 1991; Kahneman & Tversky, 2000; Mercier & Sperber, 2017) on what people actually choose has undermined models of agent rational choice. For example, in real life, people will choose outcomes that they conceive as being fairer even when, as result, they personally end up bearing additional costs or receiving lower benefits. This result has been observed in human infants, other primates, and even dogs, and is likely an evolutionary response to being a *social animal dependent upon relationships with others*. However it arises, the fact that people are not motivated to maximize benefits and minimize costs (although they obviously sometimes do) calls into question the naïve account of human behaviour that informs much health-promotion activity.

A meaningful application of such findings comes from research on incentives. Recent studies (Smith & York, 2004) show that doctors respond by providing more preventive services, such as blood pressure monitoring, when financial incentives to do so are introduced into payment schemes. Incentives can have an effect, sometimes a very large one. But interestingly, incentives only seem to work if the thing incentivized is something the person wanted to do anyway and the incentive is quite large. Here, as we noted earlier, the public health example of reducing smoking may mislead. Almost all current smokers would like either to quit or smoke less, thus smokers often welcome schemes that incentivize quitting, make continuing to smoke more costly or inconvenient, or remind people of the hazards associated with smoking. The same logic does not carry over to sugary or fatty snacks, fast food, or physical exercise.

Small incentives, or incentives to do something the person is disinclined to do for whatever reason, are much less effective in altering behaviour. Also interesting is the fact that incentives not only increase the behaviour incentivized, but also change the patterns of choice and action by the recipient across a range of other activities. In the doctor example, a physician may do more blood pressure screening, but spend less time with patients who have time-consuming mental health problems. As a result, the overall quality of care of patients may decline rather than improve. Denmark came to believe poorer people's choices of foods worsened in light of the "fat taxes" because of substitution effects and increased pressure on their food budgets.

Paradoxically, incentives may actually *decrease* the desired behaviour. Work on ethically motivated behaviour such as volunteer work on behalf of charities shows people are *demotivated* by cash incentives. Presumably their voluntary activity is valued for intrinsic reasons and the introduction of cash and other exogenous incentives undermines that internal motivation.

Incentives clearly have perverse and unintended effects as well as the desired ones. In health-promotion work, this has generally been ignored because the implicit motivational models have been either too crude or simply wrong. For reasons such as these, we need to be wary of the effects of such popular measures as taxes on sugary drinks and fatty foods. As we saw in the previous chapter, all forms of "sin tax" risk being no more than a government revenue grab in the form of a regressive tax that further harms less well-off people.

Box 13.1	Case Study ○ Incentives and Reminders Yield Perverse Result: the IDEA Clinical Trial

A high-quality randomized clinical trial produced a shocking result (Jakicic et al., 2016). Study participants equipped with fitness tracker devices (currently a $1.5-billion-dollar industry in the US) lost substantially less weight using the devices than study participants who did not use the technology. Since the devices are specifically engineered to give positive feedback, monitor progress, issue reminders, and otherwise provide motivation, the finding undermines the entire behaviourist model.

In the study, overweight people were randomized into two groups. Both groups participated in conventional programs designed to modify their diets and increase their physical activity. One group was fitted with, and trained in the use of, fitness trackers; the other was not. After an 18-month intervention, the fitness tracker group lost 5.3 fewer pounds than the control group (7.7 pounds versus 13.0 pounds).

"Rational Behaviour" and Information

Another set of problems arises from treating people as agents whose decisions will improve (and become "freer") in light of increased information. This can readily be seen by looking at the principle of fully informed consent in health care.

The gold standard in health care is "fully informed consent," which respects the autonomy of the patient by providing detailed information about the proposed procedure and its risks and potential benefits. The idea is to overcome the information asymmetry between a health care expert, such as a doctor, and a patient by equipping the patient with a similar level of information as the doctor. That way, it becomes more the patient's choice and not the doctor's. But several recently discovered real-world features corrode the gold standard of care.

First, some patients do not want to know (and often are not able to understand fully) the implications of all the alternative treatment modalities. Not all women, for example, want their doctors to discuss the options of breast cancer treatment and go into all the risks and benefits; they would rather the doctors choose what they think is the best treatment option. In other words, they trust the judgment of their doctors. Second, more information generally leads to complexity and indecision, rather than the "fully informed decision" anticipated. A doctor discussing the merits and demerits of a PSA screening test for prostate cancer will, if honest, expose the contradictory evidence and the substantial risks associated with screening, making it very difficult for the average man to decide. Third, and more fundamentally, patients have a range of other concerns like the care burden imposed on family members, what other people will think of their choice, how fair or appropriate an option is given their familial and other life circumstances, and the good will and ongoing relationship they have with their health care providers.

So, why do we persist in seeking "fully informed consent" in our hospitals? The simple and accurate answer is: to mitigate the liability of the health care provider by answering the potential legal charge of assault (doing something to someone without their legal consent). The autonomous agency concept, as it plays out in today's hospitals, is misleading, not only for patients with limited capacity, such as those with dementia or the acutely ill, but for many capable patients as well. One reason is that it is not irrational to place faith in others and to act on trust; denying this is not only individualistic, but also mistaken. Another is that more information does not make decision making easier, but often makes it more difficult.

The health care consent example raises another related point. We usually cannot know the implications of the choices under consideration. Information and evidence are incomplete and conflicting. For example, we have all been told to drink fluids even when we are not thirsty, especially when we exercise. Dehydration is supposedly dangerous to our health and saps our performance. This seems plausible, and many people force-hydrate themselves in light of this information. But the advice is almost certainly wrong. Recent meta-analyses show that more people, especially athletes, are harmed by over-hydration than by dehydration. Performance athletes (and students writing exams) do better when *moderately dehydrated* than when fully hydrated. Most people would be better off if they rarely drank fluids except when they are thirsty (Heneghan et al., 2012). The point of the example is that health-related information is notoriously unreliable. Moreover, the balance of evidence shifts as researchers conduct more, and better studies. We really do not know if people would be healthier if they ate less carbohydrate or smaller amounts of animal protein or cut back on their salt intake. (We do know most should cut back on their calories!) In the end, the best advice is to eat only when hungry, drink only when thirsty, avoid things we know are poisonous (alcohol, tobacco), eat a wide variety of foods, and get at least some exercise daily. The rest is mostly unproven, provisional, subject to change.

This in no small part helps explain why "healthy lifestyles" provide so little health advantage in terms of disease, disability, and life expectancy.

Moreover, the general population experiences "information overload." The media's widespread and often misleading reporting on health matters creates the impression that everything is potentially harmful. The average person is confronted by many sources vying for his or her attention and demanding action. Many people retreat into indifference or, worse, the irrational, obtaining information from celebrities, quacks, or dodgy Internet sites.

The costs of acquiring quality information comprise only part of the problem. Information, it turns out, has a relatively small role to play in behaviour. This has been well understood by advertisers for over a century. It is far more important to influence people's attitudes than provide information. Recent research in psychology (Tavris & Aronson, 2007) demonstrates that people are not even aware of their underlying values and attitudes. For example, well-educated and liberal people, who believe themselves to be tolerant, demonstrate preferences for people who are most like themselves in terms of race, ethnicity, and social class. They harbour, unknown to themselves, racist and other prejudices that influence their choices and actions.

Some psychologists think people can train themselves through reflection to "veto" thoughts, emotions, and actions that spontaneously arise from unconscious sources; others are less sure (Kahneman & Tversky, 2000). At dispute is the extent to which we can identify our biases and inculcated inclinations and, through an act of will, block them. For example, people in the United Kingdom reacted with horror and outrage when it was discovered in 2013 that horsemeat had found its way into the food supply. The reaction appears to have arisen from the British love of horses and their regard of them as pets and companions, rather than from a sense of betrayal at the processed food industry's rather cavalier approach to what goes into their products. The former is arguably less rational than the latter. But could the knowledge that most of the world sees horses as suitable food and knowing that horse meat is leaner and probably healthier than beef affect the reaction? Probably not. What is certain is much human thought and behaviour turn out to be quasi-determined and certainly not conscious and rational. In reality, "reasons" are often after-the-fact justifications of impulses, but our self-justifications appear to us as rational and compelling (Tavris & Aronson, 2007; Mercier & Sperber, 2017).

"Rational Behaviour" and Our Brains

Neurology has also undermined the traditional view of agency. As long ago as the 1980s, neuropsychologist Benjamin Libet questioned the existence of human free will based on a series of experiments showing (he thought) that the brain determines actions *before* the person has considered what they want to do and has become aware of that decision. Activity in the brain and in motor-neuron units *precedes* consciousness. Libet's findings do not imply that people are unable to choose their own actions, a conclusion he erroneously advanced, but suggest choice is far more constrained and unconscious than naïve models of human behaviour allow. Social psychologist John Bargh shows in his program of research that much of what we experience as "choice" is actually the brain's automatic interpretation of, and reaction to, stimuli arising from our context (Bargh & Ferguson, 2000; Bargh & Earp, 2009). Daniel Wegner (2003) develops these themes in his influential book *The Illusion of Conscious Will*.

Recently, the idea of "enculturing brains" has taken root. Theorists contend that history and other forms of socially patterned practice become encoded in the brains of people participating in each particular social formation. For example, as the activities of people on a pathway to addiction become more repetitive and ritualized, the brain alters in response, modifying neural circuits and processing. Similar, albeit more subtle, processes go on due to **brain plasticity** and **neural sculpting** as a result of all of our ongoing activities. Thus, we would expect people who have lived different lives, had different pursuits, and engaged with people of different backgrounds to have functionally different brains. Those particular forms of brain activity, unique to the social history (the life course) and current context of the person, have been demonstrated empirically. Systematic differences in brain organization and function can be detected in brain scans. Moreover, those neural patterns are broadly predictive of choices and behaviour, including our health-relevant behaviour (Roepstorff, Niewöhner, & Beck, 2010).

"Rational Behaviour" and Sociology

Social patterning of behaviour also draws from a robust theoretical tradition in sociology, beginning with Durkheim. Modern theorists, perhaps best represented by Anthony Giddens, have resolved the problem of crude determinism and reframed the agency/structure problem. In works such as *The Constitution of Society* (1984) Giddens argues that human action is "enstructured."

According to Giddens, human action is intentional and goal directed, but we arrive at our understandings of what is possible and how best to attain it through the social institution of language, our interactions with others, and our place in a variety of social institutions ranging from our families and workplaces to the broader social and economic structures of our society. In reality, we do not see free action on one hand and a range of determined outcomes arising from structural social forces on the other, but rather an interaction of agency and structure, individuals and their social contexts—"enstructuration." It is thus a mistake, Giddens warns us, to regard human action as "caused" by social variables such as early life circumstances. But it is equally a mistake to think that individuals freely choose what they do or refrain from doing. Moreover, structures do not merely provide opportunities and constraints—an example being the model of opportunity structures we discussed in the section on neighbourhoods. The very meaning of our lives and our actions is derived from structures. Much of our behaviour makes sense to us and to others only in the context of those specific structures. The values, beliefs, and interests we incorporate in our decision making, as well as our decision-making processes, are grounded in our everyday context. That context, of course, depends on our social position.

It is important to see that the profound understanding arising from enstructuration does not deny free will. It does not entail that people have no choice or imply all their behaviour is determined. But enstructuration does undermine the idea of personal choice based on information, current capabilities, and estimates of costs and benefits. In a way, that should come as no surprise because, as we have seen, empirical studies routinely show that the rational behaviour model underlying much of traditional psychology and economics (as well as traditional health promotion) is wrong. In the real world, people do not act based on evidence, personal values, and anticipated costs and benefits. Instead, people are engaged in an exquisite dance between themselves as individuals and their social and environmental context.

Some Implications for Health Promotion and Public Policy

The recognition of patterning of behaviour by social variables calls into question the common belief that people choose how they behave and that hence they are personally responsible for their behaviour. The assumption of personal responsibility leads to two common conclusions about people who are "acting badly" by, for example, smoking. They "misbehave" either because they do not know any better (the stupid hypothesis) or they misbehave because they are irresponsible (the feckless hypothesis). The social response takes the dual form of education about the harms of tobacco use and regulations such as smoking bans. But it turns out that virtually no one thinks smoking is harmless or that gaining a lot of weight is a good thing. People are not stupid, and it is paternalistic and offensive to contend that they are. Moreover, regulation against recklessness or irresponsibility raises some special problems. Regulation might produce the desired result with regard to simple actions that are easy to monitor, such as smoking or seatbelt use, but it is hard to see how prohibitions would work well elsewhere. How would we go about regulating eating behaviour or amounts of exercise for example? Moreover the feckless hypothesis, contending that people are irresponsible or needlessly reckless, leads to coercion, which is then regarded by the target group as an assault on them. Working-class and Indigenous smokers reacted with understandable fury when middle-class policy-makers banned smoking in bingo halls. A hostile reaction is predictable when the target group regards the offending behaviour as part of what defines them—clubbing and pubbing among undergraduate students, for example. Health initiatives can thus be perceived as unwelcome, elitist intrusions into personal freedoms.

Paradoxically, strategies intended to reduce risk may actually increase the likelihood of bad health outcomes through licensing dangerous behaviour. For example, mandatory seatbelt legislation led to people driving faster and more recklessly. Likewise mandatory use of bicycle helmets is linked to riskier riding practices (Phillips, Fyhri, & Sagberg, 2011). Potentially worse: people thinking they are doing something good for their health, like going to the gym or taking a vitamin or a supplement, is associated with risk compensation such as heavier smoking among smokers and heavier drinking among drinkers (Chiou, Wen, Wu, & Lee, 2011). Activity and diet regimes may be linked to overeating through the same mechanism of risk compensation.

The Example of Smoking

The profile of the typical over-30, male smoker in Canada, the United States, the United Kingdom, and Australia is a man who is unemployed or works in low-paid employment, or is a prisoner, a mental health patient, or homeless. A typical over-30, female smoker is unemployed or works in low-paid employment and is a sole-support parent. But under the age of 25, a significant proportion of men and women of all types and social classes smoke.

More lower-class youth, measured by education or income of their families, take up smoking than upper-class youth. That is really no surprise because more lower-class youth come from families who smoke and live in neighbourhoods were smoking is still the norm and cigarettes are readily available. But uptake is not the best predictor of adult smoking. Smoking correlates more strongly with adult social position than position of origin. A downward social trajectory, experiencing lack of success and moving into closer association with others who are less well-off, contributes to smoking uptake in adulthood. That, more than family of origin, explains the high smoking rates among the marginalized such as prisoners, the homeless, and the mentally ill.

But more important than smoking uptake is smoking cessation. The big difference between well-off people and less well-off people is not so much in their rates of smoking uptake but rather in their rates of quitting. The vast majority of affluent people who take up smoking in their teens and early 20s quit by the time they are 30. In the UK, for example, nearly 50 per cent of affluent men over the age of 35 once smoked, but less than 15 per cent still do. About 70 per cent of poor men in the UK once smoked and over 60 per cent still do (Office for National Statistics, 2011). In part because the long-term damage to health from smoking is negligible if the smoker quits by age 30, the UK death rate from smoking is five times higher for poor men than rich ones.

Because all smokers now know the risks of smoking and all are now exposed to a broad range of measures from punitive pricing to smoking bans, the obvious question is "Why do so many people, mostly less well-off, persist in smoking?" As we saw, the big problem is with cessation. Presumably, family, friends, colleagues, and neighbours better support more-affluent people in their efforts to quit. Moreover, many places where less-affluent people gather and socialize remain places where smoking is accepted and normal, whereas the opposite is true of the places frequented by the more affluent. Affluent people also enjoy better access to counselling support, nicotine replacement therapy, and cessation drugs such as bupropion (Zyban).

Box 13.2   Case Study ○ Clustering of Behaviours

People who smoke usually drink more alcohol, exercise less, and eat more calorie-dense foods than people who do not smoke. Adolescents who use illicit drugs are more likely to engage in risky sex, smoke, and drive dangerously. Due to underlying social causes, risk factors cluster. For that reason, health-behavioural interventions, which typically target a single risk factor such as smoking, *even if they succeed in influencing that single risk factor*, are unlikely to affect a significant change in health.

Given the clustering of health behaviour, how should we design public health initiatives?

Substance Misuse

Substance misuse is strongly influenced by individual-level determinants, including education, income, security of employment, housing, race, gender, social support, and cognitive and emotional regulatory status from fetal and early childhood development. Especially important are fetal alcohol syndrome and adverse childhood experiences, both of which are strong predictors of adolescent and adult substance misuse. Meso (intermediate) -level factors, such as the characteristics of the household and neighbourhood in which the person is situated, are also significant. Macro-level factors, such as the prevalence of alcohol and drug use in society as a whole; laws and policies affecting the availability and cost of alcohol and drugs; and broad features like social disorder, rising inequality, and rapid social change also play a part. Because substance use is so strongly influenced by social factors, it is seen as a social rather than a health problem.

As noted earlier with respect to women, drinking, and their health (Chapter 6), some populations today are subjected to significant health harms from alcohol. Drinking alcohol is the leading cause for hospitalizations in Canada, not just from alcohol-related physical injuries, but also from overdose and liver and brain damage. Deaths associated with binge drinking have skyrocketed in the United Kingdom and Canada, particularly among adolescent girls. The causes are obscure but are clearly social.

Currently, the issue receiving the most attention in Canada and the United States is the "opioid crisis." Deaths are now epidemic, with over 3000 Canadians predicted to die from overdoses in 2017 (see Table 13.1). The crisis is actually several overlapping epidemics. In the Maritime provinces, opioid misuse usually takes the form of prescription drug abuse, the drugs are mostly oral, and the users are predominantly middle-aged women. In BC, opioid abuse usually takes the form of using heroin laced with fentanyl, the drugs are mostly injected, and the users are mainly 29- to 40-year-old men. Both epidemics are nation-wide, but with different combinations of drugs and drug-delivery modalities. Most deaths, almost 80 per cent, involve using more than one drug, most commonly alcohol and opiates, but also marijuana, prescription drugs, and cocaine. Two streams of opioid misuse have merged: about 20 per cent of users began with pain medication prescriptions; the rest began with alcohol and illicit street drugs.

Intensive public awareness campaigns and outreach workers among homeless drug users have not made any apparent difference. Users are well aware of the risks, and in BC users report seeking drugs containing the dangerous and unpredictable fentanyl because of the intensity of the high. Making naloxone (a drug that blocks narcotics, reversing an overdose) widely available has, like effective anti-virals in the case of HIV, encouraged

Table 13.1 Deaths from Opioids: Canada, January to August 2017

Province/Territory	Number of Deaths
Yukon	6
Northwest Territories	5
Nunavut	0
British Columbia	978
Alberta	586
Saskatchewan	64
Manitoba	69
Ontario	865
Quebec	140+
New Brunswick	29
Nova Scotia	53
Prince Edward Island	5
Newfoundland	16

Source: Health Canada, 2017. https://www.canada.ca/content/dam/hc-sc/documents/services/publications/healthy-living/opioids-map-eng.pdf

users to be *less* concerned about safety. Public health advocates in BC are now recommending de-criminalizing injection drugs (to make their potency and quality consistent) and expanding safe-injection sites—i.e., making it easier and safer for drug users to keep using. The federal government has rejected this advice, fearing that it might encourage even wider drug use in the population. Crackdowns on doctors over-prescribing opioids have dangerous side effects. In particular, people misusing prescription drugs, instead of stopping use, turn to more dangerous street drugs. Approaches to the crisis, as we have seen in other areas such as diet and obesity, must be multi-factoral and long-term, not reaches for "quick fixes." Elements of a drug strategy include harm reduction (safe injection sites, distribution of naloxone, decriminalization of drug use, supervised provision of methadone, and other substitutes), stricter limits on and better monitoring of prescribing and dispensing addictive pain medications, and improved access to drug addiction treatment centres. Implementation of such a policy must be in close consultation with the users themselves and involve the coordinated efforts of public health, the police, emergency health responders, and social services.

Why the US and Canada are experiencing such a serious increase in drug use and adverse health outcomes associated with prescription and illicit narcotics is unclear. The economy in both countries is improving and unemployment is trending downwards. But marginalization of less well-off people has worsened, inequality has increased, and the effects of racism and colonization are strongly felt by First Nations people who disproportionately make up drug users in western Canadian urban centres. The roots of the epidemic are plainly social and economic, but identifying factors amenable to change, at least in the short term, is far from easy.

In 2018, Canada is in the process of legalizing the use of cannabis. While helping with some challenges, such as the role of organized crime and the variable quality of street drugs sold, legalization creates new ones. In particular, there are concerns about the use of cannabis increasing dramatically and the potential for more youth to use cannabis more intensively. Also, the issue of second-hand smoke from smoking cannabis has activated anti-smoking advocates, who fear the public use of cannabis will pose as much threat to the health and comfort of non-smokers as tobacco once did. At the time of writing, Calgary is considering a bylaw that would prohibit smoking anything in any public place in the city; that, in turn, has upset medical users of cannabis who argue that smoking the drug is their right. The health effects of cannabis use remain controversial; smoking it does lung damage analogous to smoking tobacco, and heavy use is associated with cognitive and mental health problems. Further, there are mounting concerns about impaired driving. Cannabis intoxication is harder for law enforcement to detect and more difficult to prosecute under impaired driving laws. Should cannabis use substantially increase once legalized, driving under its influence could become a significant public health threat. What seemed in 2015 to be a simple harm reduction measure had, by mid-2018, turned into a complex nest of health-related concerns.

Healthy Lifestyles

Before leaving the subject of health-related behaviours, it is worth saying a few words about healthy lifestyles. The idea of a healthy lifestyle arose in the nineteenth century. The Victorian middle class and their counterparts in Europe and America came to see "dirt and disorder" to be reflections of character flaws, notably lack of self-respect, sloppy habits, and laziness. Alcohol consumption and sexual activity outside of the "normal" (limited to procreation within the bonds of marriage), were similarly labelled as degenerate, reflecting bad character. The goal was to live a life of self-discipline, modesty, scrupulous hygiene, and moral decency—a good and healthy lifestyle. In addition to discipline, that lifestyle ought to avoid poorly ventilated interior spaces (with their "bad air" and risk of pestilence) and include vigorous outdoor exercise, such as horse riding and hiking in the countryside. Later, in the mid-1800s, urban walking for exercise and the velocipede (cycling) became popular middle-class activities. Outdoor parks (mostly commercial ventures charging fees) with walking paths, rowing ponds, cycling tracks, and games areas opened in affluent neighbourhoods across the United Kingdom and Western Europe.

Box 13.3   Case Study ○ Fashionable Exercise

Recreation and increased physical activity became major preoccupations in Victorian England and Scotland. The extent of innovation and the effort to commercialize public interest in outdoor recreation can be seen in developments such as the Royal Patent Gymnasium, a pleasure park built in the 1850s for the affluent in Edinburgh's posh New Town district. The park, one of many built in British cities, included rowing ponds, running tracks, outdoor gymnastic equipment, and the earliest example of a public cycling track.

This old idea has made quite a spectacular return. Recently, some Canadian cities have installed outdoor gym equipment in public parks.

How probable is it that such initiatives will improve public health and fitness? Who are the likely users/beneficiaries?

Students may find the historical antecedents interesting. The history of Kennington Park in London provides a good example of the confluence of ideas of urban outdoor pursuits, leisure, sport, and health. It is available at www.vauxhallandkennington.org.uk/kpark-sports.pdf.

Sources on Scotland's Royal Patent Gymnasium include the following:
www.scotlandmag.com/magazine/issue46/12009418.html
www.edinphoto.org.uk/0_adverts/0_adverts_entertainments_-_royal_patent_gymnasium_background.htm

Middle-class charities and churches took it upon themselves to deliver, with considerable vigour, the healthy lifestyle message to those who were less scrupulously clean, engaged in a broader range of sexual activities, lived in more crowded conditions, drank more alcohol, and were inclined to rest rather than exercise in their leisure—i.e., the urban poor. The coercive forces of government were mobilized to improve the behaviour of, and generally "to better," the lower classes.

By the end of the nineteenth century, views of discipline, hygiene, and exercise took a decidedly militaristic turn. In England, Robert Baden-Powell, founder of the para-military Boy Scouts organization, stressed outdoor exercise, "manliness," sexual restraint, non-smoking, and alcohol abstinence. Military jostling between England and Germany helped foster a broader fetish for male physical fitness, power, and highly defined muscles. Urban gymnasia and swimming pools sprouted up. This was to transform into a true cult of physical fitness, outdoor exercise, sport, and athletics under the Nazis in Germany. From preschool onwards, German boys and girls in the 1930s were enrolled in sports and fitness youth groups that emphasized strength, endurance, and self-denial.

The United States went through similar trends, but, being America, it added a distinctive commercial element. In the nineteenth century, entrepreneurs like Kellogg emerged. John Kellogg (1852–1943) was, by all accounts, an amazing man. A doctor and surgeon, he was also a tremendous self-promoter, showman, and key proselytizer for the Seventh Day Adventist Christian fundamentalist movement. Many of his ideas—jogging or cycling every morning, vegetarianism, anti-smoking, avoidance of caffeine and alcohol, and "taking care of our colon" by eating lots of high-fibre cereals and having regular colonic irrigations (Kellogg favoured daily yogurt enemas)—have stayed with us, even though most are seriously misguided. Nevertheless, Kellogg is something of a poster boy for a healthy lifestyle, at least American style. (For a sympathetic account of John Kellogg and his healthy-living ideas, see http://naturalhealthperspective.com/tutorials/john-kellogg.html.)

Most American lifestyle gurus were anti-smoking, anti-drinking, religious zealots who got into the business of selling what they claimed to be health foods, ranging from Kellogg's cereals to Coca-Cola. Religious agitation for lifestyle reform culminated in efforts in the 1920s to ban alcohol sales in the United States altogether. Ever since, in the US, there has been a tight alignment between organized efforts to regulate "unhealthy" behaviour and commercial promotion of health foods, supplements, and diet therapies.

By the end of the 1960s, the cults of fitness, nutrition, and outdoor activity sank below the tide of affluence, car culture, fast food, and faith in medicine to overcome disease and disability. But in the 1970s four factors led to a comeback:

- recognition of the rising importance of chronic disease;
- diminishing faith in medicine to solve health-related problems;
- a strengthening cultural link between consumption patterns and who we are;
- the rise of consumerism and the closely related "self-help" movement.

The term "healthy lifestyle" came to refer to a number of elements: self-control, taking responsibility for your own state of health, seeking out healthy foods, and engaging in regular vigorous physical exercise, such as jogging. Consumption patterns remained central—from choices of foods and food providers, brands of athletic shoes, clothing, equipment, and fitness club memberships, to alternative health care and dietary supplements.

Adopting a lifestyle is a process of securing an identity. A **lifestyle** is a medley of practices embraced by a person as a statement of who he or she is (Giddens, 1991). Just as with the Victorians, those who adopt healthy lifestyles today are predominantly upper-middle- and upper-class people, and just like their predecessors, they see their set of choices to be virtuous. However, as we have seen throughout the book, healthy behaviours are only contingently and contextually linked to meaningful health outcomes, and we must be careful not to equate healthy lifestyles with healthy living in the sense that the person's health will actually be substantially better in consequence. Mostly, as we have learned, health depends on circumstances, not self-discipline and consumption patterns.

Box 13.4   Case Study ○ Nudging

As was pointed out in the first chapter, voluntary efforts to change individual behaviour through education, counselling, and support groups have not proven very successful. The systematic failure of diet programs marketed to women is a case in point. Very few women lose much weight, and those who do almost invariably put it back on.

Coercive regulatory approaches, such as those that were adopted (in most places) with regard to motorcycle helmets, use of seatbelts, and smoking in public places, do work, but they raise civil rights issues. Conservative voters and politicians generally regard coercive measures to be inappropriate.

Quasi-coercive approaches, such as punitive pricing through the special taxes, have been applied to tobacco and alcohol products (and proposed for junk foods and sugary drinks). But such coercive regulation and punitive pricing have limited applicability. Those strategies only apply to specific behaviours or products. We might be able to reduce consumption of sugary sodas through special taxes (provided they were set high enough), but we are unlikely to be able to devise a taxation regime that would move people away from all energy-dense foods. Coherence is also a problem. How can we tax "junk foods" like burgers but not tax high-salt, high-fat foods such as cheese (a food that is heavily subsidized in Europe and the Americas)? How can we deal with the fact that bottles of unsweetened fruit juice contain more sugar than cans of Coke?

An attractive idea was floated in the book *Nudge: Improving Decisions about Health, Wealth and Happiness* (Thaler & Sunstein, 2008). According to its authors, the behaviour of people can be changed by subtle incentives or cues. For example, using a simple system of colour coding such as green, amber, and red (traffic-light coding) consumers could be cued into whether a product was a healthy food choice. Or, to take another example, governments could provide incentives to supermarkets to feature fruit and vegetables near the checkouts instead of candy and potato chips. Simple, subtle, and non-coercive methods could be adopted to facilitate long-term changes in people's behaviour.

As one might expect, politicians, especially those on the right, quickly adopted Thaler and Sunstein's ideas. Richard Thaler became a special advisor to the British Conservative Party and the **nudge theory** was officially written into Conservative Party policy. Thaler also became an advisor to the US government.

A special committee of the British House of Lords was struck to review the evidence in support of nudge theory and the prospects of using such simple, non-coercive techniques to shape people's health behaviour. The committee reviewed hundreds of briefs and expert research reports. Its chair, Julia Newberger, reported in the summer of 2011 that nudges in the right direction do not hold substantial promise of changing public behaviour (Day, 2011). It remains to be seen whether the British and American governments stick to rolling out nudge-related policies in the face of the evidence that they will not work.

In September 2011, McDonald's restaurants announced a voluntary program in the United Kingdom. The fast-food chain, alongside KFC and Burger King, became one of the first to post calorie counts for menu items nationwide. (Subway, Domino's Pizza, Nando's, and Pizza Express refused to join.)

continued

The idea is to nudge people away from higher-calorie choices such as chicken nuggets and milkshakes to lower-calorie ones such as salads without dressing. A similar initiative in New York failed to influence consumer choices, except perhaps at the margin. That is quite understandable because people go to McDonald's precisely to eat something filling, satisfying, and cheap—i.e., high-fat/high-sugar items.

McDonald's and PepsiCo (owner of Frito-Lay and Gatorade) are at the forefront of voluntary anti-obesity initiatives inspired by nudge theory because they are highly motivated to preclude compulsory regulatory measures. Thus we find PepsiCo is a charter partner in the US Healthy Weight Commitment Foundation, a bit of a surprise for a maker of sugar drinks and potato chips until we reflect on the company's motives. We noted that Coca-Cola is a central figure in Canadian physical activity and sport promotion. The situation looks a lot like the voluntary measures tobacco makers took in the 1970s and 1980s in their effort to forestall regulation by governments. Remember, the principal sponsor of sports in Canada, the United States, and the United Kingdom used to be cigarette makers.

"Nudging" starts to look a bit like a refuge for scoundrels. Yet it might have a legitimate role if applied as part of more sophisticated, multi-pronged strategy. What might such a strategy look like if the goal is to support healthier eating?

Theoretical Considerations

The shaping of health-related behaviour is a complex and controversial field. Theorists in the social epidemiology tradition tend toward modern efforts to bridge the divide between agency and structure. In this chapter, we discussed the influence of Anthony Giddens. Other important theorists are Pierre Bourdieu and Roberto Unger.

Bourdieu (1984) developed the concept of "habitus." According to Bourdieu, individuals are best construed as agents occupying a field, a complex set of roles and relationships constituting a social domain. Each agent must accommodate himself or herself to the roles and relationships demanded by his or her position in the field. In so doing, individuals internalize a set of expectations for how they must operate within the given social domain. Those relationships and their outward expression in terms of habitual behaviour evolve over time into the habitus. According to this analysis, we can expect to find repertoires of attitudes and behaviours associated with different social positions. Tastes, pastimes, and attitudes will systemically differ from one social location (an upper-class person in Rosedale, Toronto) to another (a Haitian immigrant in Montreal). A good deal of recent health research ranging from health-behavioural work to health human geography has been based on Bourdieu's theorization.

Social theorist Roberto Unger (1987) is important because he shows a way out of strict determinism. While it is true that human behaviour is enstructured, individuals nevertheless may be able to transcend their context. Unger contends that the social arrangements that structure human thought and action are themselves human artifacts and thus the idea that human behaviour is "determined" relies on what he calls "false necessity." Individuals may not be able to change the structures that condition their thinking and behaviour, but collectives—people acting collaboratively—can. Less oppressive and restrictive social structures are possible, and striving for democratization, greater social equality, better education, and less concentration of ownership can free up capacity for human thought and action—i.e., be emancipatory. The idea is especially important to health promotion because it opens the door to empowerment, the notion that progressive political forces at the community level may create possibilities for community development. A more supportive, egalitarian and open community fosters individual freedom and human rights and preconditions for healthier choices and individual well-being. Unger's idea of empowerment holds a central place in much of today's thinking about fostering healthier communities. It highlights, once again, the link between population health and social justice.

Summary

Because health-relevant behaviours are socially patterned, cluster, and follow the social gradient, health behaviour reinforces and expands the differences we see in people's health based on their incomes, education, and social position. Typical behaviour plays an amplifying role in terms of the eventual health outcomes. But differences in health behaviour cannot explain the big differences in health outcomes. For example, there is virtually no difference in the health of low-educated Americans who live a healthy lifestyle compared to their low-income counterparts who do not. But there are big differences between low-educated Americans living a healthy lifestyle and high-educated Americans also living a healthy lifestyle. Twenty-one per cent of Americans who have not completed high school and who have unhealthy lifestyles report their health as very good or excellent compared to 27 per cent of Americans who have not completed high school and have healthy lifestyles report their health as very good or excellent. The difference is a mere 6 per cent between those with and those without healthy lifestyles. But if we compare the non-high–school completers with healthy lifestyles to college graduates with healthy lifestyles, we find a 48 per cent difference. Twenty-seven per cent versus 75 per cent report their health as very good or excellent (Braveman, Egerter, & Barclay, 2011).

The findings reported in 2011 by the Robert Wood Foundation are consistent with research evidence going back to 1990, when Mildred Blaxter showed that healthy lifestyles made no difference to the health of less well-off people (Blaxter, 1990). The big differences in health arise from the resources people have and the contexts in which they live and work, not their lifestyles.

This chapter attempted to draw out some implications for health promotion. In particular, we must remain cognizant of the limitations of efforts to change health-relevant behaviour through education, incentives, punitive measures, and regulation. Not only is human behaviour deeply entrenched and difficult to modify, it is formed through and reinforced by the life history of the individual and his or her current context. Patterns of behaviour reflect deeper social structures and processes and may even be incorporated into our neural "wiring." It follows that efforts to change the context in which people grow up and live their adult lives must not be neglected if we are serious about changing the patterns of behaviour in ways that are more supportive of human health. Education and changing incentive structures will affect behaviour only at the margins, and then in ways that are unlikely to be sustainable or meaningful in terms of significant health outcomes. Plainly we should attempt to do more.

Critical Thinking Questions

1. A leading American science writer, Leonard Mlodinow, claims in his book *Subliminal: How Your Unconscious Mind Rules Your Behaviour* (New York: Random House, 2012) that our preferences and choices are shaped by our context and life experience, although we experience our behaviour as conscious and deliberate. For example, women are much more likely to give personal contact information to strange men if the men lightly touch the woman's hand or wrist when asking for their telephone number or email address. Or to take another example, studies repeatedly show that people prefer the taste of Pepsi over Coke (in blind tasting tests) but more often choose Coke when grocery shopping because they believe Coke tastes better. In yet another example, Mlodinow reports shoppers buy Italian wine when a wine shop plays Italian music and French wine with a wine shop plays French music; yet the customers—when asked about their choices—report being unaware of the music and produce other reasons (which they genuinely believe) for the choices they made. How should these and related discoveries be incorporated into the design of public health interventions?

2. There is a close connection between lifestyle and marketing because lifestyles are, at their centre, consumption patterns—choices of clothes, music, and leisure pursuits. A huge and highly profitable fitness and health industry has been erected on the foundations of a "healthy lifestyle." How might the idea of healthy lifestyle be exploited in a more positive direction by health-promotion policy and programs?

3. Why have interventions targeting obesity focused on exercise and activity levels rather than on food and nutrition? What are the prospects of restoring more balance to public health interventions? Can individual-level behavioural interventions make much difference? If not, what are the principal alternatives?

Annotated Suggested Readings

An excellent book, one that is accessible to undergraduate students, is B. Simons-Morton, K. Mc-Leroy, and M. Wendel's *Behaviour Theory in Health Promotion Practice and Research* (Burlington, MA: Jones & Bartlett Publishers, 2012). The book discusses ecological perspectives, multi-level health promotion, learning and behavioural change, theories of motivation, social marketing, and community capacity building.

G. Williams (2003) provides an accessible review of the issues of structure, context, and agency in his article "The Determinants of Health: Structure, Context and Agency," *Sociology of Health and Wellness*, 25: 131–54. Williams is particularly successful in showing the relationship between the determinants of health perspective and sociological theorization of belief and behaviour.

For a more conventional, individual-level approach to health-related behaviours, students can consult the recent Robert Wood Foundation briefing paper "What Shapes Health-Related Behaviours?" available at www.rwjf.org/content/dam/farm/reports/issue_briefs/2011/rwjf70442

Jonah Berger's book *Invisible Influence* is an accessible and entertaining account of how our "choices" and "decisions" are a product of a host of influences of which we are unaware. *Invisible Influence: The Hidden Forces that Shape Behaviour*, Toronto: Simon & Shuster, 2016.

Annotated Web Resources

"Nudge, the Animation"
www.youtube.com/watch?v=jsy1E3ckxlM
The Rothman School prepared an animation to explain the foundations of behavioural economics underlying "nudge theory."

Behaviour and Health Research Unit
www.bhru.iph.cam.ac.uk
Students may wish to browse the excellent website organized by the Behaviour and Health Research Unit at the University of Cambridge. The website offers a portal into current research on diet, physical activity, smoking, and alcohol consumption. The review paper "Judging Nudging" is also available at this site. Their website has lots of resources on questions ranging from alcohol use to diet to smoking.

"Hidden Influence of Social Networks"
www.ted.com/talks/nicholas_christakis_the_
        hidden_influence_of_social_networks
The video "Hidden Influence of Social Networks" covers the topic of social influence on our attitudes and behaviour.

Opioid-Related Harms in Canada
https://www.cihi.ca/sites/default/files/document/
        opioid-harms-chart-book-en.pdf
The Canadian Institute for Health Information (CIHI) released the first major report on opioid harms in Canada on 15 September, 2017.

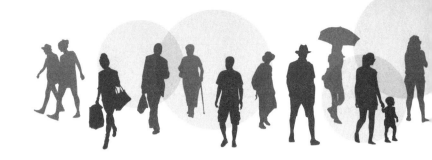

14 The Politics of Population Health

Objectives

By the end of your study of this chapter, you should be able to
- recognize the strong bonds linking population health, public policy, and politics;
- appreciate how globalization and neo-liberal ideology can harm a population's health;
- see how apparently unrelated activities—such as demands for corporate accountability, strengthened human and civil rights, and better environmental stewardship—have implications for population health.

Models of Health

The book began with a discussion of levels of analysis. Throughout, we distinguished between the individual as the unit of analysis—the individual level—and collective levels of analysis—population, place, and social class.

Different levels of analysis yield different models of health. At the individual level, we explored the biomedical model of agent and host. Health in the biomedical understanding is the absence of disease, whereas ill health arises from the interaction of host characteristics of age, sex, and genes with environmental variables and health-related behaviours. A closely related variant is the behavioural model, which shifts attention to lifestyle understood as choices the individual makes. Health in the behavioural model is functionality, a desirable state arising from choosing more exercise over less, better foods over worse, and less stressful situations over more stressful ones. The behavioural model, while recognizing that individual choices are bounded by opportunities and education, construes health-relevant behaviour as chosen by individuals. Arising from these two individual-level models are the familiar approaches to improving health: health care services, health education, and efforts to modify health-relevant behaviour through incentives, regulation, and the like.

In contrast, a contextual approach considers attributes of the population, the place, and the social, economic, cultural, and political structures in which the individual is embedded. As we have seen throughout the book, adopting this stance drives a different view of human health. Good or bad health arises from the interaction among determinants that operate on more than one level. Individual, household, social network, place, community, and class variables interact, collectively determining individual well-being. This does not mean that medical and behavioural variables are unimportant; rather, it means that those variables can only be understood properly and their impact assessed correctly within a broader, multi-level framework.

In addition to expanding explanatory power, a multi-level approach has other important implications. In particular, it has policy and political implications. If determinants of human health cannot be reduced to individual-level variables, such as personal attributes and choices, then pursuing health as a goal requires collective (i.e., political) action. Hence, public health thinking that has been informed by multi-level analysis, from Engels and Virchow in the nineteenth century to Sir Michael Marmot in the twenty-first, is associated with demands for fundamental social reform.

It helps to look at a specific example. The biomedical approach calls for reducing the incidence of diabetes by placing people on blood sugar medication (such as glucose-reducing drugs like Metformin) and instructing people to shift their dietary choices away from sugary foods toward ones with low glycemic indices. The behavioural approach calls for strategies to incentivize physical exercise and penalize choosing high-energy foods. The two approaches are compatible with each other and neither disrupts the societal status quo.

But if the epidemics of diabetes and obesity are driven by the current structure and practices of agri-business, the corporate food industry, commodity markets, the transportation industry, and urban design, then the biomedical and functional approaches will be, at best, of some small benefit, only at the margins. Modifying the individual risk profile, as Rose argued, is mostly palliative. It will not slow the rising incidence of obesity and diabetes in liberal regime populations. Table 14.1 illustrates the approaches to health using the example of obesity.

Table 14.1   Causes and Treatment of Obesity

Approach to Health	Determinants	Prevention/Treatment
Biomedical	Genetic predisposition Energy inputs/outputs Low or high birth weight	Gene therapy Drugs Surgery
Behavioural	Inactivity Excess consumption of high-energy foods	Increase minutes of moderate to vigorous exercise Change diet to low glycemic index foods
Population (Multi-level social epidemiology)	Industrial food production Subsidies, taxation regime Corporate advertising and promotion	Community-based food policies Regulation of food industry Improved working conditions, income, housing, and community amenities

Source: Adapted from Birn, Pillay, & Holtz, 2009, p. 148.

Models of Health and Political Ideologies: Sir Michael Marmot vs the Robert Wood Johnson Foundation

Marmot and Bell (2010) wrote a commentary on the report from the Robert Wood Johnson Foundation's (RWJF) Commission to Build a Healthier America (2009), a parallel exercise to Marmot's report *Fair Society, Healthy Lives* (2010). While, to quote Marmot and Bell, "the prestigious RWJF commission has put socio-economic inequalities firmly on the political agenda" (Marmot & Bell, 2010, p. S73), the RWJF's position repeatedly collapses back into a biomedical and behavioural model. Marmot and Bell speculate that the authors chose to go with the status quo (attributing health to personal choice and, in spite of their radical socio-economic analysis, coming up with hackneyed recommendations like encouraging physical activity and teaching people about healthier diets) because they sought political approval from conservative US policy-makers. But the critical difference between *Fair Society, Healthy Lives* and the RWJF report is that the former condemns arrangements in the contemporary United Kingdom as unjust.

Marmot's key message is that population-level health differences arise from social inequalities, not from the fault of individuals. Thus, reducing health inequalities is a matter of social justice. His evidence shows that the distribution of the bases for good health—education, employment, income, housing, and personal safety—are far more significant factors in determining a population's health than health care services and conventional public health activities. Because health determinants such as income and employment opportunities are mal-distributed in the UK, existing social conditions create an unfair pattern of advantage and disadvantage, Marmot concludes that the UK, an unfair society, is a sick society precisely because of its unjustified social and economic inequalities. Thus, in Marmot's view, the UK is in need of substantial reform. In contrast, the RWJF report implies that the US requires no more than modest, incremental improvements. The reasons for the difference between Marmot and the RWJF go deeper than pandering to US public opinion and Marmot being braver. There is a link between existing social, political, and economic arrangements, how human health is understood (in general), and who and what is responsible for bad health (in particular). That link is **ideology**.

Individual-Level Models of Health and Liberal Ideology

Biomedical thinking is heavily conditioned by the marketplace in health care. Doctors, pharmacists, drug companies, and manufacturers of diagnostic and treatment equipment—health care providers generally—are purveyors of services and goods in a free market economy. Apart from a few marginalized professionals such as those who work in public health, health care is about marketing services and goods to individuals. Medical research

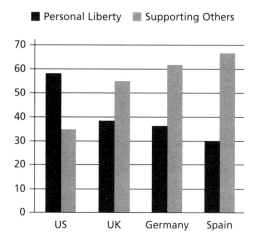

Figure 14.1 Which Is More Important: Supporting Those in Need or Freedom to Pursue One's Personal Goals?

Source: Adapted from Pew Center, 2011.

in support of health care is conducted at the molecular and cellular level at the lab bench or at the individual level in clinical work with a view to marketing cures. Billions of dollars are at stake with the sale of compounds that purport to modify risk factors and, more dubiously, health outcomes. Over 10 per cent of the overall economy and 1 in 10 jobs in advanced, capitalist countries like Canada, the United States, the United Kingdom, and Australia (all liberal regimes) are committed to the production and sale of health care services and goods to individuals. Plainly that level of activity and the concentrations of wealth and power associated with it affect deeply our political, social, and economic institutions. They also profoundly affect how we think about our health. This is especially evident in the United States, where the health care market is less regulated than in Canada, the UK, and Australia and the preponderance of health care financing, as well as its provision, remain in private hands.

Behavioural thinking aligns strongly with liberal ideology, which in turn aligns with the nature of the market economies of the liberal regime world. Liberal societies, led by the US, emphasize liberty above all else and characterize individuals who are not compelled to do something (i.e., are free of interference from the government) as at liberty to choose whatever is in their best interests. This is the key defence for having a more or less unregulated (by government) market in goods, services, and labour. In liberal ideology, the freedom to choose is not regarded as constrained by social position, income, education, labour-market conditions, and the like. A person is free to improve his or her social position, it is believed, in just the same way as he or she is free to choose shoes or hairstyle. It all comes down to what a person wants and how much effort they are prepared to put into getting it. Social patterning of choice, the person's capacity to choose, and the capability to act meaningfully to achieve what he or she has chosen, is ignored.

Ideology is ubiquitous and runs deep. Only around 37 per cent of Americans and about 40 per cent of Canadians think people's income and social position are mostly matters of luck, whereas about 60 per cent of Danes believe luck is the principal determinant (see Figure 14.2). As Figure 14.2 shows, a population's willingness to contribute to the

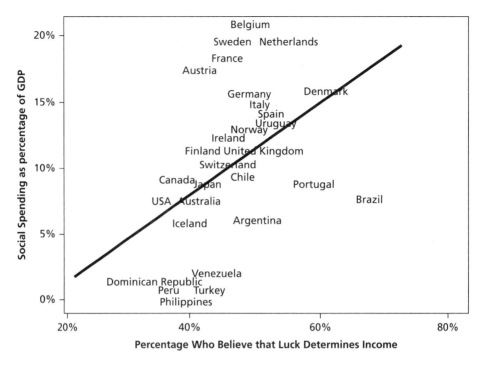

Figure 14.2 The Ideology of Redistribution
Source: Alesina & Angeletos, 2005.

welfare of others is heavily influenced by whether or not people believe their social position to be deserved, attained by effort, or simply a consequence of good or bad fortune.

A worldwide survey showed that Canadians and Americans are the least likely to believe that people's social position and life prospects are mostly determined by forces outside of their own control. More than two-thirds of Germans think success in life is determined by forces outside individuals' control, but only one-third of Americans agree (Pew Research Center, 2011). Among wealthy US Republicans, 80 per cent see themselves as authors of their own success (Taylor, 2008). Americans, almost uniquely in the world, attribute financial success to hard work. But they are surely mistaken. If a person's cognitive ability, emotional regulation, ability to plan, physical stamina, resilience, and persistence are all determined by the health of his or her mother and the conditions of his or her upbringing—facts now established through recent epidemiological and neurological research—luck surely has a great deal to do with ultimate social position. Increasingly, Canadians, Americans, and Britons who were not lucky enough to be born into affluent families face lifelong difficulties and sub-optimal health.

The liberal regime world of which Canada is a part is characterized by (a) faith in free markets, (b) suspicion of governments, and (c) low taxes and a low level of public services. Those views have intensified since the 1980s with the rise of consumerism and **neo-liberalism,** a political movement originating in the US and UK that seeks to shrink the size of government, reduce regulation of corporations and markets, and cut taxes. In contrast, Northern European countries (social democratic regimes) embrace a **solidarity** principle—people see themselves as linked to others with their welfare tied to the health and welfare of the other members of their communities. The principle of solidarity underlies collective community action, demands on government to create fairer social and economic arrangements, stricter regulation of corporations and markets, and, of course, higher and more progressive taxes. Solidarity also underlies efforts to support more vulnerable individuals and families through more robust social welfare measures, child care, and health care services.

Thus the differences between individual-level models of health and collective ones are not just theoretical but also practical and highly political. Liberal, individualist market-driven societies, especially ones dominated by health care corporations and private health care providers, will be hostile to collective models of health, whereas more solidaristic societies will be horrified by the belief that health arises from personal virtue or individual effort.

The evidence presented in this book shows that it is impossible to untangle the features driving bad health outcomes from social structures and deep, social injustices ranging from exploitative wages and working conditions, systematic environmental degradation, profit-driven agri-business, social exclusion, gender inequality, and racism. Those conclusions are too strong to stomach for the RWJF. Thus, in the end, the commissioners returned to the liberal regime default position: health is ultimately a personal responsibility, a function of healthy choices.

Globalization and Human Health

Hutton (2012) characterizes modern Canada, the US, the UK, and Australia in the following fashion:

> The pursuit of individual advantage trumps obligations to others and the upholding of what society holds in common. Taxes are what little people pay. State (public) schools are for the *hoi poloi*, not us. Companies are only legal constructs to be bought and sold as casino chips—not social institutions that create wealth in a complex iterative relationship with the society around them. Banks can lend indiscriminately, secure that losses will be socialized and gains privatized. Trade unions only inhibit the autonomy of management and qualify shareholder rights.

Sharp reductions in personal and corporate taxes and the shift from progressive to regressive income and consumption taxes have exacerbated the trend toward increasing inequality in the liberal regime world (apart from Australia, where income policies have mitigated the effect). The ease with which money may be moved around the world, a new feature arising not only from technology but also from deregulation of financial transactions, has led to the rich stashing an estimated 20 to 30 *trillion* dollars in offshore tax havens in order to avoid taxes altogether (Stewart, 2012). Alongside this, wages for lower- and middle-income people have either stagnated since 1980 or actually declined, whereas employment and unearned income for high-income people have risen astronomically. The downward pressure on the health and well-being of middle- and lower-income earners in the liberal regime world is thus enormous.

In the United States, a country with slumping health and well-being amid rising affluence, social class now leads race as the primary determinant of health (Putnam, 2000; Hutton, 2012). Residential segregation by income has worsened across America; the proportion of poorer people living among poor people and the proportion of richer people living among richer people have steadily risen since 1980 (Fry & Taylor, 2012). The life prospects for lower- and middle-class children in liberal regime countries have diverged sharply due to growing differences in nutrition, housing, neighbourhoods, and schools. Affluent parents are investing in their children like never before, reflected in, among other things, a flight from public schools to private ones—a trend that has been described as "a mortal threat" to community solidarity (Hutton, 2012). Not surprisingly, social mobility has sharply declined in Canada, the United States, the United Kingdom, and Australia. For millions of middle- and lower-income people, social and economic conditions can no longer be expected to improve over their lives. Continuing cuts to publicly funded health, social, and housing services and government policies of privatization, turning hitherto public services into private, for-profit ones, compound the other impacts of social and economic change.

These are all the effects of bad policy. Prioritizing the pursuit of corporate profit based on assumptions that those profits will be invested into a growing, sustainable economy that will provide a sustainable tax base for governments is a grossly unjust approach based on a set of dangerous delusions. Deregulation, undermining labour unions and employment standards, relaxing environmental regulation, cutting taxes, turning public assets over to private control, and promoting global free trade have interacted to create a class of super-rich and, simultaneously, a toxic soup of environmental and social degradation and unhealthy workplaces. In short, chronic ill health, premature death, and blighted lives can, in substantial part, be attributed to the application of neo-liberal, pro-market thinking to public policy.

We will conclude the discussion of population health and politics by looking at the effects of neo-liberalism and globalization, first on environmental determinants of health, second on food security and nutrition, and finally on the world of employment.

Globalization, Carbon Emissions, and Climate Change

Rapidly rising production and consumption associated with globalization and the corporate promotion of a consumer culture lie behind the enormous rise in carbon emissions into the atmosphere (see Table 14.2). Canada and the US are the worst offenders, mostly due to "Big Oil," the energy sector. Because of the power of the oil corporations, and, in Canada's case, the growing dependence on energy exports to keep the country solvent, Canada and the US have collaborated to undermine global efforts to reduce CO_2 emissions. In Canada's case, many jobs are tied to the oil sands and much foreign income to energy exports, fracking, oil sands expansion and pipeline projects receive political support despite evidence of environmental harms and longer-term unsustainability.

Dependence on private automobile use, partly a function of public transportation infrastructure and urban design, constitutes part of the problem. The use of

Table 14.2 World CO_2 Emissions (Billion Metric Tons) by Region

Region	1990	2004
North America	11.4	13.5
Northern and Western Europe	5.8	6.9
Japan and South Korea	4.1	4.4
Former Soviet Union	1.5	2.2
Asia	9.8	13.5
Middle East	0.7	1.3
Africa	0.6	0.9
Central and South America	0.7	1.0
Total	21.2	26.9

Source: Adapted from Birn, Pillay, & Holtz, 2009. Figure 10.1 from p. 477. Adapted from US Department of Energy, 2007, p. 74.

heavy transport trucks, container ships, oil tankers, and air freight for the worldwide transmission of commodities within the globalized, consumption-driven economy is a bigger part of the problem. For example, despite intense efforts to improve fuel economy, load more efficiently, and avoid "empty running" (trucks moving without being fully loaded), heavy transport vehicle CO_2 emissions increased by about 10 per cent between 1990 and 2004 (McKinnon, n.d.). Extravagant use of fossil fuels through air travel contributes significantly to atmospheric carbon. For example, the 2012 "11-day international Copenhagen Climate Change Conference in Denmark generated 41,000 tons of CO_2. US delegates alone produced enough CO_2 to fill 10,000 Olympic swimming pools" (Kolich, 2013).

Rising temperatures and associated changes in ice cover and weather patterns, now firmly linked to dumping CO_2 into the air, are disrupting world food production. Both agriculture and fisheries have suffered. For example, the collapse of the Canadian Pacific sockeye salmon run is now believed to be the result of warming oceans. Australia, one of the world's major grain producers, has suffered chronic drought for most of the past decade, as has Russia. In 2012, Canada and the US saw grain and forage crops devastated by high temperatures and low rainfall. Much of West and Central Africa are locked in drought and famine. Timing of the monsoon, affected by climate change, caused floods in 2013 that decimated agricultural production in India and Bangladesh, turning them into food importers for the first time in decades.

Global warming has also caused severe weather events, ranging from deadly hurricanes and cyclones, to flooding and mudslides, to deaths from heat and dehydration. Insect vector diseases have become more widespread, including West Nile virus in Canada and the US and malaria and dengue fever elsewhere, because breeding conditions for biting insects have been improved by warming. Forests and food crops are also threatened by insect pests. The loss of much of Canada's boreal forest to pine beetles is another example of the effects of global warming. The implications of climate change, of course, will get much worse without urgent international action. Should the Arctic continue to warm, which is highly probable, global warming will accelerate due to the loss of reflective snow and ice. The addition of fresh water from melting will desalinate the northern seas, affect sea life throughout the complex ocean systems, alter sea currents (and consequently worldwide weather), as well as flood substantial areas densely populated by people. The human-health consequences are nothing short of catastrophic.

Once again, the results we see are the consequences of bad policy. Failure by the Canadian and US governments to regulate the transport and oil industries and otherwise act to reduce the atmospheric carbon burden is reckless and harms the health and well-being of this, as well as future, generations.

Globalization, Food Security, and Nutrition

Climate change combines with speculation on the commodity futures and financial markets to drive up global food prices, sparking a food crisis in 2007–08 and severe shortages and sharp price rises in the summer of 2012. Ironically, the multi-national oil industry plays another role in the food crisis in addition to global warming. Corporate manipulation of oil prices in the lead-up to the 2012 food crisis had three effects on food: (1) the costs of producing and transporting foods rose due to rising fuel costs; (2) fertilizers, which are mostly made from petroleum products, became more costly; and (3) worries about oil prices and the security of supply led the US government to subsidize biofuel production. Government incentives pulled up to 40 per cent of available corn out of the food chain and into ethanol production, exacerbating food shortages and jacking up grain prices. The nutritional status of millions of people was compromised by these events, including lower-income people in the liberal regime world. Now, paradoxically, the sudden drop in oil prices has not led to a reduction in the cost of fertilizer nor to abandonment of the bio-fuel subsidies; instead, it has led to profligate use of energy and a return to US auto makers and consumers preferring huge pickups and SUVs over smaller, more efficient vehicles.

In Chapter 11 we touched upon the complex nature of food production, distribution, and sales, processes that have been increasingly corporatized over the past 50 years. Most animal- and plant-sourced food is now produced by agri-business using large-scale industrial production methods, "factory farming." The impact is mixed. For consumers, the cost of foodstuffs is lower, but for the environment the consequences of fertilizer and pesticide runoff, contamination of waterways and aquifers, soil depletion, extravagant water use, and release of CO_2 and methane into the atmosphere are dire. The production system, combined with government subsidies, yields relatively cheap sugars, fats, carbohydrates, and red meats but relatively expensive fruit, vegetables, and nuts. Corporatized food production also poses several public health risks ranging from the contamination of drinking water by E. coli and cryptosporidium (from cattle), to novel strains of virus (from factory farming of ducks, chickens, and pigs). Chapter 12 discusses some of those risks.

Distribution and sales of food in the liberal regime world are dominated by major food distributors and retailers. A key consequence is that local producers of fruit and vegetables often cannot recoup their cost of production because of the low prices the supermarkets demand. Profits are concentrated in the hands of the retailers. In consequence, orchard lands in Canada's Okanagan valley and Niagara peninsula are no longer dedicated to apple, soft fruit, and vegetable production for the Canadian market. They now specialize in (mainly multi-national corporate-owned) alcohol production.

Corporate food producers vie for shelf space in supermarkets, and the prime display areas are reserved for high-profit convenience foods, cosmetics, and household products. Adult consumers and their children are barraged by advertising, all for manufactured items high in energy yield but low in nutrition. And as we noted in Chapter 11, governments are loath to regulate the food industry on either the production or the retail end. The policy response is meek: some labelling requirements, voluntary codes, and other soft—and generally ineffectual—measures. The contrast between Canada and the US and the European Union or Japan, with their more stringent food standards and price regulation, is stark.

The World of Work

Recall from Chapter 9 that employment conditions are a major driver of human health. Recent research confirms much of what has been argued throughout the book, particularly the importance of policy shaping the social, cultural, and economic institutions that mediate the distribution of health-relevant resources, especially access to income. Countries that offer higher levels of social protection for, and encourage solidarity among, their citizens (the coordinated market economies of Europe and Japan), do much better in health- and life-expectancy terms than countries that encourage individualism and consumerism (the liberal market economies of Canada, the United States, and the United Kingdom). One of the areas in which **coordinated market economies** (CMEs) and **liberal market economies** (LMEs) diverge is regulation of the labour market.

CMEs, such as Germany and the Netherlands, have more highly regulated wages and benefits, more standardized working conditions, shorter working hours, guaranteed paid-leave provisions and pensions, and more generous unemployment insurance and job-training benefits than do LMEs, such as Canada and the US. The difference in health outcomes arising from the two approaches is significant. In CMEs, the unemployed are much less likely to suffer adverse health effects or premature death than their counterparts in LMEs (McLeod, Hall, Siddiqi, & Hertzman, 2012). The health profile of lower-educated individuals is much closer to that of higher-educated people in CMEs than LMEs. In other words, CMEs have a flatter health gradient and better overall population health than LMEs, partly because CMEs more actively address low wages, poor working conditions, and unstable employment that contribute to the gaps in the health status of people.

LMEs are closely associated with flexible employment versus standard employment, meaning that more people are part-time or contract workers rather than permanent full-time employees. Flexible employment, especially where hours, wages, and benefits are insecure, is associated with a raft of adverse health outcomes "including poor self-rated health, musculoskeletal disorders, injuries, and mental health problems" (Kim et al., 2012).

Workers in precarious employment in CMEs have health profiles comparable to workers in more secure work, whereas workers in precarious employment in LMEs are severely compromised. Again, the approach in CMEs of ensuring continuity of income through well-developed unemployment insurance programs reduces the gap in health between groups of workers and interrupts the process of accumulation of risk, thereby flattening the health gradient.

LMEs, because of limited government regulation of working conditions and the priority given to consumption and profit, are associated with shift work. Shift work begets shift work: once a portion of the labour force is working unconventional hours, other parts of the economy are led to do likewise, especially food stores, pharmacies, fast-food outlets, and gas stations. The proportion of the population working outside of the old 9-to-5 norm grows. One-third of Canadians are now employed in shift work (Vyas et al., 2012).

Shift work disrupts the normal circadian rhythm. Blood pressure, hormone levels, appetite, and blood sugar levels are all affected. Social life and engagement with family, friends, and the broader social network are also disrupted by shifts, especially rotating shifts. So too are habits: shift workers find it difficult to have sit-down meals of wholesome foods and, in consequence, eat more convenience and junk food than non-shift workers. All of this exacts a large health toll. Shift workers are 23 per cent more likely to have a heart attack than non-shift workers (Vyas et al., 2012). Or put another way, over 7 per cent of heart attacks in Canada and nearly 2 per cent of strokes can be attributed to shift work (Vyas et al., 2012). Most of this burden of preventable disease comes from modifiable practice. Adverse health effects may be mitigated though worksite improvements (e.g., canteens, exercise facilities, rest breaks), more sensible scheduling of work, and simply avoiding the proliferation of 24/7 services. But those changes require collective action though employee associations and reforms to public policy, both of which will be stiffly resisted by corporate interests in the liberal regime world.

Population Health and Politics

While this is a book about health, it moves toward a close in this final chapter discussing politics. That is not an accident. As Virchow once said, "politics are nothing but medicine on a larger scale" (quoted in Mackenbach, 2009). Like Virchow, contemporary social epidemiologists think our current health problems arise mostly as a result of poor public policies stemming from a democratic deficit: the absence of fair, accountable, participatory mechanisms that foster human rights and personal development. While large-scale reform leading to just institutions is not a near-term probability, striving for fairer treatment of mothers and their children, greater gender equity, less social exclusion and racism, more inclusive and supportive communities, better environmental stewardship, more accountable government and corporations, fairer employment practices, and physical and social environments more conducive to human activity is possible. Doing so is our surest path—in fact, our only path—to improving population health.

Pursuing an agenda of securing human rights and economic sustainability is precisely what Virchow argued 165 years ago. Fortunately, some societies have learned the lesson, countries like Norway and the Netherlands and, to some extent, Australia. Unfortunately, some societies, and Canada ranks among them, have not, at least until very recently. While Toba Bryant and colleagues (Bryant, Raphael, Schrecker, & Labonté, 2011) rightly characterized Canada as "a land of missed opportunity for addressing the social determinants of health," there remain grounds for optimism. Voices expressing support for goals other than relentless economic exploitation of natural and human resources have grown louder, especially since the global economic crisis of 2008.

Since the first edition of this book in 2014, a great deal has changed for the better in Canada (albeit for the worse in the US). Toba Bryant's lament is far less fitting. Environmental reviews in Canada are now more robust, and much more inclusive of populations such as First Nations affected by proposals for mines, pipelines, and other developments. Courts and federal government policy now make it clear that the long-term interests of people in terms of health and sustainability trump short-term financial gain. In 2015, Canada's newly elected federal government committed itself to a healthy public policy, gender equity, reconciliation with Indigenous peoples and closing the health gap between them and other Canadians, and fairer tax policy. The 2016 federal budget brought the promise of $8.5 billion in additional spending on Indigenous issues, as well as tax and other measures to improve the financial circumstances of Canadian families with children. The 2017 budget brought commitments for spending on affordable housing, and the 2018 budget funds greater labour force participation and pay equity for women, as well as more generous parental leave provisions. Ottawa is also working with provinces to improve support for young children and mothers, and to create programs to make essential health care more accessible to Canadians. Provincially, a government committed to community development and a sustainable economy was elected in Alberta (also in 2015), followed by an electoral upset with a similar outcome in BC in 2017. Meanwhile, progressive municipalities right across Canada are pursuing healthier community initiatives, from parks and recreation, to affordable housing, to dealing with homelessness, to bike paths and public transit. Most important is the change in the attitudes and mobilization of the public. Youth, in particular, are more interested in politics and public policy, turning out in greater numbers in elections and participating in advocacy organizations seeking social justice, better environmental protection, and more sustainable approaches to economic development. Many European countries are further down this path than Canada, notably Norway. Even in the US, despite a major setback at the federal level, many states and municipalities are moving forward on a population health agenda. China is reining in pollution, planting millions of trees, and working to improve the safety and quality of the food supply. A sustainable worldwide trend, albeit one that is still weak, is underway. There are, then, as this second edition of *Social Determinants of Health* nears completion in 2018, reasons to be optimistic.

Annotated Suggested Readings

An excellent review of how Canada has failed to put learning about population health into practice is provided in the article "Canada: A Land of Missed Opportunity." (Bryant, T., D. Raphael, T. Schrecker, and R. Labonté (2011) Canada: A Land of Missed Opportunity for Addressing the Social Determinants of Health, *Health Policy*, 101(1): 44–58).

Public Health, Ethics, and Equity (S. Anand, F. Peter, and A. Sen editors, Oxford: Oxford University Press, 2006) is an excellent book that deals explicitly with the connection between justice and public health. Part I contains essays on health equity and why equity should be an ethical and political concern. Part II deals with the relationship between health inequities and social injustice.

It is difficult to find a better, more comprehensive treatment of the subject of health and social justice than the reader *Health and Social Justice, Politics, Ideology and Inequity in the Distribution of Disease* (R. Hofrichter, editor, San Francisco: John Wiley, 2003). Essays range from public health as social justice, to ideology and public policy, to the health implications of globalization and a consumer culture.

For a specifically Canadian take on ideology, public policy, poverty, and avoidable ill health, consult D. Raphael's *Poverty and Policy in Canada: Implications for Health and Quality of Life*, especially Part IV: Public Policy and Poverty (Toronto: Canadian Scholars' Press, 2007).

Annotated Web Resources

Improving Equity in Health by Addressing Social Determinants
http://wp.globalhealthequity.ca/wp/
wp-content/uploads/2012/03/
Improving_Equity_in_Health_by_
Addressing_Social_Determinants.pdf
This presentation made by T. Schrecker and associates at the World Conference on Social Determinants of Health in 2011 covers the important concept of health as a function of resources and place in the context of globalizing forces.

Globalization and Health Equity
www.globalhealthequity.ca
A wealth of resources on globalization and health can be found at the website for The Globalization and Health Equity Research Unit.

"Is Globalization Dangerous to Our Health?"
www.youtube.com/watch?v=wYolKGXfvoo
Dr Bezruchka, a professor in Public Health and Community Medicine at the University of Washington, outlines in the video "Is Globalization Dangerous to Our Health?" the implications of globalized corporate trade for the health of Americans and those living in poorer countries in the world.

Glossary

association The probability of occurrence of one characteristic or event is linked to the probability of another characteristic or event. Also known as *correlation*.

asymptotic A curvilinear relationship in which, as values get higher, the relationship between the variables approaches zero.

attachment and regulation By "attachment," sociologist Émile Durkheim meant ties to other people. Attachment as a social-science measure estimates the degree of interaction among people and the quality of that interaction. By "regulation," Durkheim meant the exercise of social control over the individual—i.e., the extent to which a person is governed by group and societal norms and expectations. Regulation is at least partly a function of integration; the more integrated a person is into a group, the more likely he or she is to reflect group beliefs, values, and behaviour.

attachment theory The theory that holds that infants and toddlers must bond with some significant other (usually their mothers) in order to develop a secure sense of self.

Barker hypothesis The hypothesis that contends that early development (fetal stage and first few months of life) has lifelong implications for health and life expectancy (see **latent effects**). In particular, Dr Barker and colleagues have tested the relationship between infants small for their gestational age and incidence of disease in middle and later life.

behavioural variant Version of risk factor model that emphasizes behaviour and lifestyle factors as key determinants of health. (See **risk factor analysis/model**.)

biomedical variant Version of risk factor model that emphasizes agent and biological variables as key determinants of health. (See **risk factor analysis/model**.)

birth cohorts The component of a population born in a specified period which is then followed up for a lengthy period of time, often decades.

body mass index (BMI) A measure calculated by dividing weight in kilograms by height in metres squared (kg/m^2). A value under 18.5 is considered underweight, 18.5–24.9 desirable, 25–29.9 overweight, and over 30 obese. The measure has been criticized for failing to take into account fat/muscle ratio and differences in skeleton mass.

brain plasticity (or **neuroplasticity**) The capacity of the brain to reorganize itself in response to experience and learning.

BSE Bovine spongiform encephalopathy is a fatal degenerative neurological disease found in cattle, caused by misshaped proteins called prions, similar to Creutzfeldt–Jakob disease in humans, and transmissible to people who eat infected meat.

buffering A buffering variable is one that reduces the effect that would occur if the variable was absent. In the case of **Roseto**, Pennsylvania, it has been argued that strong social support buffered the effects of smoking and overeating, reducing the impact of those risk factors on heart disease incidence.

case-control studies An observational study method comparing a group who have a disease with a group (controls) who do not.

causation A *sufficient cause* precedes an effect, and its occurrence inevitably leads to the same result. A *necessary cause* is required to generate the effect, but the same outcome may be caused by different events—i.e., there may be several independent causes. A cause may be either sufficient or necessary, or both.

clinical epidemiology The attempt to make predictions about individual patients based on evidence derived from population-based studies such as clinical trials of treatments.

collinearity A situation in which several predictive variables are highly correlated with one another, making it difficult to ascertain the relative importance of each. For example, education, income, a high-quality job, and a good neighbourhood are closely associated with one another.

conflate To fuse two things together; in logic it means confusing two things by inappropriately merging their meanings or properties together.

conflict theory In its original form, a social theory that contends that groups with more resources will use their advantage to exploit less privileged groups. A broader version has entered the literature, holding that groups help to maintain their identity by adopting exclusionary practices and cultivating negative views of non-group members.

confounded relationship A potentially causal relationship is confounded when the real causal agent is closely associated with some other variable that appears to the underlying cause but, in fact, is spurious. The classic example is believing that chemicals used in hairdressing cause cancer, based on the exposure of hairdressers to chemicals known to be potential carcinogens and the elevated rates of cancer among hairdressers. The confounder in this case is smoking. Closer examination shows that hairdressers are not only exposed to chemicals but are also more likely to smoke than the general female population. Once we control for smoking, the causal relationship between the chemicals and cancer disappears.

contact theory Essentially the obverse of **conflict theory**, it is based on the assertion that more frequent contact with people unlike the members of one's own group enhances acceptance.

conventional model of health and disease This model assumes that health-relevant outcomes are a consequence of the interaction between variables associated with resilience/vulnerability (such as age and genetic inheritance) and biological and behavioural variables (such as exposure to pathogens, toxins, and level of exercise). The **biomedical** and the **behavioural variants** of **risk factor analysis/model** are the two main examples.

coordinated market economies (CMEs) A feature of countries in which government plays an active role in managing the labour market and the level of economic investment. Both **conservative regimes** like France and **social democratic regimes** like Sweden have coordinated market economies, meaning that the government is a partner with corporations and labour unions in managing economic activity; **liberal regimes** like Canada and the United States do not (they are **liberal market economies**).

critical developmental junctures A concept in biology that refers to the timing and sequencing of key physiological developments.

cross-sectional study Cross-sectional studies examine the relationship (association) between two or more variables in a defined population at a single point in time.

crude death rates An estimate of the proportion of people who died within a given period, usually a year, normally calculated by counting all deaths over the year and dividing by the mid-year population.

cultural safety Adopting the cultural stance of the client in order to make health care services more appropriate and accessible.

cumulative effects The outcome when many variables "add up" or "pile up" either in combination with another variable or over time. For example, the duration of smoking (years smoked) or unemployment (length of period without work) matter a great deal to the eventual health outcome. Or, to take an example of cumulative effect from a combination of variables, smoking is far more dangerous to health in combination with exposure to dust or fine fibres. It is always important to consider the combination of risks over time.

dangerous ecology A term characterizing neighbourhoods where vulnerable people such as the elderly and disabled are at high risk of neglect due to weak social integration.

demand–control model An occupational health model that considers the level of demand made on the worker and the amount of control he or she has over the pace and content of the work.

demographic transition Falling death rates in a population associated with rising affluence yielding first rapid population growth followed by declining birth rates. Eventually, as wealth continues to rise, death and birth rates will come into balance, both at very low levels.

deprivation amplification Bad conditions at the neighbourhood level magnify the impact of low income and low education at the individual level.

disordered neighbourhoods Poorly functioning, unsafe neighbourhoods measured by the amount of graffiti, vandalism, crime, and level of public services.

distal determinants Macro-level variables such as culture, social, and economic conditions affecting an entire population, and historical variables, with broad effects, often mediated through **intermediate** and **proximal determinants**. The legacies of colonization and efforts by the dominant culture to assimilate Indigenous people are examples of distal determinants impacting on Canadian Indigenous health.

dose response A relationship in which a change in the duration, intensity, or concentration of an exposure directly correlates to a change in the likelihood of a biological response. For example, heavier smoking for a longer period of time amounts to a greater dose and the expected dose response would be more lung disease.

ecological fallacy A logical error that arises when conclusions are drawn about individuals based on the characteristics of the population to which to those individuals belong.

effort–reward model This model (also known as the effort–reward imbalance model) postulates that job demands that are disproportionate to the intrinsic (job satisfaction) and extrinsic (praise, earnings) rewards attached to the work generate health-damaging stress. Poor-quality jobs such as unskilled labour, serving in bars and restaurants, and assembly-line work often involve large imbalances between the work expected of the employee and the rewards she or he receives.

emotional lability Excessive, poorly controlled emotional reactions, and sudden mood changes, usually associated with brain injury, brain developmental issues, and psychiatric disorders.

epidemiologic transition Falling rates of infectious, parasitic, and nutritional diseases and rising prominence of chronic diseases associated with growing affluence.

epidemiology Study of the patterns, causes, and effects of various health-related features in a population. (See **clinical epidemiology; social epidemiology**.)

epigenetics The study of differences in gene expression that arise from factors other than changes in the underlying DNA sequence; the attempt to answer questions as to why the **phenotype,** the observable characteristics of the animal or person, may differ even if the DNA remains stable.

experimental study A study design under which all the conditions are under the control of the researcher.

fetal alcohol spectrum disorder (FASD) Refers to a range of mild to severe effects caused by prenatal exposure to alcohol, including physical anomalies, cognitive deficits, and behavioural and learning difficulties.

food insecurity The risk of avoidable health problems associated with diet due to lack of resources required to secure an adequate, nutritious supply of food on a regular, ongoing basis.

fuel insecurity Also known as "fuel poverty," the risk of avoidable health problems associated with exposure to cold and damp due to lack of money to pay for electricity, natural gas, or fuel oil required for domestic heating.

gender A range of physical and behavioural characteristics associated with social roles that signify "masculine" and "feminine" (i.e., distinguish socially between men and women).

generalizability The characteristic of findings being capable of reliable reproduction in similar studies. Will the same results arise in studies of different populations?

GINI coefficient A widely used measure of income inequality where "0" is assigned to a hypothetical population that shares everything equally and "1" is assigned to a population where one individual has everything. Real-world countries range from very equal scores of around 0.20 to very unequal ones with scores of around 0.50.

gradient in health The near universal finding that health and life expectancy improve and disease incidence falls as income, education level, quality of job, or quality of neighbourhood rise. For example, a more affluent person, other things being equal, will be healthier than a less-affluent person; a person living in a better neighbourhood will enjoy better health than someone living in a worse neighbourhood.

harm reduction A policy or program designed to lessen the negative impact of a health-related behaviour.

Head Start The name given to the US program designed to provide early childhood education and support to deprived children and their families; now used to refer to any early childhood intervention intended to improve the developmental trajectory of disadvantaged children.

health adjusted life expectancies (HALEs) Only years spent in good health are counted in calculating life expectancy. The disability adjusted life year (DALY) is a related measure that discounts years of life spent disabled.

health inequalities Patterned differences in disease incidence, disability, and life expectancy between sub-populations.

health inequities Patterned differences in disease incidence, disability, and life expectancy between sub-populations that arise from conditions that can be changed by collective action, such as changes in public policies.

Health Utilities Index (HUI) A technique for measuring and comparing health-related quality of life through aggregating the results of questionnaires evaluating such dimensions of life as pain, mobility and emotional state.

healthy immigrant effect The observation that immigrants are usually healthier than *both* the populations they left and the populations they join. For example, Hispanics arriving in the US from Mexico are healthier than average Mexicans of the same age and gender *and* healthier than average Americans of the same age and gender. The reason appears to be self-selection—i.e., only the healthiest people choose to emigrate to a new country.

herd immunity The resistance of a given population to the spread of an infectious agent.

host and agent The relevant host in the case of human health is us, the person. Agents are the things that operate upon us, such as toxins and pathogens. Some forms of epidemiology treat the context in which the host lives as "an agent"; for example, we might treat certain workplaces as "toxic" because of the strain they engender in workers.

ideology A system of beliefs and values that justifies a particular outlook and approach to social and political issues.

incidence The number of new cases that arise in a specified population in a specific period of time. The incidence rate is the number of new cases arising divided by the duration of the defined period. It is an expression of disease risk (probability) in the population. (See **morbidity; prevalence**.)

independent relationship Two or more variables (independent variables) are associated causally with an outcome (a dependent variable), but the independent variables are not associated with each other. For example, asbestos fibre and smoking are both associated with lung disease, but asbestos exposure and smoking are independent of one another.

infant mortality The deaths of children less than one year old is generally regarded as a reliable summative measure of the health of a population combined with the availability and quality of health care.

informal care Care provided by a person such as a family member or friend without financial compensation.

intermediate determinants Meso-level variables such as organizations and social contexts that play a role in determining the health of individuals. The qualities of schools, available health care, neighbourhoods, and family structures are examples. One way in which such structures can directly affect health is by facilitating or impeding access to health-relevant resources.

isostrain An occupational health term referring to isolated, low-social-support, high-strain work, such as public transit work.

latent effects Outcomes that manifest later in life from events or circumstances that occurred earlier. The **Barker hypothesis** is one famous example.

liberal market economies (LMEs) Refers to countries with limited-government involvement in economic development, labour markets, and relationships between employers and their employees, such as the US, Canada, and the United Kingdom (Australia less so because of labour market intervention by the Australian Commonwealth government). (See **coordinated market economies**.)

liberal regimes Countries that place high value on personal liberty and rights. Consequently, they leave most social and economic activity to non-governmental organizations such as voluntary organizations and corporations, and avoid, to the extent practicable, the regulation of social and economic affairs. The concept was advanced by Esping-Andersen in his 1990 typology of modern capitalist societies. The United States, Canada, United Kingdom, and Australia are the principal examples.

life expectancy The average number of years members of a given population can be expected to live given that current mortality (death) rates apply.

lifestyle The mode of living or typical way of life of an individual or group; an expression of identity.

materialist hypothesis The contention that most differences in health between groups can be explained by differences in capabilities, opportunities, and access to resources.

mediated relationship A relationship that exists when a third variable plays a key role between two other variables. For example, how a person was parented (independent variable) affects his or her competence as a parent (dependent variable). A mediating variable is self-efficacy. In other words, one's parents' approach to parenting affects one's sense of self-efficacy, which in turn affects capacity and competence to parent one's own children.

medical model A focus on the biological or physical aspects of disease or disability.

metabolic syndrome A constellation of precursors to serious disease including central obesity, elevated blood pressure, and insulin resistance.

methodologically individualist Any approach that attempts to explain social phenomena by the choices and behaviours of discrete individuals.

morbidity Any departure from a normal state, such as illness or disability. It is often used, not quite correctly, as a synonym for "disease." (See **incidence; prevalence**.)

morbidity paradox The observation that women appear to have more sickness and disability than men but that they nevertheless live longer.

neo-liberalism An ideology that emerged in the 1970s and 1980s that holds governments should minimize tax and regulatory burden on individuals and corporations, reduce public services in favour of for-profit corporate services, and promote economic growth through encouraging trade and consumerism.

neo-materialist hypothesis The contention that public services, public amenities (such as parks), public policies (such as approach to taxation), and social contexts (such as neighbourhoods) have important distributive effects on health-relevant resources available to individuals.

network capital The amount of informational and other instrumental social support made available to an individual through the social networks in which he or she is embedded.

neural sculpting The brain's destructive process of "pruning" or eliminating pathways that are not in use. It is one aspect of **neuroplasticity**.

nudge theory A proposed alternative to regulation and health education that relies on providing cues to people through indirect suggestions (such as product location or packaging) that alter motivation and choice.

nutrifluff Media articles that hype the health benefits of a particular food, food component, or dietary supplement.

nutritional insecurity The inability to secure on a consistent basis the micronutrients (vitamins, minerals) from nutritious foods required to maintain optimum health.

observational study A study design in which the researcher has no control over the conditions but observes without intervention.

odds ratio The ratio of two odds, odds being the ratio of the probability of occurrence to that of non-occurrence; also known as *relative odds*. It is a way of comparing the odds of getting a disease if exposed to a factor versus the odds of getting the same disease if not exposed to that factor.

Organisation for Economic Co-operation and Development (OECD) A group of the 32 most affluent countries.

pathway effects In the life-course health literature, refers to one set of events or context setting the stage for subsequent developments. Early childhood conditions, for example, partially determine success in school, future employment opportunities, future income, and housing, etc.

phenotype The observable characteristics of a biological entity.

political economy The social science that studies the relationships between individuals and the community and markets and the government.

population The people sharing some characteristic, such as residing in a particular place or belonging to a particular ethnic or racial group; a population born in the same time period is referred to as a **cohort.**

population attribute A characteristic of a group of people that does not apply to each and every individual making up that group. A statistic such as an average—for example, average blood pressure for a group of people—is a population attribute and may not equate to the blood pressure of all or even any of the individuals making up the group.

premature mortality The calculation of potential years of life lost before age 70.

Preston curve The cross-sectional relationship between different countries' life expectancy and per capita income that forms a concave curve that increasingly "flattens" as incomes rise.

prevalence A simple count of the number of cases in a population at a point in time. It may be expressed as the number of cases divided by the population and therefore appear to be a rate similar to incidence. However, it is not a rate, and nothing regarding risk of becoming a case can be inferred from prevalence data. (See **morbidity; incidence**.)

preventive medicine A form of medical practice that attempts to reduce the risk of a disease occurring (prophylaxis), as opposed to treating a disease that has already occurred. It also includes attempts to identify disease processes early in the natural history of a disease in order to intervene earlier, based on the assumption that earlier treatment is more effective.

primary care The usual first point of contact by people seeking health care; the source of everyday care needs. In Canada, family doctors and emergency departments provide most primary care.

programming In the life-course health literature, refers to an earlier event or context "writing something into a person's biology" that plays out later in life. The theory of fetal origins of disease and disability in later life is an example.

progressive universalism An approach through which programs and services are made available for everyone on equal terms and conditions, but additional support is also made available for those with special needs.

prophylactic/prophylaxis Preventive measures.

prospective cohort studies A group of individuals with one or more similar characteristics is enrolled or recruited at one point in time then followed over time with respect to one or more outcomes of interest in order to determine which factors contribute to those outcomes. For example, the British Millennium Cohort Study is a cohort (group under study) made up of all children born in the United Kingdom in the year 2000. The outcomes of interest are diseases and disabilities. Data on the children's socio-economic conditions, education, BMI, activity levels, immunization status, and a host of other variables are consistently collected over time for every member of the cohort. Such "longitudinal" studies are required to determine the relationships among variables and the direction of causality.

protective health effect Any impact that reduces the risk of adverse outcome associated with a risk factor. For example, exercise may reduce the risk of coronary heart disease associated with high blood pressure.

proximal factors (proximal determinants) Micro, individual-level variables that impact on health. Examples are exposures to pathogens or toxins, diet, and activity level.

psychogenic dwarfism A growth and intellectual developmental disorder leading to short stature, cognitive problems, and **emotional lability**, that arises from extreme emotional deprivation or stress in early life.

psychosocial hypothesis The joint contentions that (a) psychological states arise in interaction with social environments, and (b) those psychological states have biological implications. For example, a work environment with many competing demands and limited-worker control may give rise to emotional stress, which in turn may elevate cortisol levels, which can give rise to damage to arterial linings, thereby elevating risk of coronary heart disease.

psychosomatic illness A physical condition such as pain or immobility arising from emotional factors such as stress, anxiety, or depression.

random selection Allocation of individuals to study groups by means that ensure (a) the two groups are comparable for purposes of a valid experiment, and (b) no bias in their selection has been introduced into the study.

recall bias Error due to problems of recall or differential recall of past events.

relative risk The ratio of the risk of disease in populations exposed to a factor to the risk of unexposed populations.

residualism The policy belief that society is better off when only very limited public support is provided to individuals and everyone is expected to rely upon their own resources, with some assistance from private sources such as family, charities, and churches.

resilience A biological entity's capacity to resist injury or disease.

restrictive diets Diets that radically limit calories or substantially reduce or eliminate specific foods, food groups or food components (fats, carbohydrates, etc.).

risk factor analysis/model A reductionist approach to determining the probability of disease or death by calculating the potential impact of agent variables (pathogens, toxins), biologic marker variables (blood pressure, blood-lipid profile), and behavioural variables (exercise, sexual habits) on an individual. (See **biomedical variant; behavioural variant**.)

risk factors Variables that contribute to the probability of an adverse health outcome.

Roseto effect A finding that a high level of social support within a group has **protective health effects**.

SARS Severe acute respiratory syndrome, caused by a coronavirus that crossed the species barrier (*zoonosis*) from farmed birds to humans in southern China in 2002, becoming a *pandemic* (worldwide epidemic).

secondary transfer effects Intergroup contact influences not only attitudes toward the group encountered but also attitudes toward others who are different from oneself.

secular change Long-term trends (usually understood as over more than five years) in beliefs, values, and behaviour.

sex Biological characteristics typical of males and females.

significance An estimate in statistics regarding the probability of the result not occurring purely by chance, usually expressed as a P-value. The relationship between two things, for example a certain diet and heart attack, may be statistically significant but not clinically significant. In other words, two things may be related in a real way, not merely by chance, but may still not be important from a health perspective.

social capital Collective benefits arising from co-operative attitudes and practices, grounded in trust and reciprocity.

social care The provision of services to people in need of care or protection, particularly those with a disability, emotional and mental issues, addictions, or problems related to aging.

social cohesion The extent to which bonds form among members of a group and between groups.

social democratic regimes Countries where **solidarity** forms a key value and hence governments pursue policies aimed at assisting all citizens to achieve as affluent and successful a life as possible. Universal programs and steeply progressive taxation typify these countries, which include the Nordic countries of Western Europe. The concept was advanced by Esping-Andersen in his 1990 typology of modern capitalist societies.

social epidemic The rapid spread through a population of symptoms by a process of emotional contagion within a social network—for example, an entire school becoming ill when one or few children are exposed to an unusual smell.

social epidemiology The attempt to determine the causes of health differences between sub-populations of people.

social exclusion A process of excluding members of a group from normal interaction and sharing of benefits.

social facts Values, norms, and social structures that are capable of constraining individual behaviour.

social influence Effects on personal choice arising from a wish to please others, fear of sanctions, and peer pressures to conform.

social patterning of behaviour The (usually unconscious) determination of behaviour by contextual factors such as place in a social network; the characteristics of one's neighbourhood; and the norms and structures of one's workplace, class, and social position.

social networks An individual's number of contacts and frequency of interaction with them. Contacts can be mapped, showing the relationship among the members of groups and deriving measures of extent and frequency of contact (network analysis).

social support Characteristics of social interaction that are potentially helpful to the individual, such as emotional support (empathy and caring) and instrumental support (assistance, providing information, and guidance).

solidarity A perceived community of interest that gives rise to the sense that one's own social position, success, or failure is linked to that of others in one's society (associated with the cultures of Northern Europe).

susceptibility The degree to which a biological entity is vulnerable to the threat posed by a risk factor.

swine and avian influenzas Strains of influenza that are zoonotic, i.e., can cross the species barrier from pigs or birds to humans. Influenza viruses are capable of rapid transformation and mutation, and several strains of virus are common (and contagious between) pigs and various birds, especially chickens and ducks.

targeting Aiming a policy, program, or therapy at those deemed to be in greatest need or at highest risk of adverse outcomes.

thalidomide scandal Thalidomide is a drug that was marketed between 1957 and 1962 to control nausea and other unpleasant symptoms in early pregnancy. The drug proved to be *teratogenic*—capable of inducing major deformities in the fetus. As a result, tens of thousands of babies were born without limbs or with severely malformed ones. Drug testing was substantially strengthened following the scandal, and doctors have become much more cautious about prescribing medication during pregnancy.

universalism An approach that makes policies, programs, or interventions available to all members of society irrespective of putative level of need or risk. (See **progressive universalism**.)

validity Literally, "truth value." "Construct validity" refers to how accurately a measure reflects the true nature of the thing being measured. "Content validity" refers to how comprehensively and appropriately a measure captures the relevant dimensions of a phenomenon. "Criterion validity" refers to how strongly a measure associates with other measures—for example, an IQ test with performance on an exam. A study is considered valid if its results align with what has already been established to be true, if it is free of biases and errors, and if it yields predictions that are true.

References

Introduction

Australian Institute of Health and Welfare. (2011). *Life expectancy and mortality of Aboriginal and Torres Strait Islander people.* Retrieved from http://www.aihw.gov.au/publication-detail/?id=10737418927

Centers for Disease Control and Prevention. (2013). *CDC health disparities & inequalities report—United States, 2013.* Retrieved from http://www.cdc.gov/minorityhealth/CHDIReport.html

Coburn, D., Denny, K., Mykhalovskly, E., McDonough, P., Robertson, A., & Love, R. (2003). Population health in Canada: a brief critique. *American Journal of Public Health, 93*(3), 392–396.

Commission on Social Determinants of Health. (2008). *Closing the gap in a generation: Health equity through action on determinants of health.* Geneva: World Health Organization.

Esping-Andersen, G. (1990). *Three worlds of welfare capitalism.* Cambridge: Polity Press.

Health Canada. (1986). *Achieving health for all: A framework for health promotion.* Retrieved from http://www.hc-sc.gc.ca/hcs-sss/pubs/system-regime/1986-frame-plan-promotion/index-eng.php

Kawachi, I., Subramanian, R., & Ameida-Filho, N. (2002). A glossary for health inequalities. *Journal of Epidemiology and Community Health, 56*(9), 647–652.

Marmot, M. (2010). *Fair society, healthy lives. The Marmot Review.* Retrieved from http://www.marmotreview.org/AssetLibary/pdfs/Reports/Fair-SocietyHealthyLives.pdf

McKeown, T. (1972). An interpretation of the modern rise in population in Europe. *Population Studies, 27*(3), 345–382.

National Health and Welfare (1974). *A new perspective on the health of Canadians: A working document.* Retrieved from http://www.hc-sc.gc.ca/hcs-sss/com/fed/lalonde-eng.php

Or, Z. (2000). *Determinants of health in industrialized countries.* OECD Economic Studies, No. 30. Retrieved from http://www.ppge.ufrgs.br/giacomo/arquivos/eco02072/or-2000.pdf

Public Health Agency of Canada. (2012). What is the population health approach? Retrieved from http://www.phac-aspc.gc.ca/ph-sp/approach-approche/index-eng.php

Public Health Agency of Canada. (2013). Social determinants of health and health inequalities. Retrieved from https://www.canada.ca/en/public-health/services/health-promotion/population-health/what-determines-health.html

Raphael, D. (2004). *Social determinants of health, Canadian perspectives.* Toronto: Canadian Scholars' Press.

Rostron, B.L., Boies, J.L., & Arias, E. (2010). Education reporting and classification on death certificates in the United States. *Vital and Health Statistics, 2*(151), 1–16.

Statistics Canada. (2010). *Health of first nations living off-reserve, Inuit and Métis adults in Canada: The impact of socio-economic status on inequalities in health.* Statistics Canada Health Research Paper Series. Retrieved from http://www.statcan.gc.ca/pub/82-622-x/82-622-x2010004-eng.pdf

Statistics Canada. (2012). Life expectancy healthy and total by income, 2005–07. Retrieved from http://statcan.gc.ca/camsim/a26?lang=eng&id=1020122&p2=46

World Health Organization (WHO). (2007). Health of indigenous peoples. Retrieved from http://www.who.int/mediacentre/factsheets/fs326/en

World Health Organization (WHO). (2018). Ottawa charter for health promotion. Retrieved from http://www.who.int/healthpromotion/conferences/previous/ottawa/en

Chapter 1

Australian Institute of Health and Welfare. (2012). *Diabetes.* Retrieved from http://www.aihw.gov.au/diabetes

BabyCenter. (n.d.). Popular baby names by year. Retrieved from http://www.babycenter.com/babyNameYears.htm

Barr, H., Britton, J., Smyth, A., & Fogarty, A. (2011). Association between socioeconomic status, sex and age at death from cystic fibrosis in England and Wales (1959–2008): A cross-sectional study. *British Medical Journal, 343.* doi:10.1136/bmj.d4662

Belsky, D., Caspi, A., Houts, R., Cohen, H., Corcoran, D., Denese, A., Harrington, H., Israel, S., Levine, M., Schaefer, J., Sugden, K., Williams, B., Yashin, A., Poulton, K., & Moffit, T. (2015). Quantification of biological aging in young adults. *Proceedings of the National Academy of Sciences of the United States of America.* doi:10.1073/pnas.1506264112

Blaxter, M. (1990). *Health and lifestyles.* London: Routledge.

de Looper, M. & Lafortune, G. (2009). Measuring disparities in health status and in access and use of health care in OECD countries. *OECD Health Working Papers, 43.* doi:10.1787/18152015

Demers, A., Kalrouz, S., Adlaf, E., Gilksman, L., Newton-Taylor, B., & Marchand, A. (2002). Multilevel analysis of situational drinking among Canadian undergraduates. *Social Science and Medicine, 55*(3), 415–424.

Diabetes Canada. (n.d.). Diabetes Statistics in Canada. Retrieved from https://www.diabetes.ca/how-you-can-help/advocate/why-federal-leadership-is-essential/diabetes-statistics-in-canada.

Evans, R. & Stoddart, G. (1990). Producing health, consuming health care. *Social Science and Medicine, 31*(12), 1347–1363.

Fave, M-J., Lamaze, F., Soave, D., Hodgkinson, A., Gauvin, H., Braut, V., . . . Awadalla, P. (2018, March 6) Gene-by-environment interactions in urban populations modulate risk phenotypes. *Nature Communications, 9.* doi:10.1038/s41467-018-03202-2

Gryzybowski, S. & Allen, E. (1999). Tuberculosis 2. History of the disease in Canada. *Canadian Medical Association Journal, 160*(7), 1025–1028.

Hallmayer, J. (2011). Genetic heritability and shared environmental factors among twins with autism. *Archives of General Psychiatry, 76*, 1095–1102. doi:10.10011archgenpsychiatry.2011.76

Hooper, L., Summerbell, C., Thompson, R., Sills, D., Roberts, T., Moor, H., & Davey Smith, G. (2011, July 6). Reduced or modified dietary fat for preventing cardiovascular disease. *Cochrane Database of Systematic Reviews, 7.*doi:10.1002/14651858.CD002137.pub2

Kalrouz, S., Gilksman, L., Demers, A., & Adalf, E. (2002). For all these reasons, I do . . . drink: A multilevel analysis of contextual reasons for drinking among Canadian undergraduates. *Journal of Studies on Alcohol and Drugs, 63*(5), 600–608.

Kaplanis, J., Gordon, A., & Shor, T. (2018, March 1). Quantitative analysis of population-scale family trees with millions of relatives. *Science.* doi:10.1126/science.aam9309

Kitsios, G. & Kent, D. (2012). Personalized medicine: Not just in our genes. *British Medical Journal, 344.* doi:10.1136/bmj.e2161

Krieger. N. (2008). Proximal, distal, and the politics of causation: What's level got to do with it? *American Journal of Public Health, 98*(2), 221–230.

Krieger, N. (2013). History, biology, and health inequities: Emergent embodied phenotypes and the illustrative case of the breast cancer estrogen receptor. *American Journal of Public Health, 103*(1). doi:10.2105/AJPH.2012-200967

Maibach, E., Abrams, L., & Marosits, M. (2007). Communication and marketing as tools to cultivate the public's health: A proposed "people and places" framework. *BMC Public Health.* doi:10.1186/1471-2458-7-88

Marmot, M., Syme, S., Kagan, H., Kato, H., Cohen, J., & Belsky, J. (1975). Epidemiological studies of coronary heart disease and stroke in Japanese men living in Japan, Hawaii and California. Prevalence of coronary and hypertensive heart disease and associated risk factors. *American Journal of Epidemiology, 102*, 514–525.

McGrail, K., van Doorslater, E., Ross, N., & Sanmartin. C. (2009). Income-related health inequalities in Canada and the United States: A decomposition analysis. *American Journal of Public Health, 99*(10), 1856–1863.

Michels, K. & Willet, W. (2009). The women's health initiative randomized controlled dietary modification trial: A post-mortem. *Breast Cancer Research and Treatment, 114*(1), 1–6.

Ministry of Health Labour and Welfare. (2018). Japan national health and nutrition survey. Retrieved from http://www.mhlw.go.jp/seisakunitsuite/bunya/kenkou/kenkounippon21/en/eiyouchousa/koumoku_syokukin_chousa.html

Montgomery, K. (n.d.). *The demographic transition.* St Louis: University of Missouri Saint Louis Geography Department. Retrieved from https://woc.uc.pt/antropologia/getFile.do?tipo=2&id=363.

Moynihan, R., Doust, J., & Henry, D. (2012). Preventing overdiagnosis: How to stop harming the healthy. *British Medical Journal, 344.* doi:10.1136/bmj.e3502.

Obomsawin, R. (2012). Medical miracle or masterful mirage. *Alternative-Doctor.com.* Retrieved from http://www.alternative-doctor.com/vaccination/obomsawin.html

Ohinmaa, A., Jacobs, P., Simpson, S., & Johnson, J. (2004). The projection of prevalence and cost of diabetes in Canada: 2000 to 2016. *Canadian Journal of Diabetes, 28*(2), 1–8.

Or, Z. (2000). *Determinants of health in industrialized countries.* OECD Economic Studies, No. 30. Retrieved from http://www.ppge.ufrgs.br/giacomo/arquivos/eco02072/or-2000.pdf

Pearce, N., Foliaki, S., Sporie, A., & Cunningham, C. (2004). Genetics, race, ethnicity and health. *British Medical Journal, 328*(7447), 1070–1072.

Preston, S. (1975). The changing relationship between mortality and the level of economic development. *Population Studies, 29*(2), 231–248.

Rose, H. & Rose, S. (2012). *Genes, cells and brains: The Promethean promises of the new biology.* London: Verso.

Sapolsky, R. (2017). *Behave.* New York: Penguin.

Silventoinen, K., Kaprio, J., Lahelma, L., & Koskenvuo, M. (2000). Relative effect of genetics and environmental factors on body height: Differences across birth cohorts among Finnish men and women. *American Journal of Public Health, 90*(4), 627–630.

Springer, K., Stellman, J., & Jordan-Young, R. (2011). "Beyond a catalogue of differences: A theoretical frame and good practice guidelines for researching sex/gender in human health." *Social Science and Medicine, 74*(11), 1817–1824. doi:10.1016/j.socscimed.2011.05.033

Taylor, R., Ashton, K., Moxham, T., Hooper, L., & Ebrahim, S. (2011). Reduced dietary salt for the prevention of cardiovascular disease. *Cochrane Database of Systematic Reviews, 7*. doi:10.1002/14651858.CD009217

Unemployed and single? Who are Britain's smokers? (2013, 26 September). *The Guardian.* Retrieved from http://www.theguardian.com/news/datablog/2013/sep/26/unemployed-single-britain-smokers-uk-cigarette-statistics

Wilson, L. (1990). The historical decline of tuberculosis in Europe and America: Its causes and significance. *Journal of the History of Medicine, 45*, 366–396.

World Bank. (2012). Male and female smoking prevalence, world. Retrieved from http://data.worldbank.org/indicator/SH.PRV.SMOK.MA and http://data.worldbank.org/indicator/SH.PRV.SMOK.FE

World Health Organization (WHO). (2005). *Preventing chronic diseases: A vital investment.* Retrieved from http://www.who.int/chp/chronic_disease_report/contents/part1.pdf

Chapter 2

Advisory Board. (2013). Mayo clinic IDs the top ten reasons for doctors' visits. Retrieved from https://www.advisory.com/daily-briefing/2013/01/22/study-ids-the-top-10-reasons-for-doctors-visits

Andrae, B., Andersson, T., Lambert, P., Kemetti, L., Sifverdal, S., Strander, B., Ryd, W., Dillner, J., Thornberg, S., & Sparen, P. (2012) Screening and cervical cancer care: Population-based cohort study. *British Medical Journal, 344.* doi:10.1136.bmj.e900

Canadian Mental Health Association. (2017). Barriers to service access. Retrieved from http://www.cmha.ca/public_policy/access-to-services-2/#.Wabgz60ZNBw

Canadian Institute for Health Information. (2017). Health spending. Retrieved from https://www.cihi.ca/en/health-spending

Cassels, A. (2012). *Seeking sickness: Medical screening in the misguided hunt for disease.* Vancouver: Greystone Press.

Citizens' Advice. (2015). A very general practice. Retrieved from https://citizensadvice.org.uk/Global/Citizens/Advice

Davidson, A. (2004). Dynamics without change: continuity in Canadian health policy. *Canadian Public Administration, 43*(3), 251–279.

Dehghan, M., Mente, A., Zhang, X., Swaminathan, S., Lei, W., Mohan, V., . . .vGupta, R. (2017). Association of fats and carbohydrate intake with cardiovascular

disease and mortality in 18 countries from five continents (PURE): A prospective cohort study. *Lancet, 390*(10107), 2050–2062. doi:10.1016/S0140-6736(17)32252-3

Evans, R. (1986). *Strained mercy.* Toronto: Butterworth-Heinemann.

Evans, R. & Stoddart, G. (1990). Producing health, consuming health care. *Social Science and Medicine, 31*(12), 1347–1363.

Gionet, L. & Roshanafshar, S. (2015). Select health indicators of First Nations people living off reserve. Statistics Canada, catalogue no. 82-624-X. Retrieved from https://www150.statcan.gc.ca/n1/pub/82-624-x/2013001/article/11763-eng.htm

Godlee, F. (2016). Statins: We need an independent review. *British Medical Journal, 354.* doi:10.1136/bmj.i4992

Goldacre, B. (2012). *Bad pharma: How drug companies mislead doctors and harm patients.* Toronto: McClelland & Stewart.

Guyatt, G., Devereaux, P., Lexchin, J., Store, S., Yalnizyan, A., Himmelstein, D., . . . Batnagar, N. (2007). A systematic review of studies comparing health outcomes in Canada and the US. *Open Medicine, 1*(1), 227–236.

Hennessy, D., Sanmartin, C., Ronksley, P., Weaver, R., Campbell, D., Manns, B., . . . Hemmelgam, B. (2016). Out of pocket spending on drugs. *Health Reports* (Statistics Canada). Retrieved from http://www.statcan.gc.ca/pub/82-003-x/2016006/article/14634-eng.pdf

Ioannidis, J. (2005, August 30). Why most published research findings are false. *PLOS Medicine.* doi:10.1371/journal.pmed.0020124

Law, M., Cheng, L.,Dhalla, I, Heard, D., & Morgan, S. (2012). Effect of cost on adherence to prescription medications in Canada. *Canadian Medical Association Journal, 184*(3), 297–302. doi:10.1503/cmaj.111270

Makary, M. & Daniel, M. (2016). Medical error—the third leading cause of death in the US. *British Medical Journal, 353.* doi:10.1136/bmj.2139 Centers for Disease Control and Prevention. (2010). Prescription drug use continues to Increase: U.S. prescription drug data for 2007–2008. Retrieved from https://www.cdc.gov/nchs/data/databriefs/db42.htm

Rabin, R.K. (2018, March 17). Federal agency courted alcohol industry to fund benefits of moderate drinking. *New York Times.* Retrieved from https://www.nytimes.com/2018/03/17/health/nih-alcohol-study-liquor-industry.html

Romanow, R. (2002). *Building on values: Commission on the future of health care in Canada.* Retrieved from http://www.publications.gc.ca/site/eng/237274/publication.html

Soril, L., Adams, T., & Phipps-Taylor. (2017). Is Canadian healthcare affordable? A comparative analysis of the Canadian healthcare system from 2004 to 2014. *Healthcare Policy, 13*(1), 43–58. doi:10.12297/hcpol.2017.25192

UBC Therapeutics Initiative. (2014). *Statins: Proven and associated harms*. Retrieved from https://www.ti.ubc.ca/2014/05/28/statins-proven-and-associated-harms

Welch, G., Schwartz, L. & Woloshin, S. (2011). *Overdiagnosed: Making people sick in the pursuit of health*. Boston: Beacon Press.

Wootton, D. (2006). *Bad medicine: Doctors doing harm since Hippocrates*. Oxford: Oxford University Press.

Chapter 3

Black, D., Morris, J., Smith, C., & Townsend, P. (1980). *Inequalities in health: Report of a working group*. London: DHSS.

Cassel, J. (1976). The contribution of the social environment to host resistance. *American Journal of Epidemiology, 104*, 107–123.

Christakis, N. & Allison, P. (2006). Mortality after hospitalization of a spouse. *New England Journal of Medicine, 354*, 7.

Clandola, T., Ferrie, J., Sacker, A., & Marmot, M. (2007). Social inequities in self-reported health in early old age: Follow-up of prospective cohort study. *British Medical Journal, 334*(7601), 990. Dunn, J., Burgess, B., & Ross, N. (2005). Income distribution, public service expectations and all-cause mortality in US states. *Journal of Epidemiology and Community Health, 59*(9), 768–774.

Kuper, H. & Marmot, M. (2003). Job strain, job demands, decision latitude, and the risk of coronary heart disease within the Whitehall II study. *Journal of Epidemiology and Community Health, 57*(2), 147–153.

Malleson, A. (2005). *Whiplash and other useful illnesses*. Montreal: McGill-Queens University Press.

Marmot, M. (2010). *Fair society, healthy lives. The Marmot Review*. Retrieved from http://www.marmotreview.org/AssetLibary/pdfs/Reports/FairSocietyHealthyLives.pdf

Marmot, M., Rose, G., Shipley, M., & Hamilton, P. (1978). Employment grade and coronary heart disease in British civil servants. *Journal of Epidemiology and Community Health, 32*(4), 244–249.

Martikainen, P. & Valkonen, T. (1996). Mortality after the death of a spouse in relation to duration of bereavement in Finland. *Journal of Epidemiology and Community Health, 50*(3), 264–268.

McGrail, K., van Doorslater, E., Ross, N., & Sanmartin. C. (2009). Income-related health inequalities in Canada and the United States: A decomposition analysis. *American Journal of Public Health, 99*(10), 1856–1863.

Office for National Statistics (UK) (2011). *Trends on life expectancy by the national statistics socioeconomic classification 1982–2006*. Retrieved from https://www.ons.gov.uk/peoplepopulationandcommunity/birthsdeathsandmarriages/lifeexpectancies/methodologies/trendsinlifeexpectancybynationalstatisticssocioeconomicclassification1982to2006qmi

Rose, G. (1985) Sick individuals and sick populations. *International Journal of Epidemiology, 14*(1), 32–38.

Rose, G. & Arthur, G. (2008). *Rose's strategy of preventive medicine: The complete original text*. New York: Oxford University Press.

Ross, N., Wolfson, M., Dunn, J., Berthelot, J., Kaplan, G., & Lynch, J. (2000). Relation between income inequality and mortality in Canada and the United States: Cross sectional assessment using census data and vital statistics. *British Medical Journal, 320*, 898–902.

Ross, C. & Mirowsky, J. (1999). Refining the association between education and health: The effects of quantity, credential and selectivity. *Demography, 36*(4), 445–461.

Susser, M. & Susser, E (1996). Choosing a future for epidemiology 1. Eras and Paradigms. *American Journal of Public Health, 86*, 668–673.

Susser, M. & Susser, E. (1996). Choosing a future for epidemiology 2. From black boxes to Chinese boxes. *American Journal of Public Health, 86*, 674–677.

Syme, S. (1996). Rethinking disease: Where do we go from here? *Annals of Epidemiology, 6*, 463–468.

Townsend, P. & Davidson, N. (1982). *Inequalities in health: The Black Report*. Hermondsworth: Penguin.

Turcotte, M. (2011). Intergenerational education mobility. University completion in relation to parents' education level. *Canadian Social Trends (Statistics Canada), 92*. Retrieved from https://www150.statcan.gc.ca/n1/pub/11-008-x/2011002/article/11536-eng.htm

Wilkinson, R. (1986). Socioeconomic differences in mortality: Interpreting the data in their size and trends. In R. Wilkinson (Ed.), *Class and health* (pp. 88–114). London: Routledge.

Wilkinson, R. (1996). *Unhealthy societies: The affliction of inequality*. London: Routledge.

Chapter 4

Abbott, D., Keverne, E., Bercovitch, F., Shively, C., Mendoza, S., Saltman, W., . . . Sapolsky, S. (2003). Are subordinates always stressed? A comparative analysis of rank differences and cortisol levels among primates. *Hormones and Behavior, 43*(1), 67–82.

Blakely, T., Atkinson, J., & O'Dea, D. (2003). No association of income inequality with adult mortality within New Zealand: A multi-level study of 1.4 million 25–64 year olds. *Journal of Epidemiology and Community Health, 57*(4), 279–284.

Canadian Centre for Policy Alternatives. (2013, January 28). Income inequality spikes in Canada's big cities. Retrieved from http://www.policyalternatives.ca/newsroom/news-releases/income-inequality-spikes-canadas-big-cities

Canadian Centre for Policy Alternatives. (2018). Indigenous children face deplorable poverty. Retrieved from https://www.policyalternatives.ca/newsroom/updates/indigenous-children-face-deplorable-poverty

Canadian Mortgage and Housing Corporation. (2011). Housing costs in Vancouver. Retrieved from http://www.cmhc-schl.gc.ca/en/co/buho/sune/sune_007.cfm

Conference Board of Canada. (2013). Income inequality. Retrieved from https://www.conferenceboard.ca/hcp/Details/society/income-inequality.aspx?AspxAutoDetectCookieSupport=1

Dietitians of Canada. (2010). *The cost of eating in BC, 2009.* Retrieved from http://www.dietitians.ca/Downloadable-Content/Public/BC_CostofEating_2009-(1).aspx

Deaton, A. (2003). Health, inequality and economic development. *Journal of Economic Literature*, XLI (March), 113–158.

Deaton, A. & Lubotsky, D. (2003). Mortality, inequality and race in American cities and states. *Social Science and Medicine 56*(6), 1139–1153.

Dunn, J., Veenstra, G., & Ross, N. (2006). Psychosocial and neo-material dimensions of SES and health revisited: Predictors of self-rated health in a Canadian national survey." *Social Science and Medicine, 62*(6), 1465–1473.

Durkheim, É. (1897). *Suicide: A study in sociology* (2002 edition). New York: Routledge.

Esping-Anderson, G. (1990). *Three worlds of welfare capitalism*. Cambridge: Polity Press.

Fawcett Society. (2011). Single mothers: Singled out. Retrieved from https://www.fawcettsociety.org.uk/single-mothers-singled-out

Fischer-Baum, R., Soffen, K., & Long, H. (2018, January 30). What Washington tax plans could mean for you. *Washington Post*. Retrieved from https://www.washingtonpost.com/graphics/2017/business/what-republican-tax-plans-could-mean-for-you/?utm_term=.52b7695b65d

Galloway, G. (2012, April 10). Canadians open to tax hikes to create more equal society, poll finds. *Globe and Mail*, p. A1.

Garfinkel, I., Rainwater, L., & Smeeding, T. (2010). *Welfare and welfare states: Is America a laggard or a leader?* New York: Oxford University Press.

Gesquiere, L., Learn, N., Simao, M., Onyango, P., Alberts, S., & Altmann, J. (2011). Life at the top: Rank and stress in wild male baboons. *Science, 333*(6040), 357–360.

Gravelle, H. (1998). How much of the relation between population mortality and unequal distribution of income is a statistical artefact? *British Medical Journal, 316*(7128), 382.

Hernandez-Quevedo, C., Jones, A., Lopez-Nicolas, A., & Rice, N. (2006). Socioeconomic inequalities in health: A comparative longitudinal analysis using the European Community Household Panel. *Social Science and Medicine, 63*(5), 1246–1261.

Hou, F. & Miles, J. (2005). Neighbourhood inequality, neighbourhood affluence and population health. *Social Science and Medicine, 60*(7), 1557–1569.

Humphries, K. & van Doorslaer, E. (2000). Income-related health inequalities in Canada. *Social Science and Medicine, 50*(5), 663–671.

Lavis, J., McLeod, C., Mustard, C., & Stoddart, G. (2003). Is there a gradient life span by position in the social hierarchy? *American Journal of Public Health, 93*(5), 771–774.

Lynch, J., Davey Smith, G., Harper, S., Hillemeier, M., Ross, N., Kaplan, G., & Wolfson, M. (2004a). Is income inequality a determinant of population health? Part 1. A systematic review. *Milbank Quarterly, 82*(1), 5–99.

Lynch, J., Davey Smith, G., Harper, S., & Hillemeier, M. (2004b). Is income inequality a determinant of population health? Part 2. A systematic review. *Milbank Quarterly, 82*(2), 355–400.

Kaplan, G., Pamuk, E., Lynch, L., Cohen, R., & Balfour, J. (1996). Inequality in income and mortality in the United States: Analysis of mortality and potential pathways. *British Medical Journal, 312*, 99–1003.

Kawachi, I. (1999). Social capital and community effects on population and individual health. *Annals of the New York Academy of Science, 896*, 120–130.

Kawachi, I. & Berkman, L. (2000). Social cohesion, social capital and health. In L. Berkman & I. Kawachi (Eds.), *Social epidemiology* (pp. 174–190). New York: Oxford University Press.

Kawachi, I., Kennedy, B., & Glass, R. (1999). Social capital and self-rated health: A contextual analysis. *American Journal of Public Health, 89*(8), 1187–1193.

Kawachi, I., Kennedy, B., Lochner, K., & Prothrow-Stith, D. (1997). Social capital, income inequality and mortality. *American Journal of Public Health, 87*(9), 1491–1498.

Kawachi, I., Subramanian, R., & Ameida-Filho, N. (2002). A glossary for health inequalities. *Journal of Epidemiology and Community Health, 56*(9), 647–652.

Kennedy, B., Kawachi, I., Glass, R., & Prothrow-Stith, D. (1998). Income distribution, socioeconomic status, and self-rated health in the United States: Multi-level analysis. *British Medical Journal, 317*(7163), 917–921.

Mackenzie, H. & Shillington, K. (2009). *Canada's quiet bargain: The benefits of public spending.* Toronto: Canadian Centre for Policy Alternatives.

Marmot, M. (2006). Transcript of *Unnatural Causes* film interview. Retrieved from http://www.unnaturalcauses.org/assets/uploads/file/MichaelMarmot.pdf

McGrail, K., van Doorslater, E., Ross, N., & Sanmartin. C. (2009). Income-related health inequalities in Canada and the United States: A decomposition analysis. *American Journal of Public Health, 99*(10), 1856–1863.

McGrail, K. (2007). Medicare financing and redistribution in British Columbia, 1992 and 2002. *Health Policy, 2*(4), 123–137.

McLeod, C., Lavis, J., Mustard. C., & Stoddart, G. (2003). Income inequality, household income, and health status in Canada: A prospective cohort study. *American Journal of Public Health, 93*(8), 1287–1293.

Morris, J. (2000). A minimum income for healthy living. *Journal of Epidemiology and Community Health, 54,* 885–889.

Navarro, V. (2002). A critique of social capital. *International Journal of Health Services, 32*(3), 423–432.

Numbeo. Cost of living in Vancouver. (2013). Retrieved from http://www.numbeo.com/cost-of-living/city_result.jsp?country=Canada&city=Vancouver

Organisation for Economic Co-operation and Development (OECD). (2008). *Growing unequal? Income distribution and poverty in the OECD.* Paris: Author.

Olson, L., Tang, S., & Newacheck, P. (2005). Children in the United States with discontinuous health insurance coverage. *New England Journal of Medicine, 353*(4), 382–391.

Preston, S. (1975). The changing relationship between mortality and the level of economic development. *Population Studies, 29*(2), 231–248.

Putnam, R. (1993). *Making democracy work: Civic traditions in modern Italy.* New York: Princeton University Press.

Robert Wood Johnson Foundation. (2011, March 1). Stress and health. Retrieved from https://www.rwjf.org/en/library/research/2011/03/how-social-factors-shape-health.html

Rodgers, G. (1979). Income and inequality as determinants of mortality: An international cross-sectional analysis. *Population Studies, 33*(2), 343–351.

Ross, N., Wolfson, M., Dunn, J., Berthelot, J., Kaplan, G., & Lynch, J. (2000). Relation between income inequality and mortality in Canada and the United States: Cross sectional assessment using census data and vital statistics. *British Medical Journal, 320,* 898–902.

Sapolsky, R. (1990). Stress in the wild. *Scientific American, 262*(1), 116–123.

Sapolsky, R. (2017). *Behave.* New York: Penguin.

Scoffield, H. (2012, January 2). By noon today, the super rich have made an average worker's yearly salary.

Global News. Retrieved from https://globalnews.ca/news/195004/by-noon-today-the-super-rich-have-made-an-average-workers-yearly-salary-4

Sen, A. (1999). *Development as freedom.* Oxford: Oxford University Press.

Sen, A. (2009). *The idea of justice.* London: Allen Lane.

Shibuya, K., Hashimoto, H., & Yano, E. (2002). Individual income, income distribution, and self-rated health in Japan: Cross sectional analysis of nationally representative sample. *British Medical Journal, 324(7328),* 16–19.

Statistics Canada. (2005). Income in Canada. Retrieved from http://www.statcan.gc.ca/pub/75-202-x/2005000/4154865-eng.htm

Statistics Canada. (2012, 23 March). Household debt in Canada. *The Daily .* Retrieved from http://www.statcan.gc.ca/daily-quotidien/120323/dq120323b-eng.htm

Statistics Canada. (2017a, September 13). Children living in low-income households. *Census in Brief.* Retrieved from https://www12.statcan.gc.ca/census-recensement/2016/as-sa/98-200-x/2016012/98-200-x2016012-eng.cfm

Statistics Canada. (2017b, September 13). Household income in Canada: Key results from the 2016 Census. *The Daily.* Retrieved from http://www.statcan.gc.ca/daily-quotidien/170913/dq170913a-eng.htm?CMP=mstatcan

Subramanian, S. & Kawachi, I. (2003). The association between state income inequality and worse health is not confounded by race. *International Journal of Epidemiology, 32*(6), 1022–1028.

Suomi, S. (2005). Mother–infant attachment, peer relationships, and the development of social networks in Rhesus monkeys. *Human Development, 48*(1/2), 67–79.

US Census Bureau. (2015). GINI index of money income and equivalence-adjusted income: 1967 to 2014. Retrieved from https://www.census.gov/library/visualizations/2015/demo/gini-index-of-money-income-and-equivalence-adjusted-income—1967.html

US Census Bureau. (2017) *Income and poverty in the United States: 2016.* Retrieved from https://www.census.gov/library/publications/2017/demo/p60-259.html

Wilkins, R., Berthelot, J., & Ng, E. (2002). Mortality by neighbourhood income in urban Canada from 1971 to 1996. *Health Reports (*Statistics Canada*), 13* (Supplement), 45–71.

Wilkinson, R. (1986). Socioeconomic differences in mortality: Interpreting the data in their size and trends. In R. Wilkinson (Ed.), *Class and health* (pp. 88–114). London: Routledge.

Wilkinson, R. (1996). *Unhealthy societies: The affliction of inequality.* London: Routledge.

Wilkinson, R. & Pickett, K. (2005) Income inequality and population health: A review of the evidence. *Social Science and Medicine, 62*(7), 1768–1784. doi:10.1016/j.socscimed.2005.08.036

Wilkinson, R. & Pickett, K. (2009). *The spirit-level: Why more equal societies almost always do better.* London: Allen Lane.

Wolf, M. (2011, December 23). US inequality doesn't have to be the West's roadmap. *Globe and Mail.* Retrieved from https://www.theglobeandmail.com/report-on-business/economy/economy-lab/us-inequality-doesnt-have-to-be-the-wests-road-map/article620400/

World Health Organization, Commission on Social Determinants of Health. (2008). *Health equity through action on the social determinants of health.* Retrieved from http://whqlibdoc.who.int/publications/2008/9789241563703_eng.pdf

Yalnizyan, A. (2010). *Rise of Canada's richest 1%.* Ottawa: Canadian Centre for Policy Alternatives.

Zheng, H. (2012). Do people die from income inequality of a decade ago? *Social Science and Medicine, 75*(1), 36–45.

Chapter 5

Anderson, L., Shinn, C., Fulilove, M., Scrimshaw, S., Fielding, J., & Norman, J. (2003). The effectiveness of early childhood development programs. A systematic review. *American Journal of Preventive Medicine, 24*(3), S32–S46.

Barker, D. (1998). In utero programming of chronic disease. *Clinical Science, 95*(2), 115–128.

Beswick, J. & Sloat, E. (2006). Early literacy success: A matter of social justice. *Education Canada, 46*(2), 23–26.

Bickart, K., Wright, C., Dautoff, R., Dickerson, B., & Barrett, L. (2010).Amygdala volume and social network size in humans. *Nature Neuroscience, 14*, 163–164.

Billette, J-M. & Janz, T. (2012). Injuries in Canada: Insights from the Canadian Community Health Survey. *Health at a Glance* (Statistics Canada). Retrieved from http://www.statcan.gc.ca/pub/82-624-x/2011001/article/11506-eng.htm

Blane, D., Hart, C., Davey Smith, G., Gillis, C., Hole, D., & Hawthorne, V. (1996). Association of cardiovascular disease risk factors with socioeconomic position during childhood and during adulthood. *British Medical Journal, 313*, 1434.

Borghol, N., Suderman, M., McArdle, W., Racine, A., Hallett, M., Pembrey, M., . . . Szyf, M. (2011). Associations with early life socioeconomic position in adult DNA methylation. *International Journal of Epidemiology, 41*(1). doi:10.1093/ije/dyr147

Bowlby, J. (1988). *A secure base: Clinical application of attachment theory.* London: Routledge.

Boynton-Jarrett, R., Ryan, L., Berkman, L., & Wright, R. (2008). Cumulative violence exposure and self-rated health: Longitudinal study of adolescents in the United States. *Pediatrics, 122*(5), 961–970.

Chen, E., Martin, A., & Matthews, K. (2007). Trajectories of socioeconomic status across children's lifetimes predict health. *Pediatrics, 120*(2), e297–e303.

Child care by the numbers: Safe and affordable day-care remains elusive. (2013, July 23). *CBC News.* Retrieved from https://www.cbc.ca/news/canada/child-care-by-the-numbers-1.1327893

Commission on Social Determinants of Health. (2008). *Closing the gap in a generation: Health equity through action on determinants of health.* Geneva: World Health Organization.

Doblhammer, G. & Vaupel, V. (2001). Lifespan depends on month of birth. *Proceedings of the National Academy of Science, 98*(5), 2934–2939.

Dominguez-Salas, P., Moore, S., Baker, M., Bergen, A., Cox, S., Dyer, R., Fulford, A., Guan, Y., Laritisky, E., Silver, M., Swan, G., Zeisel, S., Waterland, R., Prentice, A. & Hennig, B. (2014). Maternal nutrition at conception modulates DNA methylation of human metastalle epialleles. *Nature Communications.* doi:10.1038/ncomms4746

D'Onise, K., Lynch, J., Sawyer, M., & McDermott, R. (2010). Can preschool improve child health outcomes? A systematic review. *Social Science and Medicine, 70*(9), 1423–1440.

Essex, M., Thomas, B., Hertzman, C., Lam, L., Armstrong, J., Newmann, S., & Kobor, M. (2011). Epigenetic vestiges of early developmental adversity: Childhood stress exposure and DNA methylation in adolescence. *Child Development, 84(1).* doi:10.1111j.1467-8624.2011.01641.x

Gallagher, J. (2017, 23 August). Vaginal seeding after Caesarean section risky, warn doctors. *BBC News.* Retrieved from http://www.bbc.com/news/health-41011589

Geddes, R., Haw, S., & Frank, J. (2010). *Interventions for promoting early child development for health.* Edinburgh: Scottish Collaboration for Public Health Research and Policy.

Human Early Learning Partnership. (2005). *BC atlas of child development.* Vancouver: Human Early Learning Partnership.

Hertzman, C. & Power, C. (2003). Health and human development: Understandings from lifecourse research. *Developmental Neuropsychology, 24*(2/3), 719–744.Hertzman, C. & Power, C. (2006). A lifecourse approach to health and human development. In Heymann J., Hertzman C., Barer, M., & Evans, R. (Eds.), *Healthier societies: From analysis to action* (pp. 83–106). Oxford: Blackwell.

Himmelreich, M., Lutke, C., & Travis, E. (2017). The lay of the land: Final results of a health survey of 500 adults with FASD. 7th Annual Conference on FASD, March 1–4, 2017, University of British Columbia, Vancouver, BC.

Huber, D. & Weisel, T. (1982). Exploration of the primary visual cortex. *Nature, 299*, 515–524.

Kershaw, P., Irwin, L., Trafford. K., & Hertzman, C. (2005). *British Columbia atlas of child development.* Retrieved from http://earlylearning.ubc.ca/media/uploads/publications/bcatlasofchilddevelopment_cd_22-01-06.pdf

Krakowiak, P., Walker, C., Bremer, A., Baker, S., Ozonoff, S., Hansen, R., & Hertz-Picciotto, I. (2012). Maternal metabolic conditions and the risk for autism and other neurodevelopmental disorders. *Pediatrics, 129(5).* doi:10.1542/peds.2011–2583

Lange, S., Probert, C. & Gemel, G. (2017). Global prevalence of fetal alcohol spectrum disorder among children and youth. *JAMA Pediatrics, 171*(10). doi:10.1001/jamapediatrics.2017.1919

Loeb, S., Bridges, M., Bassok, D., Fuller, B., & Rumberger, R. (2007). How much is too much? The influence of preschool centers on children's social and cognitive development. *Economics of Education Review, 26*(1), 52–66.

Lynch, J., Law, C., Brinkmen, S., Chittleborough, C., & Sawyer, M. (2010). Inequalities in child healthy development: Some challenges for effective implementation. *Social Science and Medicine, 71*, 1244–1248.

Maguire, E. (2000). Navigation-related structural change in the hippocampi of taxi drivers. *Proceedings of the National Academy of Science, 97*(8), 4398–4403.

Marmot, M. (2010). *Fair society, healthy lives. The Marmot review.* Retrieved from http://www.marmotreview.org/AssetLibary/pdfs/Reports/FairSocietyHealthyLives.pdf

Mikkonen, J. & Raphael, D. (2010). *Social determinants of health: The Canadian facts.* Toronto: York University School of Health Policy and Management.

Mustard, J. (2007). Experience-based brain development: Scientific underpinnings of the importance of early child development in a global world. In M. Young and L. Richardson (Eds.), *Early child development from measurement to action* (pp. 35–64). Washington: World Bank.

Nigg, J. (2006). *What causes ADHD?* New York: Guilford Press.

Organisation for Economic Co-operation and Development (OECD). (2009). *Doing better for children.* Retrieved from http://www.oecd.org/document/12/0,3746,en_2649_34819_43545036_1_1_1_1,00.html.

Organisation for Economic Co-operation and Development (OECD). (2010). *Social expenditure database.* Retrieved from http://www.oecd.org/social/expenditure.htm

Palfrey, J., Hauser-Cram, P., Bronson, M., Warfield, M., Sirin, S., & Chan, E. (2005). The Brookline early education project: A 25-year follow-up study of a family-centred early health and development intervention. *Pediatrics, 116*(7), 144–152. http://pediatrics.aappublications.org/content/116/1/144?download=true

Park, M. & Kobor, M. (2014). Potential for social epigenetics for child health policy. *Canadian Public Policy, 41*(Supplement 2). doi:10.3138%2Fcpp.2014-081

Peck, N. (1994). The importance of childhood socioeconomic group for adult health. *Social Science and Medicine, 39*(4), 553–562.

Pensola, T. & Martikainen, P. (2003). Cumulative social class and mortality from various causes of adult men. *Journal of Epidemiology and Community Health 57*(9), 745–751.

Phillips, N., Hammen, C., Brennan, P., Najman, J., & Bor, W. (2005). Early adversity and the prospective prediction of depressive and anxiety disorders in adolescents. *Journal of Abnormal Child Psychology, 33*(1), 13–24.

Portales-Casamar, E., Lussier, A., Jones, M., MacIsaac, J., Edgar, R., Mah, S., . . . Kobor, M. (2016). DNA methylation signature of human fetal alcohol spectrum disorder. *Epigenetics and Chromatin, 9.* doi:10.1186/s13072-016-0074-4

Relton, C., Groom, B., St. Pourcain, M., Sayers, A., Swan, D., Embleton, N., . . . Davey Smith, G. (2012). DNA methylation patterns in cord blood DNA and body size in childhood. *PLOS ONE, 7*(3), e31821.

Reynolds, A., Temple, J., Ou, S., Arteaga, I., & White, B. (2011). School-based early childhood education and age-28 wellbeing: Effects by timing, dosage and subgroup, *Science, 333*(6040), 360–364.

Robert Wood Johnson Foundation. (2011). Exploring the social determinants of health. Issue brief: Early childhood experiences and health. Retrieved from https://www.rwjf.org/en/library/research/2011/03/early-childhood-experiences-and-health.html

Sapolsky, R. (2017). *Behave.* New York: Penguin.

Sebastian, C., Tan, G., Roiser, J., Viding, E., Dumontheil, I., & Blakemore, S. (2011). Developmental influences on the neural bases of responses to social rejection: Implications of social neuroscience for education. *Neuroimage, 57*(3), 686–694.

Siddiqi, A., Kawachi, I., Berkman, L., Hertzman, C., & Subramanian, S. (2012). Education determines a nation's health, but what determines educational outcomes? A cross-national comparative analysis. *Journal of Public Health Policy, 33*(1), 1–15.

Sloat, E. & Willms, J. (2000). The international adult literacy survey: Implications for Canadian social policy. *Canadian Journal of Education, 23*(3), 218–233.

Suomi, S. (2005). Mother–infant attachment, peer relationships, and the development of social networks in Rhesus monkeys. *Human Development, 48*(1/2), 67–79.

Swanson, S. & Colman, I. (2013). Association between exposure to suicide and suicidality outcomes in youth. *Canadian Medical Association Journal, 190(30).* doi:10.1503/cmaj.121377

Teicher, M., Anderson, C., & Polcari, A. (2012, February 13). Childhood maltreatment is associated with reduced volume in the hippocampal subfields CA#, dentate gyrys and subiculum. *Proceedings of the National Academy of Sciences.* doi:10.10.1073/pnas.1115396109

Teicher, M., Andersen, S., Polcari, P., Anderson, C., Navalta, C., & Kim, D. (2003). The neurological consequences of early stress and childhood maltreatment. *Neuroscience and Biobehavioural Reviews, 27*(1–2), 33–44.

Washbrook, E. & Waldfogel, J. (2008). Family income and children's readiness for school. *Research in Public Policy, 7,* 3–5.

World Health Organization. (2012). Social determinants of health and well-being among young people. Retrieved from http://www.euro.who.int/__data/assets/pdf_file/0003/163857/Social-determinants-of-health-and-well-being-among-young-people.pdf

Chapter 6

Centers for Disease Control and Prevention. (2016). Fact sheets: Excessive alcohol use and risks to women's health. Retrieved from https://www.cdc.gov/alcohol/fact-sheets/womens-health.htm

American Cancer Society. (2012). Tobacco use and the GLBT community. Retrieved from http://www.cancer.org/myacs/highplainshawaiipacific/areahighlights/tobacco-use-and-the-glbt-community

Baranowski, A. & Hecht, H. (2017). Gender differences and similarities in receptivity to sexual invitations. *Archives of Sexual Behaviour, 44*(8). doi:10.1007/s/0508-015-0520-6

Bauer, G., Travers, R., Scanlon, K., & Coleman, T. (2012, April 20). High heterogeneity of HIV-related sexual risks among transgendered people in Ontario, Canada: A province-wide respondent-driven sampling survey. *BMC Public Health.* doi:10.1186/1471-2458-12-292.

Bird, C. & Rieker, P. (1999). Gender matters: An integrated model for understanding men's and women's health. *Social Science and Medicine, 48*(6), 745–755.

Britt, K., & Short, R. (2012). The plight of nuns: Hazards of nulliparity. *Lancet, 379,* 2322–2323.

Canadian Cancer Society. (2010). What is cancer? Retrieved from http://www.cancer.ca/Canada-wide/About%20cancer/Cancer%20statistics.aspx?sc_lang=en

Canadian Cancer Society. (2017). Cancer statistics at a glance. Retrieved from http://www.cancer.ca/en/cancer-information/cancer-101/cancer-statistics-at-a-glance/?region=on

Council on Contemporary Families. (2015). Parenting and happiness in 22 countries. Retrieved from https://contemporaryfamilies.org/brief-parenting-happiness

Centre for Longitudinal Studies. (2017, September 20). One in four girls is depressed at age 14, new study reveals. Retrieved from http://www.cls.ioe.ac.uk/news.aspx?itemid=4646&itemTitle=One+in+four+girls+is+depressed+at+age+14%2c+new+study+reveals&sitesectionid=27&sitesectiontitle=News&returnlink=news.aspx%3fsitesectionid%3d27%26sitesectiontitle%3dNews

Crompton, S. (2011, October 13). What's stressing the stressed? Main sources of stress among workers. *Canadian Social Trends (Statistics Canada).*

Daguerre, A. (2011, July 5). How health cuts are killing women. *The Guardian.* Retrieved from http://www.guardian.co.uk/commentisfree/cifamerica/2011/jul/05/maternitypaternityrights-women

Deaton, A. & Stone A. (2014). Evaluative and hedonic wellbeing among those with and without children at home. *Proceedings of the National Academy of Science, 111*(4) 1328–1333. doi:10.1073/pnas.1311600111

Dennerstein, L., Dudley, E., Hopper, J., Guthrie, J., & Burger, H. (2000) A prospective population-based study of menopausal symptoms. *Obstetrics and Gynecology, 96*(3), 351–358. doi:10.1016/S0029-9=7844(00)00930-3

Denney, J., McNown, R., Rogers, R., & Doubilet, S. (2012). Stagnating life expectancies and future prospects in an age of uncertainty. *Social Science Quarterly, 94(2).* doi:10.111/j.1540-6237.2012.00930.x

Denton, M., Prus, S., & Walters, V. (2003). Gender differences in health: A Canadian study of psychosocial, structural and behavioural determinants of health. *Social Science and Medicine, 58,* 2585–2600.

Frieling, H., Romer, K., Scholtz, S., Mittelbach, F., Wilhelm, J., DeZwaan, M., . . . Bleich, S. (2009). Epigenetic disregulation of dopaminergic genes in eating disorders. *International Journal of Eating Disorders, 43*(7), 577–583.

Gay marriage "improves health." (2011, December 16). *BBC News.* Retrieved from https://www.bbc.co.uk/news/health-16203621

Gorman, R. & Read, J. (2006). Gender disparities in adult health: An examination of three measures of morbidity. *Journal of Health and Social Behavior, 47*(2), 95–110.

Grandi, G., Ferrari, S., Xholli, A., Cannoletta, M., Palma, F., Romani, C., . . . Cagnacci, A. (2012). Prevalence of menstrual pain in young women. *Journal of Pain Research.* doi:10.2147/JPR.S30602

Kaminsky, P., Chapman, B., Haynes, S. & Own, L. (2005). Body image, eating behaviours, and attitudes toward exercise among gay and straight men. *Eating Behaviors, 6*(3). doi:10.1016/j.eatbeh.2004.11.003

Linburg, L. & Hjern, A. (2003). Risk factors for anorexia nervosa: A national cohort study. *International Journal of Eating Disorders, 34*(4), 397–408.

Liu, H. & Umberson, D. (2008). Times they are a changin': Marital status and health differentials from 1972 to 2003. *Journal of Health and Social Behaviour, 49*, 239–253.

MacIntosh, C., Fines, P., Wilkins, R., & Wolfson, M. (2009). Income disparities in health-adjusted life expectancy for Canadian adults, 1991–2001. *Health Reports* (Statistics Canada), *20*(4). Retrieved from https://www150.statcan.gc.ca/n1/pub/82-003-x/2009004/article/11019-eng.htm

MacLennan, A., Taylor, A., Wilson, D., & Wilson, D. (2000). The prevalence of pelvic floor disorders and their relationship to gender, age, parity and mode of delivery. *British Journal of Obstetrics and Gynecology, 107*(12), 1460–1470. doi:10.111/j.1471-0528.2000.tb11669.x

Martikainen, P., Martelin, T., Nihtila, E., Majamaa, K., & Koskinen, S. (2005). Differences in mortality by marital status in Finland from 1976 to 2000: Analyses of changes in marital status distributions, socio-demographic and household composition, and causes of death. *Population Studies, 59*(1), 99–115.

McSherry, J. (1985). Was Mary, Queen of Scots, anorexic? *Scottish Medical Journal, 30*(4), 243–245.

Merz, B. (2017, April 19). Binge drinking continues to rise—particularly among women and seniors. *Harvard Women's Health Watch.* Retrieved from https://www.health.harvard.edu/blog/binge-drinking-continues-to-rise-particularly-among-women-and-seniors-2017041811603

Mulders-Jones, B., Mitchison, D., Giros, F., & Hay, P. (2017, January 31) Socioeconomic correlates of eating disorders in an Australian-based population sample. *PLOS ONE, 12*(1). doi:10.13711journal.pone.0170603

National Center for Health Statistics. (2017). *Mortality in the United States, 2016.* NCHS Data Brief No. 293. Retrieved from https://www.cdc.gov/nchs/data/databriefs/db293.pdf

Organisation for Economic Co-operation and Development (OECD). (2015, May 12). Tackling harmful alcohol use. Retrieved from http://www.oecd.org/health/tackling-harmful-alcohol-use-9789264181069-en.htm

Pearce, J. (2004). Richard Morton: Origins of anorexia nervosa. *European Neurology, 52*(4), 191–192.

Pew Research Center. (2011, May 13). *Most say homosexuality should be accepted by society.* Retrieved from http://www.pewresearch.org/pubs/1994/poll-support-for-acceptance-of-homosexuality-gay-parenting-marriage

Ramage-Morin, P. (2008). Chronic pain in Canadian seniors. *Health Reports (Statistics Canada), 19*(1), 37–52.

Reczek, C. (2012). The promotion of unhealthy habits in gay, lesbian, and straight intimate partnerships. *Social Science and Medicine, 75*(6), 1114–1121. doi:10.1016/j.socsimed.2012.04.019

Ross, C. & Bird, C. (1994). Sex stratification and health lifestyle: Consequences of men's and women's perceived health. *Journal of Health and Social Behaviour, 35*, 161–178.

Sapolsky, R. (2017). *Behave.* New York: Penguin.

Simon, R. & Barrett, A. (2010). Nonmarital romantic relationships and mental health in early adulthood: Does the association differ for women and men? *Journal of Health and Social Behaviour, 51*, 168–183.

Statistics Canada. (2009). Sexual orientation. *Health Reports, 19*(1). Retrieved from https://www150.statcan.gc.ca/n1/pub/82-003-x/2008001/article/10532/5002598-eng.htm

Statistics Canada. (2015). Same-sex couples and sexual orientation by the numbers. Retrieved from https://www.statcan.gc.ca/eng/dai/smr08/2015/smr08_203_2015

Statistics Canada. (2017, September 13). Household income in Canada. *The Daily.* Retrieved from http://www.statcan.gc.ca/daily-quotidien/170913/dq170913a-eng.htm?CMP=mstatcan

Stoving, R., Andries, A., Brixen, K., Bilenberg, N., & Horder, K. (2011). Gender differences in outcomes of eating disorders: A retrospective cohort study. *Psychiatry Research, 186*(2/3), 362–366.

Strudwick, P. (2012, November 27). "Homophobia" and "Islamophobia" are the right words for the job. *The Guardian. Retrieved from https://www.theguardian.com/commentisfree/2012/nov/27/homophobia-islamophobia-right-words-associated-press*

United Nations Development Program (UNDP). (2010). International human development indicators. Retrieved from http://hdr.undp.org/sites/default/files/reports/270/hdr_2010_en_complete_reprint.pdf

Verbrugge, L. (1985). Gender and health: An update on hypothesis and evidence. *Journal of Health and Social Behaviour, 26*, 156–182.

Violence against women worldwide "epidemic." (2013, 20 June). *BBC News.* Retrieved from http://www.bbc.co.uk/news/health-22975103

World Health Organization (WHO). (2017). *HIV/AIDS: Transgender people.* Retrieved from http://www.who .int/hiv/topics/transgender/en

World Bank. (2018). *Sex ratio at birth (male births per female births).* Retrieved from https://data.worldbank .org/indicator/SP.POP.BRTH.MF?view=chart

Wiseman, E. (2012, June 10). Uncomfortable in our skin: The body image report. *The Guardian.* Retrieved from https://www.theguardian.com/lifeandstyle/2012/ jun/10/body-image-anxiety-eva-wiseman

Young, J. (2010). Anorexia nervosa and estrogen: Current status of the hypothesis. *Neuroscience and Biobehavioral Review, 34*(8), 1195–2000.

Chapter 7

Australian Institute of Health and Welfare. (2011). Life expectancy and mortality of Aboriginal and Torres Strait Islander people. Retrieved from http://www .aihw.gov.au/publication-detail/?id=10737418927

Bailey, Z., Krieger, N., Agenor, M., Graves, J., Linos, N. & Bassett, M. (2017) Structural racism and health inequities in the USA: Evidence and interventions. *Lancet, 389,* 1453–1463.

Barth, J., Sneider, S., & von Kanel, R. (2010). Lack of social support in the etiology and the prognosis of coronary heart disease: A systematic review and meta-analysis. *Psychosomatic Medicine, 72*(3), 229–238.

Bickart, K., Wright, C., Dautoff, R., Dickerson, B., & Barrett, L. (2010). Amygdala volume and social network size in humans. *Nature Neuroscience, 14,* 163–164.

Brooks, D. (2011). *Social animal: The hidden sources of love, character and achievement.* New York: Random House.

Centers for Disease Control and Prevention. (2010). Black life expectancy, 2010. Retrieved from http://www.cdc .gov/nchs/fastats/lifeexpec.htm

Chiu, M., Austin, P., Manuel, D., & Tu, J. (2010). Comparison of cardiovascular risk profile among ethnic groups using population health surveys between 1996 and 2007. *Canadian Medical Association Journal, 182*(8), E301–E310. doi:10.1503/cmaj.091676

Christakis, N. & Fowler, J. (2009). *Connected: The surprising power of our social networks and how they shape our lives.* New York: Little, Brown.

Durkheim, É. (1897). *Suicide: A study in sociology* (2002 edition). New York: Routledge.

Egolf, B., Lasker, J., Wolf, S., & Potvin, L. (1992). The Roseto effect: A 50-year comparison of mortality rates. *American Journal of Public Health, 82*(8), 1089–1092.

Gabert-Quillen, C., Irish, L., Sledjeski, E., Fallon, W., Spoonster, E., & Delahanty, D. (2012). The impact of social support on the relationship between trauma history and posttraumatic stress disorder symptoms in motor vehicle accident victims. *International Journal of Stress Management, 19*(1), 69–79.

Helm, T. & Coman, J. (2012, June 24). Rowan Williams pours scorn on David Cameron's "big society." *The Guardian/The Observer.* Retrieved from https://www.theguardian.com/uk/2012/jun/23/ rowan-williams-big-society-cameron

Holt-Lunsted, J., Smith, T., & Layton, J. (2010, July 27) Social relationships and mortality risk. *PLOS Medicine.* doi:10.1371/journal.pmed.1000316.

Holt-Lunsted, J. & Smith, T. (2016). Loneliness and social isolation as risk factors for CVD: Implications for evidence-based patient care. *BMJ Journals: Heart, 102*(13). doi:10.1136/heartjnl-2016-310034

Hystad, P. & Carpiano, R. (2012). Sense of community-belonging and health behaviour change in Canada. *Journal of Epidemiology and Community Health, 66,* 277–283.

Jordan, J. & Neimeyer, R. (2003). Does grief counseling work? *Death Studies, 27,* 765–768.

Henry J. Kaiser Family Foundation. (2009). *Key health and health care indicators by race/ethnicity and state.* Retrieved from https://kaiserfamilyfoundation.files. wordpress.com/2013/01/7633-02.pdf

Karademas, E. (2005). Self-efficacy, social support and well-being: The mediating role of optimism. *Personality and Individual Differences, 40*(6). Retrieved from http://www.sciencedirect.com/science/article/pii/ S0191886905003910

Kawachi, I. (1999). Social capital and community effects on population and individual health. *Annals of the New York Academy of Science, 896,* 120–130.

Kawachi, I. & Berkman, L. (2000). Social cohesion, social capital and health. In L. Berkman & I. Kawachi (Eds.), *Social epidemiology* (pp. 174–190). New York: Oxford University Press.

Kawachi, I., Kennedy, B., Lochner, K., & Prothrow-Stith, D. (1997). Social capital, income inequality and mortality. *American Journal of Public Health, 87*(9), 1491–1498.

Kondo, N. (2009) Income inequality, mortality, and self-rated health: Meta-analysis of multilevel studies. *British Medical Journal, 339,* b4471. doi:10.1136/ bmj.b4471.

Kroenke, C., Kubzansky, L., Schernhammer, E., Holmes, M., & Kawachi, I. (2006). Social networks, social support, and survival after breast cancer diagnosis. *Journal of Clinical Oncology, 24*(7), 1105–1111.

Legh-Jones, H. & Moore, S. (2012). Network social capital, social participation, and physical inactivity in an urban adult population. *Social Science and Medicine, 74*(9),1362–1367. doi:10.1016/j.socscimed.2012.01.005

Navarro, V. (2002). A critique of social capital. *International Journal of Health Services, 32*(3), 423–432.

Orth-Gomer, K. & Johnson, J. (1987). Social network interaction and mortality, a six-year follow-up study of a random sample of the Swedish population. *Journal of Chronic Disease, 40*(10), 949–957.

Pager, D. & Shepherd, H. (2008) The sociology of discrimination: racial discrimination in employment, housing, credit, and consumer markets. *Annual Review of Sociology, 34*, 181–209.

Plavinski, S., Plavinskaya, S., & Klimov, A. (2003). Social factors and increase in mortality in Russia in the 1990s: Prospective cohort study. *British Medical Journal, 326*, 1240–1242.

Please explain your true values, Mr. Cameron. (2011, October 2). *The Observer* (Editorial). Retrieved from https://www.theguardian.com/commentisfree/2011/oct/02/observer-editorial-big-society-cameron

Putnam, R. (1993). *Making democracy work: Civic traditions in modern Italy.* New York: Princeton University Press.

Putnam, R. (2007). E Pluribus Unum: Diversity and community in the twenty-first century. *Scandinavian Political Studies, 30*(2), 137–174.

Sapolsky, R. (2017). *Behave.* New York: Penguin.

Schmid, K., Hewstone, M., Kupper, B., Zick, A., & Wagner, U. (2012). Secondary transfer effects of intergroup conflict: A cross-national comparison in Europe. *Social Psychology Quarterly, 75*(1), 28–51. doi:10.1177/0190272511430235

Shaw, M., Dorling, D., & Davey Smith, G. (2006). Poverty, social exclusion and minorities. In M. Marmot & R. Wilkinson (Eds.), *Social determinants of health* (pp. 196–223). New York: Oxford University Press.

Shkolnikov, V. (1997). *The Russian health crisis of the 1990s in mortality dimensions.* Cambridge: Harvard Center for Population and Development Studies, Working Paper 97.01.

Stafford, M., Newbold, B., Bruce, K., & Ross, N. (2011). Psychological distress among immigrants and visible minorities in Canada: A contextual analysis. *International Journal of Social Psychiatry, 57*(4), 428–441.

Wilkinson, R. (1996). *Unhealthy societies: The affliction of inequality.* London: Routledge.

Wilkinson, R. & Pickett, K. (2009). *The spirit-level: Why more equal societies almost always do better.* London: Allen Lane.

Wohland, P., Rees, P., Nazoo, J. & Jagger, C. (2015). Inequality in healthy life expectancy between ethnic groups in England and Wales. *Ethnicity and Health, 20*(4), 341–353. doi:10.1080/13557858.2014.921892

Chapter 8

BC community pleads for help to halt suicide epidemic. 7 suicide attempts in one week leads to calls for more services for aboriginal youths. (2007, November 22). *CBC News.* Retrieved from http://www.cbc.ca/news/canada/british-columbia/story/2007/11/22/bc-hazeltonsuicides.html

Bjerregaard, P., Young, T., Dewailly, E., & Ebbesson. S. (2004). Indigenous health in the Arctic: An overview of the circumpolar Inuit population. *Scandinavian Journal of Public Health, 32*, 390–395.

Chandler, M. & Lalonde, C. (1998). Cultural continuity as a hedge against suicide in Canada's First Nations. *Transcultural Psychiatry, 35*(3), 191–219. doi:10.1177/136346159803500202

Curry, B. (2007, January 13). Nunavut education system in a shambles, report finds. *Globe and Mail,* A7.

Dobrota, A. (2007, January 13). Optimistic fresh start has gone unrealized. *Globe and Mail, A7.*

Garner, R., Carriere, G., & Sanmartin, C. (2010). The health of First Nations living off reserve, Inuit, and Metis adults in Canada: The impact of socio-economic status on inequalities in health. Statistics Canada Health Research Working Paper Series. Retrieved from http://www.statscan.gc.ca/pub/82-622-x/82-622-x2010004-eng.pdf

Gold, S., O'Neil, J., & Van Wagner, V. (2007). The community as provider: Collaborative and community ownership in Northern maternity care. *Canadian Journal of Midwifery Research and Practice, 16*(2), 5–17.

Health Canada. (2014). *A statistical profile on the health of First Nations in Canada: Determinants of health, 2006 to 2010.* Retrieved from http://publications.gc.ca/collections/collection_2014/sc-hc/H34-193-1-2014-eng.pdf

Krieger. N. (2008). Proximal, distal, and the politics of causation: What's level got to do with it? *American Journal of Public Health, 98*(2), 221–230.

Ontario knew about mercury contamination near Grassy Narrows in 1990: Report. (2017, November 12). *CBC News.* Retrieved from https://www.cbc.ca/news/canada/thunder-bay/mercury-report-grassy-narrows-1.4399441

Reading, C. & Wien, F. (2009). *Health inequities and social determinants of aboriginal people's health.* Prince George: National Collaborating Centre for Aboriginal Health. Retrieved from https://www.ccnsa-nccah.ca/docs/determinants/RPT-HealthInequalities-Reading-Wien-EN.pdf

Schwartz, D. (2015). Truth and Reconciliation Commission by the numbers. *CBC News.* https://www.cbc.ca/news/indigenous/truth-and-reconciliation-commission-by-the-numbers-1.3096185

Statistics Canada. (2010, May 13). Study: *Aboriginal labour market update. The Daily.* Retrieved from http://www.statcan.gc.ca/daily-quotidien/100513/dq100513b-eng.htm

Statistics Canada. (2012). *Mortality rates among children and teenagers living in Inuit Nunangat. Health*

Reports2(3) . Retrieved from http://www.statcan.gc.ca/
pub/82-003-x/2012003/article/11695-eng.htm

Tasker, J.P. (2018, February 14). Trudeau promises a new
legal framework for Indigenous people. *CBC News.*
Retrieved from http://www.cbc.ca/news/politics/
trudeau-speech-indigenous-rights-1.4534679

Tasker, J.P. (2018, March 26). Trudeau exonerates
Tsilhqot'in chiefs hanged in 1864. *CBC News.* Retrieved from http://www.cbc.ca/news/politics/
pm-trudeau-exonerates-tsilhqotin-chiefs-1.4593445

Tunney, C. (2017, December 7). Liberals face funding
gap on First Nations water promise: PBO. *CBC News.*
Retrieved from http://www.cbc.ca/news/politics/
pbo-indigenous-water-boil-1.4437451

Waldram, J., Herring, D., & Young, T. (2006). *Aboriginal
health in Canada: Historical, cultural and epidemiological
perspectives.* Toronto: University of Toronto Press.

Wilson, D. & Macdonald, D. (2010). *The income gap
between Aboriginal peoples and the rest of Canada.*
Ottawa: Canadian Centre for Policy Alternatives.

Chapter 9

Aust, B. & Ducki, A. (2004). Comprehensive health promotion interventions at the workplace: Experiences with
health circles in Germany. *Journal of Occupational
Health Psychology, 9*(3), 258–270.

Beland, F., Birch, S., & Stoddart, G. (2002). Unemployment
and health: Contextual level influences on the
production of health in populations. *Social Science
and Medicine, 55*, 2033–2052.

Blouin, C., Chopra, M., & van der Hoeven, R. (2009).
Trade and social determinants of health. *Lancet,
373*(9662), 502–507.

Brady, D., Fullerton, A., & Cross, J. (2010). More than just
nickels and dimes: A cross-national analysis of working
poverty in affluent democracies. *Social Problems,
57*(4), 559–585. Retrieved from https://www.ncbi.nlm
.nih.gov/pubmed/20976971

Crompton, S. (2011, October 13). What's stressing the
stressed? Main sources of stress among workers.
Canadian Social Trends (Statistics Canada).

Commission on Social Determinants of Health. (2008).
*Closing the gap in a generation: Health equity through
action on determinants of health.* Geneva: World
Health Organization.

de Jong, J., Bosma, H., Peter, R., & Slegrist, J. (2000). Job
strain, effort-reward balance and employee well-being:
A large cross sectional study. *Social Science and
Medicine, 50*(9), 1317–1327.

Evans, G. & Carrere, S. (1991). Traffic congestion, perceived
control, and psychophysiological stress among urban
bus drivers. *Journal of Applied Psychology 76*(5), 658.

Ferrie, J. (2001). Is job insecurity harmful to health? *Journal
of the Royal Society of Medicine, 94*, 71–76.

Gallo, W., Bradley, C., Falba, T., Dublin, J., Cramer, L.,
Bogardus, L., & Kasl, S. (2004). Involuntary job loss as
a risk factor for subsequent myocardial infarction and
stroke. Findings from the Health and Retirement Survey.
American Journal of Industrial Medicine, 45, 408–416.

Hallock, K. (2011, May). Pay ratios and pay inequality.
Workspan (Cornell University Institute for Compensation Studies).

Irwin, N. (2017, September 3). To understand rising
inequality, consider the janitors at two top companies, then and now. *New York Times.* Retrieved from
https://www.nytimes.com/2017/09/03/upshot/to-
understand-rising-inequality-consider-the-janitors-
at-two-top-companies-then-and-now.html

Jin, R., Shaw, C., & Suoboda, T. (1997). The impact of
unemployment on health: A review of the evidence.
Journal of Public Health Policy, 18(3), 275–301.

Kim, I., Muntaner, C., Vahid Shahidi, F., Vives, A.,
Vanroelen, C., & Benach, J. (2012). Welfare states,
flexible employment, and health: a critical review.
Health Policy, 104(2), 99–127.

Lavis, J., McLeod, C., Mustard, C., & Stoddart, G. (2003). Is
there a gradient life span by position in the social hierarchy? *American Journal of Public Health, 93*(5), 771–774.

Marmot, M. (2010). *Fair society, healthy lives. The
Marmot Review.* Retrieved from http://www
.marmotreview.org/AssetLibary/pdfs/Reports/
FairSocietyHealthyLives.pdf

Scott, A. (2000). Shift work and health. *Primary Care,
27*(4), 1057–1079.

Snijder, C., Brand, T., Jaddoe, V., Hofman, A., Mackenbach, J., Steegers, E., & Burdof, A. (2012). Physically
demanding work, fetal growth and the risk of adverse
birth outcomes. The Generation R study. *Occupational
and Environmental Medicine, 69*(8), 543–550.

Statistics Canada. (2018). Minimum wage in Canada since
1975. *The Daily.* Retrieved from https://www150.statcan.
gc.ca/n1/pub/11-630-x/11-630-x2015006-eng.htm

Substance Abuse and Mental Health Services Administration. (2015). *Results from the 2015 National Survey
on Drug Use and Health: Detailed tables.* Retrieved
from https://www.samhsa.gov/data/sites/default/files/
NSDUH-DetTabs-2015/NSDUH-DetTabs-2015/NS-
DUH-DetTabs-2015.pdf

Thorpe, A., Owen, N., Neuhaus, M., & Dunstan, D. (2011).
Sedentary behaviors and subsequent health outcomes
in adults: A systematic review of longitudinal studies,
1996–2011. *American Journal of Preventive Medicine,
41*(2), 207–215.

Turcotte, M. (2011, August 24). Commuting to work:
Results of the 2010 General Social Survey. *Canadian
Social Trends (Statistics Canada).* Retrieved
from https://www150.statcan.gc.ca/n1/pub/11-
008-x/2011002/article/11531-eng.htm

Van der Doef, M. (1999). The job demand-control model and psychological wellbeing: A review of 20 years of empirical research. *Work and Stress, 13*(2), 97.

Voss, M., Nylen, L., Floderus, B., Diderichsen, F., & Terry, T. (2004). Unemployment and early cause-specific mortality: A study based on the Swedish twin registry. *American Journal of Public Health, 94*(12), 2155–2161.

Chapter 10

Alini, E. (2017, August 1). The Vancouver homebuyer tax is one year old. Here's what Canada can learn from it. *Global News.* Retrieved from https://globalnews.ca/news/3636579/vancouver-foreign-homebuyers-tax-one-year-anniversary

Blaxter, M. (1990). *Health and lifestyles.* London: Routledge.

Boardman, J. (2004). Stress and physical health: The role of neighborhoods as mediating and moderating mechanisms. *Social Science and Medicine, 58,* 2473–2483.

Brody, G., Ge, X., Conger, R., Gibbons, F., & Murray, V. (2001). The impact of neighborhood disadvantage, collective socialization, and parenting on African American children's affiliations with deviant peers. *Child Development, 72*(4), 1231–1246.

City of Vancouver. (2017). *Housing characteristics fact sheet.* Retrieved from http://vancouver.ca/files/cov/housing-characteristics-fact-sheet.pdf

Cohen, A., Marsh, T., Williamson, S., Golinelli, D., & McKenzie, T. (2012). Impact and cost-effectiveness of family fitness zones: A natural experiment in urban public parks. *Health and Place, 18,* 39–45.

Crisis. (2011). Crisis policy briefing: Housing benefit cuts, July 2011. Retrieved from http://www.crisis.org.uk

Commission on Social Determinants of Health. (2008). *Closing the gap in a generation: Health equity through action on determinants of health.* Geneva: World Health Organization.

Diez Roux, A., Markin, S., Arnett, D., Chambless, L., Massing, M., Nieto, F., Sorlie, S., Szklo, M., Tyroler, H., & Watson, R. (2001). Neighborhood of residence and incidence of heart disease. *New England Journal of Medicine, 34*(5), 99–106.

Duncan, C., Jones, K., & Moon, G. (1996). Health-related behaviour in context: A multilevel modeling approach. *Social Science and Medicine, 42*(6), 817–830.

Frankish, C., Hwang, S., & Quantz, D. (2005). Homelessness and health in Canada: Research lessons and priorities. *Canadian Journal of Public Health, 96*(Supplement 2), S23–S29.

Frohich, K., Potvin, L., Chabut, P., & Lorin, E. (2002). A theoretical and empirical analysis of context: Neighbourhoods, smoking and youth. *Social Science and Medicine, 54*(9), 1401–1417.

Gennetian, L., Sciandra, M., Sanbonmatrsn, L., Ludwig, J., Katz, L., Duncan, G., Kling, J. & Kessler, R. (2012). Long-term effects of Moving to Opportunity on youth outcomes. *Cityscape, 14*(2), 137–168. Retrieved from https://scholar.harvard.edu/lkatz/publications/long-term-effects-moving-opportunity-youth-outcomes

Heath, G., Parra, D., Sarmiento, O., Andersen, L., Owen, N., Goenka, S., Montes, F., & Brownson, R. (2012). Evidence-based intervention in physical activity: Lessons from around the world. *Lancet, 389*(9838). Retrieved from http://dx.doi.org/10.1016/S0140-6736(12)60816-2

Heath, G., Brownson, R., Kruger, J., Miles, R., Powell, K., & Ramsey, L. (2006). The effectiveness of urban design and land use and transport policies and practices to increase physical activity: A systematic review. *Journal of Physical Activity and Health, 1,* S55–S71.

Hertzman, C. & Power, C. (2006). A lifecourse approach to health and human development. In Heymann J., Hertzman C., Barer, M., & Evans, R. (Eds.), *Healthier societies: From analysis to action (pp. A599–A602).* Oxford: Blackwell.

Hou, F. & Miles, J. (2005). Neighbourhood inequality, neighbourhood affluence and population health. *Social Science and Medicine, 60*(7), 1557–1569.

Hwang, S. (2001). Homelessness and health. *Canadian Medical Association Journal, 164*(2), 229–233.

Jacobs, D., Clinckner, R., Zhou, J., Viet, S., Marker, D., Rogers, J., . . . Friedman, W. (2002). The prevalence of lead-based paint hazards in US housing. *Environmental Health Perspectives, 110*(10), A599–A602.

Kayha, D. (2011). Rising energy costs causing fuel poverty deaths. *BBC News.* https://www.bbc.com/news/business-15359312

Kawachi, I., Kennedy, B., & Glass, R. (1999). Social capital and self-rated health: A contextual analysis. *American Journal of Public Health 89*(8), 1187–1193.

Klinenburg, E. (2002). *Heat wave: A social autopsy of disaster in Chicago.* Chicago: University of Chicago Press.

Kohen, J., Brooks-Gunn, J., Leventhal, T., & Hertzman, C. (2002). Neighbourhood income and physical and social disorder in Canada: Associations with young children's competencies. *Child Development, 73*(6), 1844–1860.

Larimer, M., Malone, D., Garner, M., Atkins, D., Burlington, B., Lonczak, H., Tanzer, K., Ginzler, J., Clifasefi, S., Hobson, W., & Marlott, G. (2009). Health care and public service use and costs before and after provision of housing for chronically homeless persons with severe alcohol problems. *Journal of the American Medical Association, 301*(13), 1349–1357.

Lee, I., Shiroma, E., Lobelo, F., Puska, P., Blair, S., & Katzmarzyk, P. (2012). Effect of physical activity on non-communicable disease worldwide: an analysis of burden of disease and life expectancy. *Lancet, 380(9839).* doi:10.1016/S0140-6736(12)61031-9

Ley, D. & Lynch, N. (2012). *Divisions and disparities: Socio-spatial income polarization in Greater Vancouver, 1970–2005.* University of Toronto Cities Centre. Retrieved from http://neighbourhoodchange.ca/documents/2012/10/divisions-and-disparities-in-lotus-land-socio-spatial-income-polarization-in-greater-vancouver-1970-2005-by-david-ley-nicholas-lynch.pdf

Macintyre, S. & Ellaway, A. (2000). Neighbourhood cohesion and health in socially contrasting neighbourhoods: Implications for the social exclusion and public health agendas. *Health Bulletin* (Edinburgh), *58*(6), 450–456.

McMartin, P. (2012, November 22). In metro Vancouver, there are more rich, more poor and less in between. *Vancouver Sun,* . Retrieved from http://www.vancouversun.com/opinion/columnists/Pete+McMartin+Metro+Vancouver+there+more+rich+more/7597585/story.html

McMartin, P. (2016, 5 January). The high cost of misery in Vancouver's downtown eastside. *Vancouver Sun.* Retrieved from http://www.vancouversun.com/health/pete+mcmartin+high+cost+misery+vancouver+downtown+eastside/11632586/story.html

Merkin, S., Basurto-Daville, R., Karlamangla, A., Bird, N., Lurie, N., Escarce, J., & Seeman, T. (2009). Neighborhoods and cumulative biological risk profiles by race/ethnicity. *Annals of Epidemiology, 19*(3), 194–201.

Myles, J. (2017, November 11). Average rent in Toronto since 2000. *TorontoRentals.* Retrieved from https://www.torontorentals.com/blog/average-rent-in-toronto-since-2000

National Coalition for the Homeless. (2011). Retrieved from http://www.nationalhomeless.org.

Omariba, W. (2010). Neighbourhood characteristics, individual attributes and self-rated health among older Canadians. *Health and Place, 16*(5), 986–995.

Picard, A. (2016, February 15). Canada experiencing alarming growth in homelessness. *Globe and Mail.* Retrieved from https://www.theglobeandmail.com/news/national/canada-experiencing-alarming-growth-in-child-homelessness/article28756629

Pickett, K. & Pearl, M. (2001). Multilevel analyses of neighbourhood socioeconomic context and health outcomes: A critical review. *Journal of Epidemiology and Community Health, 55*(2), 111–122.

Rayner, J. (2011, October 1). Sharp rise in demand for handouts of free food. *The Observer,*. Retrieved from https://www.theguardian.com/society/2011/oct/01/families-queue-for-food-handouts

Robert, S. & Reither, E. (2004). A multilevel analysis of race, community disadvantage, and body mass index among adults in the US. *Social Science and Medicine, 59*(12), 2421–2434.

Rogot, E., Sorlie, P., & Backlund, E. (1992). Air conditioning and mortality in hot weather. *American Journal of Epidemiology, 136*(1), 106–116.

Ross, N. (2004). *What have we learned studying income inequality and population health?* Ottawa: CIHI. Retrieved from https://secure.cihi.ca/free_products/IIPH_2004_e.pdf

Ross, N., Wolfson, M., Dunn, J., Berthelot, J., Kaplan, G., & Lynch, J. (2000). Relation between income inequality and mortality in Canada and the United States: Cross sectional assessment using census data and vital statistics. *British Medical Journal, 320*, 898–902.

Seliske, L., Pickett, W., & Janssen, I. (2012). Urban sprawl and its relationship to active transportation, physical activity and obesity in Canadian youth. *Health Reports* (Statistics Canada). Retrieved from http://www.statcan.gc.ca/pub/82-003-x/2012002/article/11678-eng.pdf

Statistics Canada. (2017, October 27). Chart 7: Distribution of households that paid 30% or more of household total income towards shelter costs by census metropolitan area (CMA), 2016. *The Daily.* Retrieved from http://www.statcan.gc.ca/daily-quotidien/171025/cg-c007-eng.htm

Van Os, J., Driessen, G., Gunther, N., & Delespaul, P. (2000). Neighbourhood variance in incidence of schizophrenia. Evidence for person environment interaction. *British Journal of Psychiatry, 176*, 243–248.

Chapter 11

Ahmed, A., Richtel, M. & Jacobs, A. (2018). In NAFTA talks, US tries to limit junk food warning labels. *New York Times.* Retrieved from https://www.nytimes.com/2018/03/20/world/americas/nafta-food-labels-obesity.html

Alaimo, K., Olson, C., & Frongillo, C. (2001). Food insecurity and American school-aged children's cognitive, academic, and psychosocial development, *Pediatrics, 108*(1), 44–53.

Bausall, K. (2007). *Snake oil science, the truth about complementary and alternative medicine.* Oxford: Oxford University Press.

BC Provincial Health Services Authority. (2016). BC food security gateway. Retrieved from https://bcfoodsecuritygateway.ca

Benedictus, L. (2016, March 8). Can chocolate make you smarter? (And thinner?) (And healthier?) *The*

Guardian. https://www.theguardian.com/lifeandstyle/shortcuts/2016/mar/08/can-chocolate-make-you-smarter-and-thinner-and-healthier

Brownell, K., Farley, T., Willett, W., Popkin, B., Chaloupka, F., Thompson, J., & Ludwig, D. (2009). The public health and economic benefits of taxing sugar-sweetened beverages. *New England Journal of Medicine, 361*, 1599–1605.

Brunstrom, J., Burn, J., Sell, N., Collingwood, J., Rogers, P., Wilkinson, L., . . . Ferriday, D. (2012). Episodic memory and appetite regulation in humans. *PLOS ONE, 7*(12), e50707. doi:10.1371/journal.pone.0050707

Butler, P. (2012, November 18). Britain in nutrition recession as food prices rise and incomes shrink. *The Guardian.* Retrieved from https://www.theguardian.com/society/2012/nov/18/breadline-britain-nutritional-recession-austerity

Chouinard, H., Davis, D., LaFrance, J., & Perloff, J. (2006). *Fat taxes: Big money for small change. Working Paper 1007, California Agricultural Experiment Station.* Gianni Foundation for Agricultural Economics, University of California, Berkeley. Retrieved from http://are.berkeley.edu/~jeffrey_lafrance/working%20papers/WP-1007.pdf

Christakis, N. & Fowler, J. (2009). *Connected: The surprising power of our social networks and how they shape our lives.* New York: Little, Brown.

Dietitians of Canada. (2010). *The cost of eating in BC 2009.* Retrieved from http://www.dietitians.ca/Downloadable-Content/Public/BC_CostofEating_2009-(1).aspx

Ello-Martin, J., Ledikwe, J., & Rolls, B. (2005). The influence of food portion size and energy density on energy intake: Implications for weight management. *American Journal of Clinical Nutrition, 82*, 236S–241S.

Flegel, K., Kit, B., Orpana, H., & Graubard, B. (2013). Association of all-cause mortality with overweight and obesity using standard body mass index categories: A systematic review and meta-analysis. *Journal of the American Medical Association, 309*, 71–82.

Food insecurity in Nunavut should be considered a national crisis. (2017, May 19). *CBC News.* Retrieved from http://www.cbc.ca/news/health/food-insecurity-1.4122103

Garriguet, D. (2009). Diet quality in Canada. *Health Reports (Statistics Canada), 20*(3), 41–52. Retrieved from https://www150.statcan.gc.ca/n1/pub/82-003-x/2009003/article/10914-eng.htm

Hamer, M. & Stamatakis, E. (2013). Overweight and obese cardiac patients have better prognosis despite reporting worse perceived health and more conventional risk factors. *Preventive Medicine, 57(1).* doi:10.1016/j.ypmed.2013.02.012

Health Canada. (2008). Household food insecurity in Canada. Retrieved from http://www.hc-sc.gc.ca/fn-an/surveill/nutrition/commun/insecurit/index-eng.php

Health Canada. (2014). A statistical profile on the health of First Nations in Canada: Determinants of health, 2006–2010. Retrieved from https://www.canada.ca/en/indigenous-services-canada/services/first-nations-inuit-health/reports-publications/aboriginal-health-research/statistical-profile-health-first-nations-canada-determinants-health-2006-2010-health-canada-2014.html

Health Canada. (2018). *Health Canada releases the results of voluntary efforts to reduce sodium in processed foods.* Retrieved from https://www.canada.ca/en/health-canada/news/2018/01/health_canada_releases-resultsofvoluntaryeffortstoreducesodiuminp.html

Hooper, L., Summerbell, C., Thompson, R., Sills, D., Roberts, T., Moor, H., & Davey Smith, G. (2011). Reduced or modified dietary fat for preventing cardiovascular disease. *Cochrane Database of Systematic Reviews*, issue 7, article no. CD002137. doi:10.1002/14651858.CD002137.pub2

Jones, A., Veerman, J. & Hammond, D. (2017). *Health and economic impact of a tax on sugary drinks in Canada.* University of Waterloo Faculty of Applied Sciences. Retrieved from https://www.diabetes.ca/getattachment/Newsroom/Latest-News/Will-a-sugary-drinks-levy-benefit-Canadians/The-Health-and-Economic-Impact-of-a-Sugary-Drinks-Tax.pdf.aspx

Kirkpatrick, S. & Tarasuk, V. (2008). Food insecurity is associated with nutrient inadequacies among Canadian adults and adolescents. *Journal of Nutrition, 138*(3), 604–612.

Langlois, K. & Garriguet, D. (2011). Sugar consumption among Canadians of all ages. *Statistics Canada, Health Reports, 22*(3). Retrieved from https://www150.statcan.gc.ca/n1/pub/82-003-x/2011003/article/11540-eng.htm

Michelle Obama on new book. (2012, May 29). *Good Morning America.* Retrieved from https://abcnews.go.com/GMA/video/michelle-obama-book-american-grown-16448732

Mooney, J., Haw, S., & Frank, J. (2011). *Policy interventions to tackle the obesogenic environment.* Edinburgh: Scottish Collaboration for Public Health Research and Policy.

Morland, K. & Filomena, S. (2007). Disparities in the availability of fruits and vegetables between racially segregated urban neighborhoods. *Public Health and Nutrition 10*(12), 1481–1489.

Morland, K., Wing, S., Diez Roux, A., & Poole, C. (2002). Neighborhood characteristics associated with the location of food stores and food service places. *American Journal of Preventive Medicine, 22,* 23–29.

Mytton, O., Gray, A., Rayner, M., & Rutter, H. (2007). Could targeted food taxes improve health? *Journal of Epidemiology and Community, 61*(8), 689–694.

Nestle, M. (2007). *Food politics.* Berkeley: University of California Press.

Neumark-Sztainer, D., Wall, M., Guo, J., Story, M., Haines, J., & Eisenberg, M. (2006). Obesity, disordered eating, and eating disorders in a longitudinal study of adolescents: How do dieters fare 5 years later? *Journal of the American Dietetics Association, 106*(4), 559–568.

Organisation for Economic Co-operation and Development (OECD). (2010). *Obesity and the economics of prevention: Fit not Fat.* Retrieved from http://www .oecd.org/els/health-systems/obesity-and-the-economics-of-prevention-9789264084865-en.htm

Organisation for Economic Co-operation and Development (OECD). (2011). *Obesity and the economics of prevention: Fit not Fat—Canada key facts.* Retrieved from http://www.oecd.org/document/14/0,3343 ,en_2649_33929_46038670_1_1_1,00.html

Powell, L., Slater, S., Mirtcheva, D., Bao, Y., & Chaloupka, F. (2007). Food store availability and neighbourhood characteristics in the United States. *Preventive Medicine, 44*(3), 189–195.

Public Health Agency of Canada. (2011). *Obesity in Canada.* Retrieved from http://www.phac-aspc.gc.ca/ hp-ps/hl-mvs/oic-oac/index-eng.php

Rose-Jacobs, R., Black, M., Casey, P., Cook, J., Cutts, D., Chilton, M., . . . Frank, D. (2008). Household food insecurity–associations with at-risk infant and toddler development. *Pediatrics, 121*(1), 65–72.

Sacks, G., Veerman, J., Moodie, M., & Swinburn, B. (2010). Traffic light nutrition labeling and junk food tax: A modeled comparison of cost-effectiveness for obesity prevention. *International Journal of Obesity 35*(7), 1001–1009. doi:10.1038/ijo.2010.228

Sacks, G., Rayner, M., & Swinburn, B. (2009). Impact of front-of-pack traffic light nutrition labeling on consumer food purchases in the UK. *Health Promotion International 24(4),* 344–352.

Scottish Government. (2008). *The Scottish Health Survey 2008.* Retrieved from http://www.scotland.gov.uk/ Publications/2009/09/28102003/0

Shohaimi, S., Welch, A., Bringham, S., Luben, R., Day, N., Wareham, N., & Khaw, K. (2004). Residential area deprivation predicts fruit and vegetable consumption independently of individual educational level and occupational social class. *Journal of Epidemiology and Community Health, 58*(8), 686–691.

Singh, S., Midha, S., Namrata, S., Yogendra, K. & Promod, K. (2008).

Dietary counseling versus dietary supplements for malnutrition in chronic pancreatitis: A randomized controlled trial. *Clinical Gastroenterology and Hepatology.* doi:10.1016/j.cgh.2007.12.040

Statistics Canada. (2015, March 25). Food insecurity in Canada, 2007–2012. *The Daily.* https://www150.statcan. gc.ca/n1/daily-quotidien/150325/dq150325a-eng.htm

Swindell, W.R. (2012). Dietary restriction in rats and mice: A meta-analysis and review of the evidence for genotype-dependent effects on lifespan. *Ageing Research Review, 11*(2), 254–270.

Tandon, P., Zhou, C., Chan, N., Lozano, P., Couch, S., Glanz, K., . . . Saelens, B. (2011). The impact of menu labeling on fast-food purchases for children and parents. *American Journal of Preventive Medicine, 41*(4), 434–438.

Tarasuk, V., Fitzpatrick, S., & Ward, H. (2010). Nutrition inequities in Canada. *Applied Physiology Nutrition and Metabolism 35*(2), 172–179.

Tiffin, R. & Arnoult, M. (2011). The public health impacts of a fat tax. *European Journal of Clinical Nutrition, 65*(4), 427–433.

Vozoris, N. & Tarasuk, V. (2003). Household food insecurity and poor health. *Journal of Nutrition, 133,* 120–127.

Willsher, K. (2012, November 12). France's "Nutella amendment" causes big fat international row. *The Guardian.* Retrieved from https:// www.theguardian.com/world/2012/nov/12/ france-nutella-amendment-international-row

Chapter 12

Borenstein, S. & Bajak, F. (2017, August 29). Houston drainage grid "so obsolete it's just unbelievable." *CBC News.* Retrieved from http://www.cbc.ca/news/world/ houston-harvey-drainage-1.4267585

Carrington, D. (2017, September 6). We are living on a plastic planet. *The Guardian.* Retrieved from https:// www.theguardian.com/environment/2017/sep/06/ we-are-living-on-a-plastic-planet-what-does-it-mean-for-our-health

Chensheng, L., Warchel, K., & Callahan, R. (2014). Sub-lethal exposure to neonicotinoids impaired honey bees winterization before proceeding to colony collapse disorder. *Bulletin of Insectology, 67*(1), 125–130.

Harvard School of Public Health. (2017). Environmental chemicals can harm fertility. Retrieved from https:// www.hsph.harvard.edu/news/hsph-in-the-news/ environmental-chemicals-may-harm-fertility

Health Canada. (2014). Safety of plastic containers (revised 2017). Retrieved from https://www.canada .ca/en/health-canada/services/chemical-substances/ fact-sheets/safety-plastic-containers-common-ly-found-home.html?=undefined&wbdisable=true

Huelskoetter, T. (2015). Hurricane Katrina's health care legacy. Center for American Progress. Retrieved from https://www.americanprogress.org/issues/healthcare/reports/2015/08/20/119670/hurricane-katrinas-health-care-legacy

International Institute for Sustainable Development. (2017). Equity and a healthy planet. Retrieved from https://www.iisd.org/library/equity-and-healthy-planet-iisd-annual-report-2016-2017

Irwin, N. (2017, September 3). To understand rising inequality consider the two janitors at two top companies then and now. *New York Times*. Retrieved from https://www.nytimes.com/2017/09/03/upshot/to-understand-rising-inequality-consider-the-janitors-at-two-top-companies-then-and-now.html

Johnson, L. (2017, August 27). Thousands of Atlantic salmon escape fish farm near Victoria after nets damaged. *CBC News*. Retrieved from https://www.cbc.ca/news/canada/british-columbia/atlantic-salmon-released-cooke-aquaculture-1.4257369

Kelly, A. (2017). Millions of tropical sea creatures invade waters off BC coast. Retrieved from http://www.cbc.ca/news/canada/british-columbia/tropical-sea-creatures-blooming-bc-1.4164883

Kelman, I. (2017) Don't blame climate change for hurricane Harvey, blame society. *Real Clear Science*. Retrieved from http://www.realclearscience.com/articles/2017/08/29/dont_blame_climate_change_for_hurricane_harvey_disaster_blame_society_110375.html

Looper, M. (n.d.). *Factors affecting milk composition of lactating cows*. University of Arkansas Division of Agriculture. Retrieved from https://www.uaex.edu/publications/pdf/FSA-4014.pdf

Mckie, R. (2017, September 3). Cod and haddock go north due to warming UK seas. *The Guardian*. Retrieved from https://www.theguardian.com/environment/2017/sep/02/fish-conservation-foreign-species-uk-waters-climate-change

Pighin, D., Adriana, P., Chamorro, V., Paschetta, F., Cunzolo, S., Godoy, F., Messina, V., Pordominogo, A., & Grigioni, G. (2016). A contribution of beef to human health: A review of animal production systems. *Scientific World Journal*. doi:10.1155/2016/8681491

Pollan, M. (2006). *The Omnivore's dilemma*. New York: Penguin.

Salvadori, M., Sontrop, J., Garg, A., Moist, L., Suri, R. & Clark, W. (2009). Factors that led to the Walkerton tragedy. *Kidney International Supplement, 112*, S33–S34. doi:10.1038/ki.2008.616

Chapter 13

Bargh, J. & Earp, B. (2009). The will is caused, not free. *Dialogues, Society of Personality and Social Psychology, 24*(1), 13–15.

Bargh, J. & Ferguson, M. (2000). Beyond behaviorism. On the automaticity of the higher mental processes. *Psychological Bulletin, 126*, 925–945.

Blaxter, M. (1990). *Health and lifestyles*. London: Routledge.

Bourdieu, P. (1984). *Distinction: A social critique of the judgement of taste*. Cambridge: Harvard University Press.

Braveman, P., Egerter, S., & Barclay, C. (2011, March 1). *What shapes health-related behaviors?* Robert Wood Johnson Foundation. Retrieved from https://www.rwjf.org/en/library/research/2011/03/what-shapes-health-related-behaviors---.html

Champion, V. & Skinner, C. (2008). The health belief model. In K. Glanz, B. Rimer, & K. Viswanath (Eds.), *Health behavior and health education, theory and practice* (pp. 75–94). San Francisco: Wiley.

Chiou, W-B., Wen, C., Wu, W., & Lee, K. (2011). A randomized experiment to examine unintended consequences of dietary supplement use among daily smokers: Taking supplements reduces self-regulation of smoking. *Addiction, 106*(12), 2221–2228. doi:10.1111/j.1360-0443.2011.03545.x

Christakis, N. & Fowler, J. (2009). *Connected: The surprising power of our social networks and how they shape our lives*. New York: Little, Brown.

Chuang, Y., Cubbin, C., Ahn, D., & Winkleby, M. (2005). Effects of neighborhood socioeconomic status and convenience store concentration on individual level smoking. *Journal of Epidemiology and Community Health, 59*(7), 568–573.

Day, E. (2011, July 17). A nudge in the right direction won't run the big society. *The Observer*. Retrieved from https://www.theguardian.com/society/2011/jul/17/julia-neuberger-nudge-big-society

Demers, A., Kalrouz, S., Adlaf, E., Gilksman, L., Newton-Taylor, B., & Marchand, A. (2002). Multilevel analysis of situational drinking among Canadian undergraduates. *Social Science and Medicine, 55*(3), 415–424.

Giddens, A. (1984). *The constitution of society*. Cambridge: Polity Press.

Giddens, A. (1991). *Modernity and self-identity: Self and society in the late modern age*. Cambridge: Polity Press.

Heneghan, C., Gill, P., O'Neil, B., Lasserson, D., Thake, M., Thompson, M., & Howick, J. (2012). Mythbusting sports and exercise products. *British Medical Journal, 345*, e4848. doi:10.1136/bmj.e4848

Jakicic, J., Davis, K., Rogers, R., King, W., Marcus, M., Helsel, D., Rickman, A., Wahed, A. & Belle, S. (2016). Effect of wearable technology combined with a lifestyle intervention on long-term weight loss: The IDEA randomized clinical trial. *Journal of the American Medical Association, 316*(11), 1161–1171. doi:10.1001/jama.2016.12858

Kahneman, D. & Tversky, A. (2000). *Choices, values and frames.* New York: Cambridge University Press.

Mercier, H & Sperber, D. (2017). *The enigma of reason.* Cambridge: Harvard University Press.

Office for National Statistics. (2011). Smoking behaviour and attitudes. Retrieved from http://www.statistics.gov.uk/STATBASE/Product.asp?vlnk=1638

Phillips, R., Fyhri, A., & Sagberg, F. (2011). Risk compensation and bicycle helmets. *Risk Analysis, 31*(8), 1187–95.

Roepstorff, A., Niewöhner, J., & Beck, S. (2010). Enculturing brains through patterned practices. *Neural Network, 23*(8–9), 1051–1059.

Rosenstock, I. (1974). Historical origins of the health belief model. *Health Education Monographs, 2*(4), 328–335.

Smith, P. & York, N. (2004). Quality incentives: The case of UK general practitioners. *Health Affairs, 23*(3), 112–118.

Tavris, C. & Aronson, E. (2007). *Mistakes were made (but not by me). Why we justify foolish beliefs, bad decisions, and hurtful acts.* Orlando: Harcourt Books.

Thaler, R. & Sunstein, C. (2008). *Nudge: Improving decisions about health, wealth and happiness.* Princeton: Yale University Press.

Unger, R. (1987). *Social theory: Its situation and its task.* Cambridge: Cambridge University Press.

Wegner, D. (2003). *The illusion of conscious will.* Boston: MIT.

Chapter 14

Alesina, A., & Angeletos, G-M. (2005). Fairness and redistribution. *American Economic Review, 95*(4), 960–980.

Birn, A-E., Pillay, Y., & Holtz, T. (2009). *Textbook of international health: Global health in a dynamic world.* New York: Oxford University Press.

Bryant, T., Raphael, D., Schrecker T., & Labonté, R. (2011). Canada: A land of missed opportunity for addressing the social determinants of health. *Health Policy, 101*(1), 44–58.

Fry, R. & Taylor, P. (2012, August 1). *Rise of residential segregation by income. Pew Research Center, Social and Demographic Trends.* Retrieved from http://www.pewsocialtrends.org/2012/08/01/the-rise-of-residential-segregation-by-incomeHutton, W. (2012, July 15). Born poor? Bad luck, you have won last prize in the lottery of life. *The Guardian. Retrieved from https://www.theguardian.com/commentisfree/2012/jul/15/will-hutton-social-mobility*

Kim, I., Muntaner, C., Vahid Shahidi, F., Vives, A., Vanroelen, C., & Benach, J. (2012). Welfare states, flexible employment, and health: a critical review. *Health Policy, 104*(2), 99–127.

Kolich, H. (2013). What human activities increase carbon dioxide in the atmosphere? *HowStuffWorks.*

Retrieved from http://science.howstuffworks.com/environmental/green-science/human-activities-increase-carbon-dioxide.htm

Mackenbach, J. (2009). Politics is nothing but medicine on a larger scale: Reflections on public health's biggest idea. *Journal of Epidemiology and Community Health, 63*(3). doi:10.1136/jech.2008.077032

Marmot, M. (2010). *Fair society, healthy lives. The Marmot Review.* Retrieved from http://www.instituteofhealthequity.org/resources-reports/fair-society-healthy-lives-the-marmot-review/fair-society-healthy-lives-full-report-pdf.pdf

Marmot, M. & Bell, R. (2010). Challenging health inequalities. *Occupational Health.* doi:10.1093/occmed/kqq008

McKinnon, A. (n.d.). *CO_2 emissions from freight transport.* University of Edinburgh Logistics Research Centre. Retrieved from http://www.greenlogistics.org/SiteResources/d82cc048-4b92-4c2a-a014-af1eea7d76d0_CO2%20Emissions%20from%20Freight%20Transport%20-%20An%20Analysis%20of%20UK%20Data.pdf

McLeod C., Hall P., Siddiqi, A., & Hertzman, C. (2012). How society shapes the health gradient: Work-related health inequalities in a comparative perspective. *Annual Review of Public Health, 60*(3). doi:10.1146/annurev-publhealth-031811-124603

Pew Research Center. (2011, November 17). *The American–Western European values gap.* Retrieved from http://www.pewglobal.org/2011/11/17/the-american-western-european-values-gap

Putnam, R. (2000). *Bowling alone: The collapse and revival of American community.* New York: Simon & Schuster.

Robert Wood Johnson Foundation Commission to Build a Healthier America. (2009). *Beyond health care: New directions to a healthier America.* Retrieved from https://www.rwjf.org/content/dam/farm/reports/reports/2009/rwjf40483

Stewart, H. (2012, July 21). Thirteen trillion pounds hidden from taxman by global elite. *The Guardian/The Observer. Retrieved from https://www.theguardian.com/business/2012/jul/21/global-elite-tax-offshore-economy*

Taylor, P. (2008, October 23). *Republicans still happy campers.* Pew Research Center, Social and Demographic Trends. Retrieved from http://www.pewsocialtrends.org/2008/10/23/republicans-still-happy-campers

Vyas, M., Garg, A., Iansavichys, A., Costella, J., Donner, A., Laugsand, L., . . . Hackam, D. (2012). Shift work and vascular events: A systematic review and meta-analysis. *British Medical Journal, 345*, e4800. doi:10.1136/bmj.e4800

Index